CW00926203

CLINICAL PROBLEMS IN OBSTETRIC ANAESTHESIA

CLINICAL PROBLEMS IN OBSTETRIC ANAESTHESIA

Edited by

Ian F. Russell

Consultant Anaesthetist,
Department of Anaesthesia,
Hull Royal Infirmary,
Hull,
UK

and

Gordon Lyons

Consultant Obstetric Anaesthetist,
St James's University Hospital,
Leeds,
UK

CHAPMAN & HALL MEDICAL
London · Weinheim · New York · Tokyo · Melbourne · Madras

Published by Chapman & Hall,
2–6 Boundary Row, London SE1 8HN, UK

Chapman & Hall, 2–6 Boundary Row, London SE1 8HN, UK

Chapman & Hall GmbH, Pappelallee 3, 69469 Weinheim, Germany

Chapman & Hall USA, 115 Fifth Avenue, New York, NY 10003, USA

Chapman & Hall Japan, ITP-Japan, Kyowa Building, 3F, 2–2–1
Hirakawacho, Chiyoda-ku, Tokyo 102, Japan

Chapman & Hall Australia, 102 Dodds Street, South Melbourne, Victoria
3205, Australia

Chapman & Hall India, R. Seshadri, 32 Second Main Road, CIT East,
Madras 600 035, India

First edition 1997

© 1997 Chapman & Hall

Typeset in 10/12pt Palatino by Type Study, Scarborough

Printed in Great Britain at the University Press, Cambridge

ISBN 0 412 71600 3

A catalogue record for this book is available from the British Library

Library of Congress Catalog No: 97–69102

 Printed on acid-free text paper, manufactured in accordance with
ANSI/NISO Z39.48–1992 (Permanence of Paper).

CONTENTS

CONTRIBUTORS

S. Alahuhta
Department of Anaesthesiology,
University of Oulu,
FIN-90220,
Oulu, Finland

D. Benhamou
Professor of Anaesthesiology,
Hôpital Antoine Béclère,
157 Rue de la Porte-de-Trivaux,
92141 Clamart Cedex,
Paris,
France

D.J. Birnbach
Director, Obstetric Anesthesiology,
St. Luke's-Roosevelt Hospital Center,
428 West 59th Street,
New York, NY 10019, USA

D. Bracco
Anaesthesiology Department,
University Hospital,
CH 1011 Lausanne,
Switzerland

D.J Bush
Consultant in Anaesthesia and Pain
Management,
St James's University Hospital,
Beckett Street,
Leeds LS9 7TF, UK

G. Capogna
Consultant Anaesthetist
Department of Anaesthesiology
Ospedale Generale di Zona,
"S Giovanni Calibita" Fatenbenefratelli,
Isola Tiberina,
39 00186 Roma,
Italy

D. Celleno
Consultant Anaesthetist
Department of Anaesthesiology,
Ospedale Generale di Zona,
"S Giovanni Calibita" Fatenbenefratelli,
Isola Tiberina,
39 00186 Roma,
Italy

M. Dresner
Consultant Anaesthetist,
Department of Anaesthesia,
Leeds General Infirmary,
Great George Street,
Leeds LS1 3EX, UK

H. Frizelle
Département d'Anesthésie,
Hôpital Bicêtre,
78, rue du Gal Leclerc,
94270 Le Kremlin-Bicêtre,
France

B.M. Gray
Consultant Anaesthetist,
Department of Anaesthesia,
Hull Royal Infirmary,
Anlaby Road,
Hull HU3 2JZ, UK

J. Hamza
Département d'Anesthésie Réanimation,
Hôpital Saint Vincent de Paul,
82, Avenue Denfert-Rochereau
75014 Paris,
France

K.F. Hampl
Department of Anaesthesia,
University Hospital,
Kantonsspital,
CH-4031 Basel,
Switzerland

L. Hawthorne
Research Fellow,
Obstetric Anaesthesia,
St James's University Hospital,
Beckett Street,
Leeds LS9 7TF, UK

P. Jouppila
Department of Obstetrics and Gynecology,
University of Oulu,
FIN-90220,
Oulu,
Finland

R. Jouppila
Department of Anaesthesiology,
University of Oulu,
Faculty of Medicine,
Kajaanintle 52A,
FIN-90220
Oulu, Finland

G. Lyons
Consultant Obstetric Anaesthetist,
St James's University Hospital,
Beckett Street,
Leeds LS9 7TF, UK

T.H. Madej
Consultant Anaesthetist,
Department of Anaesthesia,
York District Hospital,
Wiggington Road,
York YO3 7HE, UK

E. McGrady
Consultant Anaesthetist,
Glasgow Royal Infirmary,
84 Castle Street,
Glasgow G4 OSF, UK

H. Pargger
Department of Anaesthesia,
University Hospital,
Kantonsspital,
CH-4031 Basel,
Switzerland

A.Quinn
Lecturer,
Academic Unit of Anaesthesia,
Leeds General Infirmary,
Great George Street,
Leeds LS1 3EX, UK

N. Rawal
Department of Anaesthesiology and Intensive Care,
Örebro Medical Centre Hospital,
S-701 85 Örebro,
Sweden

I.F. Russell
Consultant Anaesthetist,
Department of Anaesthesia,
Hull Royal Infirmary,
Anlaby Road,
Hull HU3 2JZ, UK

C.C. Rout
Department of Anaesthesia,
University of Natal,
Durban,
Republic of South Africa

M.C. Schneider
Department of Anaesthesia,
University Hospital,
Kantonsspital,
CH-4031 Basel,
Switzerland

L. Swanson
Senior Registrar,
Department of Anaesthesia,
Royal Victoria Infirmary,
Queen Victoria Road,
Newcastle upon Tyne,
NE1 4LP, UK

T.A. Thomas
Consultant Anaesthetist,
Department of Anaesthesia,
Bristol Maternity Hospital,
Southwell Street,
Bristol BS2 8EG, UK

D. Thorin
Department of Obstetric Anaesthesia,
University of Lausanne,
1011 Lausanne,
Switzerland

A.Van Zundert
Lecturer, University of Antwerp, Belgium and
Vice Chairman,
Department of Anaesthesiology,
Catharina Hospital,
Michelangelolaan 2,
NL-5623 EJ Eindhoven,
The Netherlands

Y. Vial
Obstetrical Department,
University Hospital,
CH 1011
Lausanne,
Switzerland

J.J. Walker
Academic Unit of Obstetrics and
Gynaecology,
St James's University Hospital
Beckett Street,
Leeds LS9 7TF, UK

R.C. Wilson
Consultant Anaesthetist,
Department of Anaesthesia,
St James's University Hospital,
Beckett Street,
Leeds LS9 7TF, UK

FOREWORD

The twenty two chapters assembled by the editors and collaborators of this book have created an overview of obstetric anaesthetic practice in Britain and Europe. Senior staff and trainees will find it a helpful resource for steering a safe passage through the increasingly complex maze of variables that surrounds and determines the art of obstetric anaesthesia as the specialty strives towards the exponentially unattainable goal of zero adverse outcomes. During the past three decades advances in biochemistry, pharmacology, physiology and especially imaging technology have revealed increasing opportunities for good and for identifying the underlying causes of iatrogenic harm that were previously unthinkable.

Reports from international data sources indicate that certain clearly definable shortcomings run like a common thread through the causality of adverse anaesthetic outcomes, especially in obstetric anaesthetic practice. A significant proportion of these do not arise solely from a lack of knowledge of the sort addressed in this book but rather from forgetting common-sense rules of medical behaviour and the simple, anatomical, physiological and pharmacological imperatives underlying sound clinical practice. That front in the battle for safe anaesthesia can only be won by hands-on example from the leaders and teachers of the specialty, at all hours of the day and night in the 24-hour milieu in which we practice. The fine tuning of that background protective cover comes through study and discussion of focused texts such as those comprising this scholarly collection of contemporary essays.

Philip R. Bromage
Professor (Post-retirement)
Department of Anaesthesia,
McGill University,
Montreal, Canada

MATERNAL MORTALITY

1

T.A. Thomas

INTRODUCTION

Direct obstetric deaths are those resulting from obstetric complications of the pregnant state (pregnancy, labour and the puerperium), interventions, omissions, incorrect treatment, or from a chain of events resulting from any of the above. Indirect obstetric deaths are defined as those resulting from previous existing disease, or disease that developed during pregnancy and which was not due to direct obstetric causes, but which was aggravated by the physiological effects of pregnancy.

The longest running and most complete record of such obstetric deaths is the series of triennial reports on confidential enquiries into maternal deaths, which provides a record of maternal mortality in the UK from 1952 to 1993. Originally separate reports were produced for Scotland, Northern Ireland, and England and Wales. From 1985 these reports have been amalgamated into a UK report.

Information on maternal mortality had been collected in the UK prior to 1952. In 1928 the then Minister of Health, Mr Neville Chamberlain, appointed a Health Department Committee on Maternal Mortality and Morbidity. This Committee reported on 5800 maternal deaths which occurred between 1928 and 1982. The Minister of Health, as a result, asked UK medical officers of health to continue with their enquiries which had formed the basis of the Departmental Committee's report. Summaries of the medical officers' enquiries were published in annual reports 'On the State of the Public Health' for the next twenty years. By the late 1940s decreasing proportions of maternal deaths were being collected by this method; in the final few reports only about 60% of the total deaths were actually included. Because of the decrease in completeness of the record these reports had obviously become less valuable as an aid to changing and improving obstetric practice.

The present form of triennial reporting was first discussed in 1949 at the 12th British Congress on Obstetrics and Gynaecology. The Ministry of Health, the Royal College of Obstetricians and Gynaecologists and the Society of Medical Officers of Health subsequently refined the initial suggestion into a method of enquiry which combined information from the local medical officer of health, the family doctor, the midwife and the consultant obstetrician. Inclusion of an opinion from an anaesthetist is first mentioned in the 1961–1963 report and the importance of anaesthesia as a major contributor to maternal mortality is highlighted in the 1967–1969 triennial report. In the preface the chief medical officer states

Clinical Problems in Obstetric Anaesthesia
Edited by Ian F. Russell and Gordon Lyons. Published in 1997 by Chapman & Hall, London. ISBN 0 412 71600 3.

'particular attention should be called to one area where greater improvement is possible, the number of deaths attributed to anaesthesia'. He continues 'the organization of anaesthetic services in midwifery has been discussed with the joint committee of the Royal College of Obstetricians and Gynaecologists, the Faculty of Anaesthetists and the Central Midwives Board. New arrangements have been made for the review of such cases in future and the possibility of improved specialist anaesthetic services to obstetric departments is being discussed with hospital boards'. In the triennial report for the years 1970–1972 a list of regional assessors in anaesthesia appears for the first time. Further additions to the assessment of maternal deaths appeared in 1981 when regional assessors in pathology were appointed. Their specific duty, in the first instance, was to improve the quality of reporting on postmortem results. Most recently midwifery assessors have been appointed and their first input will be seen in the 1991–1993 report.

MATERNAL MORTALITY AND THE ANAESTHETIST

The role of the anaesthetist in the care of the pregnant patient has changed markedly over the years. Our specialty is now involved in many aspects of obstetric patient care, most notably:

- anaesthesia;
- analgesia;
- resuscitation;
- high dependency and intensive care;
- postoperative care;
- treatment of major haemorrhage;
- monitoring and control of blood pressure and other aspects of the cardiovascular system.

Because of this extending role, anaesthetists in many centres are involved in the care of 50% or more of patients. By the same token substandard care provided by anaesthetists may be

commented on in sections of the confidential enquiries relating to hypertension, haemorrhage, ectopic pregnancy and amniotic fluid embolism, as well as in the section devoted to anaesthesia and intensive care.

The steady improvement in maternal mortality since 1930 is probably shown most clearly by an illustration in the 1982–1984 triennial report [1] (Figure 1.1). Since 1952 anaesthesia has shown a similar, although less rapid improvement. Because of the difference in the rate of improvement between the two figures and because of the manner in which causation of death is defined in the triennial reports, anaesthesia became the third commonest cause of maternal death in 1972; a position which it maintained until 1985 (Figure 1.2). It can be seen that the number of anaesthetic deaths occurring in each triennium has decreased gradually until 1984 but much more rapidly since that date. In spite of the decreasing numbers the percentage of mortality attributed to anaesthesia actually increased slightly until 1984 and then that too fell sharply. In the 40 years that the confidential enquiries have been reporting maternal deaths, there have been a number of significant changes in the methods and techniques of anaesthesia administered to pregnant women. The introduction of endotracheal intubation as a standard method of preventing the aspiration of gastric contents appeared during the early 1960s and the use of left lateral tilt in the early 1970s. Measures to control the acidity of gastric contents began at a similar time. The use of epidural anaesthesia, and later subarachnoid anaesthesia, for many caesarean sections did not become widespread until the late 1970s and early 1980s. In the last 20 years the overwhelming majority of maternal deaths caused by anaesthesia were the result of one or other complication of general anaesthesia. There are relatively few deaths associated with either epidural or spinal anaesthesia. However, none of the figures appearing in the triennial reports show the true risk of death from any form of anaesthesia because the total number of

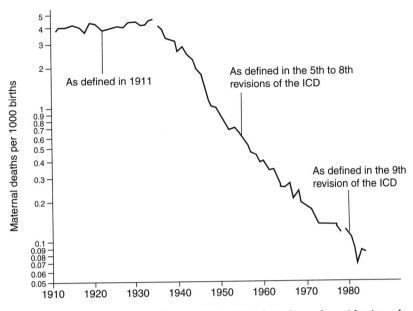

Figure 1.1 Maternal mortality (England and Wales 1911–1984) plotted on a logarithmic scale. Reproduced with permission from reference [1]. Crown copyright is reproduced with the permission of the Controller of Her Majesty's Stationery Office. *Source*: OPCS mortality statistics

anaesthetics administered to pregnant women in the UK remains unknown as does the relative proportion, or actual number, of general, epidural and subarachnoid anaesthetics. The number of caesarean sections that are carried out in the UK has risen steadily from 1970 to the present day. Good estimates of the caesarean section rate from 1970–1984 appeared in the triennial report of 1982–1984 [1]. Since that time there have been changes in the methods used to collect statistics so a degree of uncertainty remains over the annual national total number of caesarean sections. The improvement in maternal mortality associated with anaesthesia, the large difference between the number of deaths due to general anaesthesia as opposed to regional anaesthesia and the uncertainty of the denominator totals of anaesthetics and caesarean sections performed has led people to assume that the decrease in mortality is solely due to a change from general anaesthesia to regional anaesthesia. This assumption is not necessarily correct.

The safety of regional anaesthesia is not in doubt. What is being overlooked is the improvement, or decrease in risk of general anaesthesia. Using the figures available a number of conclusions can be drawn. The total number of births per triennium has remained largely unaltered for the last twenty years [3]. The proportion of deliveries by caesarean section has increased. In addition the number of women receiving one or other form of regional analgesia during their labours has also increased in the same period. It now seems possible that the actual number of general anaesthetics given has remained fairly constant, while the number of regional anaesthetics has gone up markedly [4]. In addition it is likely that general anaesthetics tend to be used more often in cases of urgent need. These latter urgent emergency cases are usually the least well prepared and most anaesthesia deaths occur in emergency cases (Figure 1.2). The combination of these facts indicates that there has been an improvement in the quality and

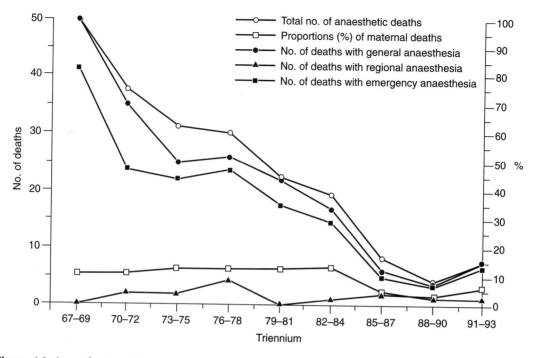

Figure 1.2 Anaesthesia and maternal death (England and Wales 1967–1984 and UK 1985–1990). Reproduced with permission from reference [2]; published by Blackwell, 1997.

safety of general anaesthesia given to pregnant patients. The improvement has occurred in parallel with a number of changes in anaesthesia services and techniques. An increasing number of sessions of experienced consultant and senior registrar time have been devoted to obstetric anaesthesia, there has been a better and more consistent approach to the control of gastric secretions, increased awareness of a need for trained assistance for the anaesthetist and a recognition that minimum standards of monitoring are the same for pregnant patients receiving anaesthesia as for any general surgical patient: the quality of monitoring is still not as uniformly high as it should be. Inexperienced trainees are still facing demands which outstrip their levels of competence and calls for senior assistance are made too late to affect outcome [5]. The fact that women are still dying from errors of endotracheal intubation shows that further improvements in anaesthesia-related mortality are possible. Between

1985 and 1993 21 patients died from complications of anaesthesia. Six of these women received general anaesthetics because they refused regional anaesthesia. In a further three women general anaesthesia was necessary because of technical difficulties with a spinal or epidural block. Judged by the details in the reports [3, 5, 6] it seems that most of these cases were not of immediate urgency and could have awaited a senior consultation. It is not possible to divine how much influence anaesthetist inexperience had in patient refusals or failures of regional anaesthesia but an experienced senior anaesthetist may have had more success in instituting regional blocks.

The acute intraoperative, or intrapartum, conduct of anaesthesia is not the limit of anaesthetic care or responsibility, however. Anaesthetists must ensure that their patients recover safely from the effects of anaesthesia. In addition they have a responsibility to prescribe and manage postpartum pain relief. The

Table 1.1 Maternal deaths in the UK 1985–1993

	1985–1987	*1988–1990*	*1991–1993*
Maternal deaths:			
Direct plus indirect	223 (9.8)	238 (10.1)	228 (9.8)
Direct	137 (6.0)	145 (6.1)	128 (5.5)
Anaesthesia deaths:			
Direct	8 (0.26)	5 (0.17)	8 (0.35)
As % of maternal deaths	4.3	2.7	6.5
'Obstetric deaths'*	8	4	7
Anaesthesia contributory	16	10	6

Rate per 100 000 maternities in parentheses.
*'Obstetric deaths' include all deaths involving a viable pregnancy and exclude cases such as ectopic pregnancy.

1988–1990 triennial report [3] says 'most anaesthetic departments now provide a postoperative pain relief service and this should be extended to cover postoperative maternity patients'. In addition this report also recommends that 'midwifery staff deputed to look after postoperative patients should be specifically trained in monitoring, the care of the airway and resuscitative procedures should be supervised by defined anaesthetists at all times'. A number of deaths in this 1988–1990 period [3] were quite clearly due to substandard postoperative care. Inappropriate use of opioids and an absence of monitoring were recorded in more than half of the ten deaths to which anaesthesia was contributory in the 1988–1990 triennium.

In the 1991–1993 report [5], the most recent, the total number of maternal deaths was lower than in 1988–1990 [3] but remained fractionally above the 1985–1987 [6] figure (Table 1.1). The mortality rate derived from these numbers was also lower in 1991–1993 than in 1988–1990 and was the same (9.8 per 100000 maternities) as in 1985–1987. The number of direct deaths known to the enquiry in 1991–1993 was less than that recorded in both the 1985–1987 and 1988–1990 triennia. The direct mortality rate therefore fell from 6.1 to 5.5 deaths per 100 000 maternities. In contrast the direct plus indirect rate fell from 10.1 to 9.8 deaths per 100000 maternities. These decreases of 10% and 3% respectively are very welcome, although the difference between the rates' improvement demands some consideration.

In the face of the overall reduction in maternal mortality a doubling of the number and rate of anaesthetic deaths was disappointing. In addition to the eight deaths directly due to anaesthesia there were six deaths to which anaesthesia was contributory and, furthermore, anaesthetists were involved in the care, at some stage, of the majority of cases of direct deaths reported in the report [5]. The rising number of caesarean section deaths together with the very considerable contribution made to maternal mortality by both haemorrhage and adult respiratory distress syndrome (ARDS) deaths give an indication of the extent of the involvement of anaesthetists and the continuing need for high-quality obstetric anaesthesia services.

ANAESTHESIA AND CAESAREAN SECTION

The total number of caesarean sections performed in the UK between 1991 and 1993 remains an unknown denominator, so caesarean section mortality rate is unclear and the 1991–1993 report [5] does not attempt to define it. An increase in caesarean section rate may explain the rise in numbers of caesarean section deaths in the 1991–1993 triennium but without denominator information this conclusion must remain uncertain. The number of general anaesthetics, epidurals and subarachnoid anaesthetics given for abdominal delivery are also unknown. What is quite clear, however, is that all caesarean section deaths attributable to anaesthetic causes are related to general anaesthesia rather than regional anaesthesia. However, in spite of an increasing number of caesarean sections being performed with regional anaesthetics the actual number of general anaesthetics given to pregnant women may not have decreased significantly [4]. Assuming a static number of general anaesthetics, an increasing number of both regional anaesthetics and caesarean sections confirms not only the overwhelming safety of regional anaesthesia but also an improvement in the quality of obstetric general anaesthesia over the period 1985–1990. A change for the worse in the case of general anaesthesia seems to have occurred in 1991–1993. The almost complete absence of any deaths in the 1982–1993 decade related to epidural or subarachnoid anaesthesia for caesarean section should encourage us to continue to recommend regional anaesthesia to parturients provided contraindications have been excluded.

The Standing Joint Committee of the Royal College of Anaesthetists (RCA) and the Royal College of Obstetricians and Gynaecologists (RCOG) hopes to begin to collect the denominator information on caesarean section numbers and the methods of anaesthesia being used. The information is to be collected with the agreement and help of the RCOG Hospital Recognition Committee and will be retrieved using the Recognition Committee's annual hospital returns. These are important denominators that will help to interpret the confidential enquiry anaesthesia data. The importance of these data will increase still further if caesarean section rates continue to climb in the UK as they have in the USA. Consultant anaesthetists with a responsibility for obstetric anaesthesia should anticipate an approach by their obstetric colleagues with requests for

Table 1.2 Anaesthesia mortality: factors contributing to death (1991–1993)

Total	8
'Obstetric' only	7
Emergency anaesthesia	6
General	5
Airway problems	4
Aspiration	2
Poor postoperative care	2
Poor fluid balance	3
Epidural	1
Anaphylaxis	2

assistance with the numbers of the various types of anaesthesia given in their unit. Knowledge of accurate totals of general anaesthetics, epidurals and subarachnoid anaesthetics given nationally would be invaluable in determining the relative safety of such procedures.

DIRECT DEATHS DUE TO ANAESTHESIA (1991–1993)

Anaesthesia in the 1991–1993 triennium [5] was responsible for eight deaths, more than in either of the preceding triennia. The greater number of deaths represented also a higher mortality rate and a larger proportion of maternal deaths than in either of the two previous triennial reports (Table 1.1). The factors contributing to these anaesthetic deaths are shown in Table 1.2.

In seven of the eight cases care was considered to be substandard. In three cases anaesthesia was given by a consultant and in five by trainees, or a 'subconsultant grade anaesthetist'. In only one of the five latter cases was a consultant anaesthetist informed of problems or difficulties in sufficient time to influence the outcome or conduct of the case. This failure to inform consultant staff stemmed from a lack of appreciation of the severity of the patient's problems and the need for senior advice or help. In addition patient monitoring was inadequate in at least six of the fatalities and high dependency or intensive care seems not to have been available when needed in four cases. Deaths from anaphylactic reactions are uncommon in any triennial period. To have two fatal anaphylactic reactions to suxamethonium in one triennium is even rarer. However, before dismissing these as rare inevitable events it should be remembered that the use of regional anaesthesia avoids the chance of this particular reaction almost entirely.

Improvements in anaesthesia related mortality in the years 1982–1990 may have lulled the specialty into a false sense of security. They may also have suggested to those responsible for the distribution of resources in health care that the obstetric anaesthesia problem had been solved. This is clearly not the case. The maintenance of a very low level of anaesthetic mortality such as that achieved in the 1988–1990 triennium is only possible if adequate resources in staffing, training, monitoring and high dependency/intensive care facilities are made available. All obstetric patients will continue to be high-risk patients when presenting for anaesthesia. The risk is greatest for emergency cases, whether planned or not and the complications of general anaesthesia are responsible for almost all fatalities. Failure to follow guidelines or protocols and seek help at an early stage was identified in most of the cases appearing in the 1991–1993 report [5]. Aspiration of gastric content was seen in only one case in this period and in this case the basic guidelines and protocols of the unit for the control of gastric secretions were not observed. The use of H_2 blocking drugs together with non particulant antacids as recommended in a number of earlier reports seems to be effective since patients correctly receiving this regimen do not appear in the confidential enquiries record for the last three reports [3, 5, 6]. The current trend to a liberal attitude which allows women to eat during labour may change this excellent record and much vigilance will be required to identify future problems.

EPIDURAL ANALGESIA (1991–1993)

One case of a death following epidural analgesia is recorded in the current report [5]. The epidural was apparently used for postpartum perineal pain. It was given without any intravenous access in place because the patient had refused the latter. Such practice ignores the most basic guidelines to safe anaesthetic practice and mars what would otherwise have been a blameless record for regional anaesthesia between 1991 and 1993. Doctors would do well to remember that they can withdraw from a case if the patient declines to accept their advice or recommendations.

HAEMORRHAGE AND ANAESTHESIA

Haemorrhage has been responsible for more maternal deaths than any other single cause since the confidential enquiries began in 1952. Women dying from obstetric haemorrhage are recorded, not only in the chapter on haemorrhage, but also in that on early pregnancy deaths (previously ectopic and abortion deaths), genital tract trauma and hypertensive disease. To appreciate the true contribution haemorrhage makes to mortality it is necessary to add together the number of mothers recorded as bleeding to death in the different chapters in the enquiry. Anaesthetists are often involved in the care of these women both because of a need for anaesthesia itself and for resuscitation. In the 1988–1990 report [3] the number of deaths from antepartum haemorrhage (APH) and postpartum haemorrhage (PPH) had risen by more than 100% from the previous triennium. In the 1991–1993 triennium [5] that number has fallen again but remains some 50% above the 1985–1987 level [6] (Table 1.3 and Table 1.4).

The last three reports [3, 5, 6] have included a number of recommendations indicating the role of anaesthetists in the treatment of obstetric haemorrhage. Some of the more cogent recommendations are blended together below to give some idea of what is expected from anaesthetists if substandard care is to be avoided.

Table 1.3 Some maternal deaths in which anaesthesia services were involved

	1985–1987	*1988–1990*	*1991–1993*
Caesarean section deaths:			
Direct	50	60	63
Indirect	22	24	35
Haemorrhage deaths	10	22	15*

*This is the total from the haemorrhage chapter only. In the 1991–93 triennium there were, in addition, at least 12 deaths from haemorrhage in other chapters and a further 14 in which haemorrhage played some part.

- 'The number of deaths from haemorrhage increased in this triennium *(1988–1990)* and substandard care was a major feature. The need for a team approach to the management of severe haemorrhage is apparently not adequately recognized.'
- 'High priority should be given to remedying any remaining deficiencies in service provision, particularly the availability of blood in smaller units. Attention should be given to the organization of staff and contingency plans to cope with sudden unexpected haemorrhage. In particular the duty anaesthetic registrar should be contacted immediately *(massive obstetric haemorrhage is diagnosed)* as in most obstetric units the anaesthetists will take over the management of the fluid replacement. Resuscitation should involve a consultant anaesthetist. Aspects of the anaesthetist's contribution to resuscitation and monitoring are highlighted. Involvement of senior experienced anaesthetists is imperative, with early adequate transfusion of blood and careful monitoring using central venous pressure lines to avoid overtransfusion.'
- 'Those units which do not have a written protocol for the management of massive haemorrhage are recommended to consider the revised guidelines provided as an annexe to Chapter 3 of the *1988–1990* report.

There is very little evidence in the 1991–1993 confidential enquiries into maternal deaths that these wise recommendations have been adopted universally.

ARDS AND ANAESTHESIA

ARDS has become a common cause of maternal mortality. It first came to prominence as a cause of maternal death in the 1985–1987 report [6]. In 1988–1990 [3], 44 women are recorded as having died from ARDS. In the most recent report [5] it is difficult to determine the total number of deaths from ARDS since the report [5] seems not to have extracted and presented this number separately. However, 104 maternal deaths occurred in intensive care units, to which the mothers had been transferred following various obstetric or anaesthetic problems It is therefore likely that the number of ARDS deaths has not declined.

HIGH DEPENDENCY AND INTENSIVE CARE

The 44 ARDS deaths in 1988–1990 [3] represent approximately 20% of direct maternal mortality, a greater proportion than either hypertensive disease or pulmonary embolism. The report concluded that 'there is a need to ensure that there is at least a properly equipped, staffed and supervised high dependency care area in every consultant obstetric unit. A nominated anaesthetist should be responsible for the care of patients in this area and all staff involved should receive regular training in postoperative care and resuscitation'. Once again the confidential enquiries have defined a standard of care of the pregnant patient which, if achieved, could produce a major improvement in maternal mortality.

Table 1.4 Number of deaths from haemorrhage and rates per million maternities, England and Wales 1973–1990 compared with UK 1985–1993

	Placenta praevia	Placental abruption	Postpartum haemorrhage	Total	Rate per million maternities
England and Wales					
1973–1975	2	6	13	21	10.9
1976–1978	2	6	16	24	13.7
1979–1981	3	2	9	14	7.3
1982–1984	2	2	3	7	3.5
1985–1987	0	4	6	10	5.0
1988–1990	5	6	10	21	10.1
United Kingdom					
1985–1987	0	4	6	10	4.5
1988–1990	5	6	11	22	9.3
1991–1993	4	3	8	15	6.4

ANAESTHETISTS' FUTURE ROLE

Anaesthetists are now involved in the care, at some stage, of the majority of patients who die of one or other pregnancy-related problem. An involvement may occur at a time when it is too late to influence care or outcome unless good communication and anticipation of risk are practised by both obstetricians and anaesthetists. When timely requests for anaesthetic assistance are received anaesthetists must be in a position to respond swiftly with full support services. They have skills in the control and modification of cardiovascular and respiratory functions which can be life-saving. However, it must be remembered that pregnancy is accompanied by many physiological changes which may themselves be complicated by pregnancy-related disease. These changes demand specialist knowledge and may make inappropriate some of the treatment regimens that may be used in non-pregnant patients. Close, timely collaboration between obstetricians, obstetric anaesthetists and intensive care anaesthetists is essential to ensure the best combination of expertise and skill if the hard core of maternal mortality in the UK is to be reduced further.

REFERENCES

1. Department of Health Report on Health and Social Subjects, Number 34 (1989) *Report on Confidential Enquiries into Maternal Deaths in England and Wales 1982–1984*, HMSO, London.
2. Holdcroft, A. and Thomas, T.A. (1997) in *Principles and Practice of Obstetric Anaesthesia*, Blackwell Scientific Publications, London (in press).
3. Department of Health, Welsh Office, Scottish Office Home and Health Department, Department of Health and Social Security, Northern Ireland (1994) *Report on Confidential Enquiries into Maternal Deaths in the United Kingdom 1988–1990*, HMSO, London.
4. Brown, G. and Russell, I.F. (1995) A survey of anaesthesia for caesarean section. *International Journal of Obstetric Anaesthesia*, **4**, 214–8.
5. Department of Health, Welsh Office, Scottish Office Home and Health Department, Department of Health and Social Security, Northern Ireland (1996) *Report on Confidential Enquiries into Maternal Deaths in the United Kingdom 1991–1993*, HMSO, London.
6. Department of Health, Welsh Office, Scottish Office Home and Health Department, Department of Health and Social Security, Northern Ireland (1991) *Report on Confidential Enquiries into Maternal Deaths in the United Kingdom 1985–1987*, HMSO, London.

PREECLAMPSIA

2

M. Dresner and J.J. Walker

INTRODUCTION

Many anaesthetists outside of regular obstetric practice are well aware that preeclampsia is an important cause of maternal morbidity and mortality, but admit to little understanding of its causes, mechanisms or management. Even obstetric anaesthetists and obstetricians must confess to an incomplete understanding of this condition. Whilst much is known about associations and pathophysiology, the causes of preeclampsia remain unknown and there is little consensus between individuals, units and nations regarding management. With this background it is unfortunately not surprising that substandard care was evident in 80% of maternal deaths due to preeclampsia in the *Report on Confidential Enquiries into Maternal Deaths in the United Kingdom 1991–1993* [1].

Preeclampsia is a disease of human pregnancy, more common amongst primipara of young age and poor socio-economic background [2]. It rarely presents before the 20th week of pregnancy, and classically manifests as a triad of hypertension, proteinuria and peripheral oedema. The primary affected organ is the placenta, threatening the foetus with increased risk of intra-uterine growth retardation, premature labour and perinatal mortality. The potential dangers facing the mother include pulmonary oedema, cerebral haemorrhage, convulsions, coagulopathy and hepatic dysfunction.

Anaesthetists who have received intensive care training are no strangers to life-threatening, multisystem disease and therefore have much to offer in the management of preeclampsia. This chapter aims to provide the background knowledge and understanding of obstetric management necessary for those wishing to become more involved in the care of preeclamptic patients. The modifications in anaesthetic procedures that are necessary in preeclampsia are also discussed.

HISTORY

Convulsions in pregnancy were referred to in ancient Egyptian, Chinese, Indian, and Greek writings, and in France in 1668 [3]. The association of frothy urine, oedema and convulsions in pregnancy was recognized in the 19th century [4, 5], but explanations of pathophysiology relied upon descriptions of the advanced disease or postmortem findings. Simpson in 1859 wrote that 'albumenuria, dropsy, and convulsions are successive effects of one common central cause – viz. a pathological state of the blood, to the occurrence of which pregnancy in some way predisposes'. Had he

Clinical Problems in Obstetric Anaesthesia
Edited by Ian F. Russell and Gordon Lyons. Published in 1997 by Chapman & Hall, London. ISBN 0 412 71600 3.

the means to measure blood pressure, no doubt he would have also commented on the incidence of hypertension. This observation was made by Vaquez in 1897 [6], who noted the regular occurrence of high systolic blood pressure in eclamptic women. The full importance of these associations was slow to be accepted.

DIAGNOSIS AND GRADING OF PREECLAMPSIA

There have been several attempts to define preeclampsia to distinguish it from other causes of hypertension in pregnancy. The term 'gestational proteinuric hypertension', coined by Davey and MacGillivray [7], is currently in favour. Differences in precise definitions and diagnostic criteria of preeclampsia will rarely significantly affect clinical management, but there is no doubt that consistency within a unit is an important prerequisite for high-quality care.

HYPERTENSION

Despite being a fundamental diagnostic criterion in preeclampsia, blood pressure assessment is less than straightforward. Whilst systolic pressure tends to be consistently reported, different measurement techniques lead to great variability in diastolic pressure. The World Health Organisation recommends that diastolic pressure should be recorded at phase IV of the Korotkoff sound (the point of muffling). However the use of phase V (disappearance of the pulse sound) is widespread in the USA and amongst many UK obstetricians and midwives [8] and it is also used by the Dinamap automated oscillotonometer. Phase V produces a reading about 5 to 10 mmHg lower than phase IV. In addition to this, the standard deviation in diastolic pressure at phase V is very high because of the hyperkinetic circulation in pregnancy, occasionally producing a reading close to zero [9]. Phase IV is therefore the best technique in pregnancy, recorded when the patient is calm, with an

appropriate cuff size and avoidance of aortocaval compression. If automated non-invasive blood pressure machines are used, they should be used all the time to allow trends to be followed. Treatment thresholds may need to be lower than when manual phase IV techniques are used.

Measuring diastolic pressure

- Use IVth Korotkoff sound (muffling)
- Use an appropriate blood pressure cuff size
- Keep the cuff level with the heart when possible
- Avoid aortocaval compression

Davey and MacGillivray define hypertension in pregnancy as two or more diastolic readings equal to or greater than 90 mm Hg at least four hours apart, or a single reading equal to or greater than 110 mm Hg.

PROTEINURIA

Davey and MacGillivray [7] define proteinuria as concentrations greater than 0.3 g/l in a 24-hour urine collection, or greater than 1 g/l in two random urine collections at least four hours apart.

Ames Multiple Reagent Strips by Bayer Diagnostics are commonly used for urinalysis by midwives. Reagent colour changes are traditionally spoken of as a number of 'pluses', for example 'four pluses of protein'. This would be written as 'protein +4'. These correlate with urine concentrations as shown in Table 2.1.

OEDEMA

Oedema is the least reliable of the diagnostic criteria for preeclampsia. It is common in normal pregnancy, yet eclampsia can occur without any oedema. Classically, normal gestational oedema is confined to the ankles and

Table 2.1 Testing for proteinuria with Ames Multiple Reagent Strips

Pluses of protein	Urine concentration (g/l)
+1	0.3
+2	1
+3	3
+4	>20

sacral area, whereas in preeclampsia it becomes generalized. This can be seen in the fingers and face, and occasionally an oedematous airway will be noted at laryngoscopy if general anaesthesia is required.

Diagnosis of preeclampsia

- Diastolic blood pressure ≥ 90 mm Hg on two readings, or
- Diastolic blood pressure ≥ 110 mm Hg on one reading

and

- Proteinuria > 3 g/l in 24 hours, or
- Proteinuria > 1 g/l in two random samples

SEVERE PREECLAMPSIA

Mild preeclampsia is managed conservatively in many units. Severe preeclampsia, however, will initiate more intensive monitoring and active treatment, so a clear definition is useful. Blood pressure criteria will vary according to the technique of measurement and should be considered on a local basis. The American College of Obstetricians and Gynecologists [10] use any one of the following criteria to define severe preeclampsia:

- systolic pressure   > 160 mm Hg
- diastolic pressure   > 110 mm Hg
- mean arterial pressure   > 120 mm Hg
- proteinuria   5 g/24 hours
                             (3+ or 4+ on dipstick)
- oliguria   < 500 ml in 24 hours

- headache or cerebral disturbances
- visual disturbances
- epigastric pain
- pulmonary oedema or cyanosis
- HELLP syndrome (haemolysis, elevated liver enzymes, low platelets)

ECLAMPSIA

If one or more grand mal convulsions, not related to other conditions, occur in preeclampsia, the diagnosis of eclampsia can be made.

THE IMPORTANCE OF PREECLAMPSIA

Although preeclampsia occurs in about 4% of pregnancies in developed countries, severe complications such as eclampsia, disseminated intravascular coagulation (DIC) and the HELLP syndrome are relatively rare. It is therefore easy to become complacent about patients with mild preeclampsia admitted for observation and bed rest on the labour or antenatal wards. However, hypertensive disorders of pregnancy are the second main cause of direct maternal deaths in the UK. Adult respiratory distress syndrome (ARDS), pulmonary oedema and cerebral haemorrhage accounted for most of the 20 deaths due to preeclampsia in the 1991–1993 triennium. Uncontrolled hypertension, convulsions and aspiration of gastric contents often precipitate the causes of death mentioned. In short, preeclampsia is a disease of treacherous nature and lethal potential that demands attentive care.

AETIOLOGY

Whatever is the cause of preeclampsia, it must explain the predisposing influences and associations. These include:

- nulliparity;
- multiple pregnancy, hydatidiform mole, diabetes, hydramnios;
- higher incidence in certain geographical areas;

- rarity of repeated problems in subsequent pregnancies.

NULLIPARITY

Preeclampsia is mostly a disease of primigravidae and a normal first pregnancy seems to protect the patient from future preeclampsia [11]. Even a previous abortion may offer some protection [12]. These statements depend upon the patient remaining with one sexual partner; a pregnancy with a new partner increases the risk of preeclampsia to that of a nulliparous woman.

These facts suggest that the disease of preeclampsia may be related to antigens or factors emanating from the foetoplacental unit. After an exposure to these antigens the mother is subsequently much less susceptible to the disease, possibly through the development of antibodies to the causative antigens. A new partner leads to new antigens and renewed risk. Thus an immunological explanation of the root cause of preeclampsia seems likely.

MULTIPLE PREGNANCY, HYDATIDIFORM MOLE, DIABETES AND HYDRAMNIOS

The strong association between hydatidiform mole and preeclampsia eliminates foetal tissue as the cause of the disease. Rapid uterine enlargement is a common factor, but polyhydramnios alone seems innocent unless it is linked to another factor [13]. The presence of large amounts of placental tissue is more likely to be responsible: twins confer a four-fold risk of preeclampsia over singletons, and diabetes mellitus doubles the incidence [14]. This would comply with an immunological mechanism, given that a large placental mass would produce a correspondingly increased immunological load.

HIGHER INCIDENCE IN CERTAIN GEOGRAPHICAL AREAS

It is extremely difficult to separate the influences of environmental factors, diet, genetics and standards of health care in explaining differences in the incidence of preeclampsia around the world. In addition to this, the reliability of reporting and accuracy of case notes is very variable. Even so, there is no doubt that the incidence and severity of preeclampsia is high in parts of the developing world and that the disease is a major cause of maternal mortality.

RARITY OF REPEATED PROBLEMS IN SUBSEQUENT PREGNANCIES

If the first pregnancy is normal, preeclampsia is rare in subsequent pregnancies [15]. This apparent protective effect of the first pregnancy can be explained in part by the immunological theories previously discussed, but the protection is not absolute. After a preeclamptic first pregnancy, the incidence in the next pregnancy has been reported to be as high as 35.4% [16]. It may be, therefore, that a normal first pregnancy is not protective, but merely demonstrates a lack of susceptibility of that particular mother and father combination.

IS PREECLAMPSIA AN IMMUNOLOGICAL DISEASE?

In normal pregnancy the mother is able to accept the paternal antigens displayed by the foetoplacental unit, and it may be that preeclampsia is caused by a failure of this mechanism. Whilst the first pregnancy seems to 'immunize' the mother against preeclampsia in future pregnancies from the same partner [17], no increase in ABO, HLA, or Y-linked compatibility has been found in couples with a preeclamptic pregnancy [18]. However, Redman *et al.* [19] showed a higher incidence of HLA homozygosity in such couples. This would increase the chances of antigen sharing between these couples which may lead to the mother failing to mount the normal immunological response to the foetoplacental unit. Several cytochemical changes linked to the immune system have been noted in preeclampsia, including lymphocyte dysfunction [20, 21], neutrophil activation [22, 23] and elevated cell adhesion molecule levels [24].

So, an immunological origin to preeclampsia seems likely, but the exact mechanism remains unclear. There may be an increased response to foetal antigens or a reduction of the appropriate suppressive effect normally seen in pregnancy. The latter theory is supported by the fact that the risk of preeclampsia is greatly increased with twins, but there is no difference in risk between homo and heterozygous twins.

The immunological interaction between mother and baby begins at implantation of the embryo. At the luteal phase of every menstrual cycle large granular lymphocytes migrate into the endometrium and, in the event of conception, remain there until the twentieth week of pregnancy. These lymphocytes respond to contact with invading trophoblasts by producing antibodies that suppress T-lymphocyte activation [25] within the uterus. As trophoblasts are known to enter the maternal circulation, this reaction could also take place systemically. It may be that insufficient production of the blocking antibodies allows a reaction between mother and placenta that lays the foundation for preeclampsia.

What complicates this picture is the fact that the placental lesion of preeclampsia is not specific, being seen also in intra-uterine growth retardation [26]. This suggests that some other aetiological component is required to convert the immunological and placental disorder into a multisystem disease.

PATHOPHYSIOLOGY

Whilst the cause of preeclampsia remains the subject of conjecture, more consensus exists about the pathophysiology. Many agree that the organ responsible for preeclampsia is the placenta, starting with **failure of spiral artery relaxation**. In normal pregnancy, placentation leads to loss of muscle and relaxation of the myometrial spiral arteries, with a resultant increase in blood flow to the foetoplacental

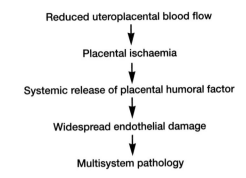

Figure 2.2 The pathophysiology of preeclampsia.

unit. In preeclampsia, two lesions compromise this adaptation. Firstly, there is a relative failure of trophoblastic invasion of the arterial walls [27], and secondly some arteries become blocked with fibrin, platelets and lipid-laden macrophages [28]. The result is uterine blood flow being reduced by up to 30–40% [29, 30]. Abnormalities of flow velocity wave forms of the uterine arcuate arteries can be detected by Doppler techniques at 18–24 weeks' gestation, before preeclampsia becomes overt [31]. Although the root cause of this phenomenon is not known, it is possible to piece together a convincing flow diagram (Figure 2.1) of the pathophysiology of preeclampsia starting from this point.

The consequence of failure of spiral artery relaxation is chronic **placental ischaemia**. Late evidence of this fact is the shrunken, calcified placenta with multiple infarcts commonly seen in preeclampsia. Histologically, these placentae show trophoblastic proliferation and syncytial knots, with blunting and clubbing of the micro villi. Proof that these placental lesions are due to ischaemia exists in the fact that similar changes can be produced *in vitro* by exposing cultured trophoblasts to hypoxia [32].

Failure of spiral artery relaxation and subsequent placental ischaemia are not confined to preeclampsia. These abnormalities are seen in intra-uterine growth retardation, when the mother can be completely healthy. In the preeclamptic woman, however, this placental dysfunction is associated with a multisystem

Table 2.2 Prostacyclin/thromboxane ratios in preeclampsia

	Thromboxane/prostacyclin ratio
Normal pregnancy	0.63
Mild preeclampsia	0.77
Severe preeclampsia	1.94

endothelial disorder [33]. It has been long postulated that a **humoral factor of placental origin** is responsible for this escalation, but still none has been isolated. It is unfashionable to use the word 'toxaemia' in relation to preeclampsia, but the idea of a systemic toxin being involved is attractive in explaining the pathophysiology of preeclampsia. It would also have therapeutic implications if such a toxin could be neutralized. However, similar ideas in intensive care medicine, such as using anti-endotoxin in Gram negative septicaemia [34] and anti-tumour necrosis factor in the systemic inflammatory response syndrome have so far proved disappointing.

Whatever is responsible for converting preeclampsia from a placental to a multisystem disorder, there is much evidence to confirm the presence of widespread **endothelial damage**. Plasma fibronectin, a cell surface glycoprotein present on trophoblasts and all endothelial tissues, becomes elevated in preeclampsia [35]. The same is true of factor VIII-related antigen [36]. A disturbance of the balance between serum prostacyclin/thromboxane provides further evidence, and the ratio (Table 2.2) between these two antagonizing eicosanoids correlates with the severity of preeclampsia [37].

A review of the roles of these two agents helps to explain the link between endothelial damage and many of the features of preeclampsia. Prostacyclin is a vasodilator and endogenous anticoagulant that plays a vital role in tissue perfusion. It exists in balance with its fellow arachidonic acid derivative, thromboxane, which causes vasoconstriction and platelet aggregation. The relative excess of thromboxane can help explain the hypertension, reduced renal perfusion and intravascular coagulation seen in preeclampsia. A widespread lesion of the endothelium also accounts for peripheral oedema, proteinuria, cerebral oedema and a susceptibility to pulmonary oedema.

CLINICAL FEATURES

Preeclampsia rarely presents before the 24th week of pregnancy, and never before the 20th week except in association with a hydatidiform mole. A common mode of presentation is asymptomatic hypertension and proteinuria at a routine antenatal check-up. The earlier in pregnancy it develops, the more likely it is to progress in severity. Despite all manner of conservative and active regimens, the disease can only be reliably terminated by ending the pregnancy. Signs and symptoms usually resolve within 48 hours of delivery. Almost every system of the body can become involved, and these are now discussed in turn.

THE CARDIOVASCULAR SYSTEM

The traditional view of the haemodynamics of preeclampsia is of hypertension due to an elevated systemic vascular resistance (SVR) [38], with a reduced intravascular volume and low central venous pressure. This was confirmed in a small series of untreated preeclamptic patients subjected to pulmonary artery catheterization [39]. However, more recent data suggest that this view is over-simplified.

Two published series of severe preeclamptics have shown normal haemodynamics in many patients, but a great heterogeneity [40, 41]. A common finding was a high stroke work index in relation to the wedge pressure, indicating a hyperdynamic left ventricle. This suggests that the hypertension of preeclampsia may be due to a hyperdynamic rather than constricted haemodynamic state in some cases [42]. However, in both these series, patients had received intravenous fluids at 75 ml/hour

Table 2.3 Studies of haemodynamics in severe preeclampsia

	Controls ref. 39 (n = 4)	Untreated preeclamptics ref. 39 (n = 10)	Treated preeclamptics ref. 40 (n = 45)	Treated preeclamptics ref. 41 (n = 41)
Diastolic blood pressure (mm Hg)	77 (70–90)	106 (100–120)	110 (65–140)	106 (74–130)
Mean arterial pressure (mm Hg)	95 (93–106)	121 (113–136)	138 (97–171)	130 (100–155)
Heart rate (b.p.m)	84 (70–90)	100 (90–130)	95 (69–129)	94 (65–122)
Pulmonary capillary wedge pressure (mm Hg)	9 (6–12)	3.3 (1–5)	10 (4–30)	8.3 (3–13)
Systemic vascular resistance dynes.s/cm^5	886 (805–1021)	1943 (1480–2580)	1496 (716–2734)	1496 (716–2734)
Cardiac index l/(min.m)^2	4.53 (3.96–4.97)	2.75 (1.97–3.33)	4.14 (2.43–5.91)	4.4 (3.1–6.2)

and magnesium sulphate prior to pulmonary artery catheterization, and some were in labour.

Some observations from studies of haemodynamics in severe preeclampsia are given in Table 2.3.

In conclusion, it may be that the untreated severe preeclamptic patient does indeed have a high SVR and is somewhat hypovolaemic. After some intravenous fluid and mild vasodilatation (such as caused by magnesium sulphate) these parameters normalize. Continuing hypertension may then be due to an inappropriately high SVR in combination with a hyperdynamic left ventricle.

THE RESPIRATORY SYSTEM

The importance of pulmonary oedema (in the form of ARDS) as a cause of death in the *Report on Confidential Enquiries into Maternal Deaths in the United Kingdom 1991–1993* [1], has already been commented on in this chapter. What are the mechanisms responsible for this potentially lethal problem?

Oedema does not occur in the normal individual because of the colloid osmotic pressure exerted by plasma proteins. In preeclampsia, plasma proteins are lost in large amounts through proteinuria and into the tissues through the damaged capillary endothelium. Low colloid osmotic pressure and a damaged pulmonary vascular endothelium thereby leave the preeclamptic patient vulnerable to pulmonary oedema. If it were it not for the relative hypovolaemia and low filling pressures discussed earlier, pulmonary oedema would presumably be more common.

Thirty-seven cases of pulmonary oedema were reported by Sibai *et al.* in 1987, giving an incidence of 2.9% in patients with severe preeclampsia [43]. Older, multiparous patients seemed at increased risk, as were those with preeclampsia superimposed on chronic hypertension. Perhaps the most important risk factor was the injudicious use of intravenous fluids, given in response to medical, surgical or obstetric complications. Thus, haemorrhage, sepsis and surgical procedures are risk factors for pulmonary oedema in preeclampsia. Pulmonary oedema was also associated with DIC in 48.6% of cases and the HELLP syndrome in 43.2%. With a perinatal mortality in this series of 53% and a maternal mortality of 10.8%, pulmonary oedema can be seen to be an extremely serious complication.

The likely consequences of pulmonary oedema in the obstetric patient are maternal hypoxia and foetal hypoxia leading to an urgent caesarean section, the need for potentially hazardous invasive monitoring, the possible need for intubation in hypoxic conditions and ventilation on the intensive care unit. This alarming list must preface any discussion of fluid balance and the management of oliguria in preeclampsia.

THE RENAL SYSTEM

It is a common misconception amongst anaesthetists that oliguria in preeclampsia is primarily due to volume depletion and poor renal perfusion, and should therefore be managed with intravenous fluids. Obstetricians tend to focus more on the intra-renal lesion of preeclampsia, and commonly argue against aggressive rehydration because of their fear of pulmonary oedema.

Because of the imbalance between prostacyclin and thromboxane, and the hypovolaemia that results from oedema and hypertension, renal blood flow and glomerular filtration rate are reduced in preeclamptic women. However, the decrements of 25–30% below values in normal pregnancy are still at or above non-pregnant levels [44]. In addition to this, there is a subset of oliguric preeclamptic women with normal or high cardiac filling pressures [45]. These facts suggest that there is little to gain and potential danger in blind, aggressive volume therapy.

There is reassurance for those anxious about a conservative approach to fluid therapy. The classic intra-renal lesion, described by Spargo *et al.* in 1959 [46] as glomerular capillary endotheliosis, consists of endothelial cell engorgement with intracellular inclusions. It is present in over 70% of primiparous women with preeclampsia, but it reverses completely after delivery [33]. Acute tubular necrosis does occur in pure preeclampsia, but it is almost always precipitated by abruption or haemorrhage, and is associated with a recovery to normal renal function [47].

In summary, pre-existing chronic hypertension, parenchymal renal disease, or acute problems that reduce renal oxygen delivery, such as haemorrhage, hypoxia, disseminated intravascular coagulation or the HELLP syndrome, are risk factors for renal failure in preeclampsia. The uncomplicated renal lesion

of preeclampsia is reversible, and oliguria and proteinuria normally resolve within 48 hours after delivery. So long as the obligatory output of about 400 ml of concentrated urine per 24 hours is produced, the risk of permanent renal damage is very low.

THE NERVOUS SYSTEM

The neurological features of preeclampsia include:

- headache;
- visual disturbances (including very rare retinal artery thrombosis and temporary cortical blindness);
- eclampsia;
- cerebrovascular accident.

Hyper-reflexia is a subjective sign of doubtful significance in preeclampsia, since reflexes are normally brisk in pregnancy.

Postmortem examination of the brains of women who have died after preeclampsia/eclampsia reveals cortical petechial haemorrhages and micro-infarcts (classically ring haemorrhage around thrombosed precapillaries). Subcortical, brain stem and small subarachnoid haemorrhages, as well as cerebral oedema are also seen. Massive, deep intracerebral haemorrhages may also be found, and are the commonest cause of death in preeclampsia. These findings are similar to those of hypertensive encephalopathy in previously normotensive individuals, and so it is tempting to assume that hydrostatic trauma is the sole mechanism of neurological damage in preeclampsia. However, as eclampsia is often associated with unremarkable blood pressures it seems likely that damage to the neurovascular endothelium is also an important factor.

ECLAMPSIA

In developing countries, which have maternal mortality rates 100–200 times higher than Europe and North America, it is estimated that 10% of maternal deaths are associated with eclampsia [48]. A UK hospital survey in 1922 reported eclampsia in 4% of hospital labours, with a case fatality of 22% [49]. Since that time, evidence from New Zealand in 1962 [50], Sweden in 1985 [51] and North America in 1990 [2], has suggested a declining incidence of eclampsia in the developed world.

The most accurate and up to date profile of eclampsia in a developed country was produced by the British Eclampsia Survey Team (BEST) in 1994 [52]. Comprehensive data from every case of eclampsia that occurred within the UK in 1992 were reviewed, revealing a national incidence of 4.9 per 10 000 maternities. Of these nearly 1 in 50 women (1.8%) died, and 35% suffered at least one major complication. Teenagers showed a three-fold higher risk over older women, and multiple pregnancies increased the risk of eclampsia six times. Of those with premonitory symptoms, the most frequent were headache (50%), visual disturbance (19%) and epigastric pain (19%). Strikingly, however, 41% had no symptoms before their first fit, and 38% had no recorded hypertension or proteinuria. Convulsions occurred antenatally in 38%, intrapartum in 18% and postpartum in 44%. In the latter group, 12% of cases occurred more than 48 hours after delivery.

Eclampsia is commonly perceived as the end of a linear progression of disease from mild preeclampsia, so convulsions are not expected until a patient has severe hypertension, proteinuria and symptoms. This view is not only incorrect, but potentially dangerous. It seems more likely that eclampsia, like the HELLP syndrome, represents a variant of the pregnancy induced endothelial disorder that is preeclampsia.

THE LIVER

Pathological changes of the liver in preeclampsia include periportal haemorrhages, ischaemic lesions, generalized swelling and even large subcapsular haematomata. Hepatic oedema causes stretching of the capsule, producing epigastric pain. This is an important

---

> **Impending eclampsia?**
>
> - Headache
> - Epigastric pain
> - Visual disturbance
>
> **BUT**
>
> - 41% with no symptoms
> - 38% with no hypertension or proteinuria

symptom, as it is one of the diagnostic criteria for severe preeclampsia.

Perhaps the most well-known hepatic aspect of preeclampsia is the HELLP syndrome.

HELLP SYNDROME

The HELLP syndrome consists of:

- Haemolysis
- Elevated
- Liver enzymes
- Low
- Platelets.

HELLP is diagnosed by an abnormal blood film, elevated bilirubin and lactate dehydrogenase. The haemolysis is microangiopathic in nature, resulting from the passage of red blood cells through small vessels with damaged intima and fibrin mesh deposits. Elevated liver enzymes result from periportal and focal parenchymal hepatic necrosis, in which large fibrinous deposits are seen within the sinusoids. Sibai regards liver enzymes above three standard deviations from the mean as significant [53]. Low platelets, below $100 \times 10^9/l$, result from DIC.

This variant of preeclampsia can follow a very aggressive course, causing foetal and maternal mortality as high as 60% and 24% respectively. In Sibai's series of 304 cases, he described the typical presentation as that of a white, multiparous patient, over 25 years old, with a history of poor pregnancy outcome.

Symptoms usually begin before 36 weeks' gestation, but postnatal presentation occurs in around 30%. Common presenting symptoms are malaise (in 90% of patients), epigastric pain (90%), nausea and vomiting (50%) and flu-like symptoms. Physical signs commonly include right upper quadrant tenderness (80%), weight gain and oedema (60%), but hypertension and proteinuria may be absent or mild. Thus the variety of signs and symptoms of the HELLP syndrome do not resemble the usual picture of severe preeclampsia. However, as rapid progression to DIC and hepatorenal failure can occur, each of these apparently non-specific signs and symptoms should be taken seriously in pregnancy.

Resolution of the condition after delivery is much more protracted than uncomplicated preeclampsia, and indeed, the patient may worsen in the first 24–48 hours [54]. Patients with platelets counts of less than $50 \times 10^9/l$, may take 11 days to reach $100 \times 10^9/l$ [55], and diuresis may be slow enough to warrant dialysis.

A milder form of this syndrome is sometimes seen, with modest alteration of liver function tests and thrombocytopenia, and regression after delivery without major sequelae is the norm. Haemolysis does not occur, leading to the eponym of the ELLP syndrome.

HAEMATOLOGY

Normal pregnancy produces a hypercoagulable state, and this can become exaggerated in preeclampsia. This is due to endothelial damage and the resultant imbalance of endothelial prostanoids towards thromboxane, causing increased platelet stickiness and vasoconstriction. Relative hypovolaemia resulting from oedema and hypertension leads to sluggish peripheral blood flow, which may add to the tendency for intravascular coagulation in preeclampsia. Consumptive coagulation can then lead to thrombocytopenia and coagulopathy.

In most patients with mild preeclampsia, platelet count and coagulation tests are normal. The incidence of thrombocytopenia (platelet count $< 150 \times 10^9/l$) is approximately 20% [56], but there is great variation between reports. It is extremely unlikely for a significant clotting abnormality to exist with platelet counts above $100 \times 10^9/l$, but below this level it is wise to perform coagulation screening. This has obvious relevance to the risk of haemorrhagic complications such as cerebral and hepatic haematoma, ante and postpartum haemorrhage, and the safe conduct of invasive surgical and anaesthetic procedures. As will be discussed later, coagulation status is an important consideration in regional analgesic and anaesthetic techniques.

MANAGEMENT OF PREECLAMPSIA

The general aims of therapy are to minimize vasospasm and improve perfusion of the uterus, placenta and maternal vital organs. Many units would add the reduction of CNS excitability to this list. Treatment will be considered under the following headings:

- the anaesthetist;
- the obstetrician;
- conservative management and general support;
- anti-hypertensive therapy;
- prevention and treatment of convulsions;
- fluid balance;
- management of HELLP syndrome.

THE ANAESTHETIST

In the vast majority of obstetric units, anaesthetists play no part in the management of uncomplicated mild preeclampsia unless epidural analgesia or caesarean section are required, only becoming further involved when life-threatening complications such as haemorrhage, convulsions or pulmonary oedema occur. To be maximally effective in this crisis role, obstetric anaesthetists must be become completely familiar with their obstetricians' management protocols and be aware of the progress of all preeclamptic patients on the labour ward.

THE OBSTETRICIAN

Ideally, preeclampsia would be prevented by the use of a safe prophylactic agent. Studies with fish oil [57] and low-dose aspirin [58] have, however, proved disappointing. In the future, improved understanding of precise causes and mechanisms of preeclampsia may provide a sound rationale for successful prophylaxis.

On diagnosing preeclampsia, the obstetrician's aim is to control the disease until the foetus is mature enough to survive delivery, whether this be normal, induced or operative. In severe early disease, it may be necessary to terminate a pregnancy before this time in the interests of the mother's safety [59].

CONSERVATIVE MANAGEMENT AND GENERAL SUPPORT

Comprehensive, multidisciplinary antenatal care is the starting point for the management of preeclampsia. In most countries with high maternal mortality from hypertensive disease, there is a poor level of antenatal care. When hypertension is suspected and proteinuria or oedema is noticed, early referral to an outpatient day-care unit is warranted. This allows for early risk assessment, counselling, and assessment of foetal growth and blood supply. Most hypertensive women can be managed as outpatients, but around 25% will require admission for further assessment and treatment.

ANTIHYPERTENSIVE THERAPY

During the 1980s, a reduction in deaths due to cerebrovascular accident in preeclampsia [1] correlated with an increased use of antihypertensive agents by obstetricians [60]. A recent meta-analysis of antihypertensive treatment has shown that early therapy reduces not only hypertensive crises but neonatal complications such as respiratory distress syndrome [61]. No single agent emerges as superior, as all have benefits and side effects.

The policy at St James's University Hospital, Leeds (SJUH) is to commence antihypertensive therapy if diastolic pressure is persistently over 100 mm Hg. Oral labetalol is the agent of first choice, with the logic that its combined alpha and beta-blocking effects will combat the elevated systemic vascular resistance *and* hyperdynamic left ventricle of preeclampsia. If necessary oral nifedipine can be added or labetalol infused intravenously. Animal experiments have shown placental blood flow to be well maintained with these drugs [62, 63].

After starting antihypertensive therapy, close monitoring of the mother using proteinuria, serum urates [64] and platelet counts [65] can give information concerning disease risk and progression. Foetal well-being should be followed with cardiotocography, ultrasound assessment of growth and liquor volume, and umbilical blood flow studies. Sixty per cent of patients are easily controlled, allowing some continuation of pregnancy. Another 30% respond to therapy, but show signs of maternal or foetal deterioration that necessitate delivery within a few days. Around 10% do not respond, requiring delivery within a few hours [66]. If the gestation is less than 34 weeks, two 12 mg doses of dexamethasone are given over 24 hours to encourage foetal lung maturity but a 48 hour delay before delivery is required for optimum effect.

PREVENTION AND TREATMENT OF CONVULSIONS

Recent evidence suggests that if a prophylactic anticonvulsant is to be used, magnesium sulphate is more effective than phenytoin [67] and should therefore be seen as the drug of first choice. However, it is far from clear who should receive prophylaxis. In the USA, most units give magnesium to all preeclamptic patients, and it is estimated that 5% of the pregnant population receive the drug as a result. Using UK figures, universal prophylaxis would lead to around 100 women receiving magnesium unnecessarily for every expected case of eclampsia. If one also considers the fact that 38% of eclamptics in the BEST survey [48] were not actually identified as preeclamptic before they convulsed, the value of prophylaxis becomes even more questionable.

A study of 228 women with severe preeclampsia found no advantage in adding magnesium to effective blood pressure control, with the sole case of eclampsia being in the magnesium group [68]. A larger study is required to confirm this. The decision to use magnesium sulphate as prophylaxis against eclampsia therefore remains difficult, and should perhaps be based on the incidence of eclampsia in the local population.

Evidence from the large, international multi-centre randomized Collaborative Eclampsia Trial [69] now clearly identifies magnesium sulphate as superior to diazepam and phenytoin in the treatment of eclampsia and prevention of reconvulsions.

MAGNESIUM SULPHATE

After many years of debate, the case for choosing magnesium for the treatment of eclampsia and prevention of reconvulsion is now overwhelming. For UK anaesthetists, midwives and obstetricians, it is now time to become familiar with a drug with which few have great experience.

Magnesium sulphate is available in the UK as a 50% solution with a shelf life of three years, and can be given i.m. or i.v. Like potassium, magnesium is principally an intracellular ion, so that after a loading infusion about 50% moves from the blood into bone and other cells within 90 minutes. About 50% of the infused dose is excreted in the urine within four hours. Intravenous infusion is the easiest technique with which to maintain a steady plasma level,

with adjustments necessary in the presence of oliguria or renal impairment.

The precise mechanism of magnesium's anticonvulsant action is unknown, but magnesium is both a CNS depressant, a cerebral vasodilator and a mild antihypertensive agent. Electroencephalographic findings are not normalized, but this is also sometimes true of conventional anticonvulsants, even when fitting has been controlled. Beneficial effects also include increased prostacyclin release by endothelial cells, increased uterine and renal blood flow, decreased renin and angiotensin converting enzyme activity, and reduced platelet aggregation [70]. Tocolysis can be useful in certain circumstances, but may prolong labour and predispose to increased blood loss after delivery. Decreased foetal heart rate variability may be seen, and neonatal neuromuscular and respiratory depression is possible. However, the Collaborative Eclampsia Trial [67] puts fears of toxicity into the correct perspective, with maternal mortality being lower in women receiving magnesium compared to diazepam or phenytoin. This difference was not statistically significant but, compared to the magnesium group, more mothers and babies from the phenytoin group were intubated and ventilated. This favourable safety record was achieved without the use of magnesium blood level measurements. Early toxicity is easily detected clinically: Table 2.4 illustrates that deep tendon reflexes are lost at magnesium blood levels well below that required to produce serious cardiorespiratory toxicity.

There are several popular regimens described [71, 72, 73]. At SJUH, the i.v. regimen used in the Collaborative Eclampsia Trial forms the basis of the magnesium protocol (Table 2.5).

FLUID MANAGEMENT

Oliguria in uncomplicated preeclampsia requires careful observation and assessment of fluid balance, but 0.4 ml/kg/hour of

Table 2.4 Clinical effects and plasma levels of magnesium

	Plasma level (mmol/l)
Normal	0.7–1.1
Therapeutic	2.0–3.5
ECG changes: increased PR interval and widening QRS complex	>3.0
Drowsiness	4.0
Absent deep tendon reflexes	5.0
Heart block	7.5
Respiratory paralysis	7.5
Cardiac arrest	13.0

concentrated urine can be tolerated without intervention. More severe oliguria or anuria requires bladder catheterization to confirm the diagnosis, a test dose of 20 mg frusemide, and if no response is obtained, central venous pressure (CVP) assessment. This approach avoids blind fluid challenges, which should be considered extremely rash. (**This is one of the very few situations when an oliguric surgical patient should receive frusemide before CVP measurement**.)

The management of oliguria is summarized in Table 2.6.

Central venous pressure correlates poorly with left ventricular end diastolic volume in preeclampsia, and the inconsistency of central haemodynamics found in various studies has been discussed earlier in this chapter. However, extreme values do give useful in-

formation. A CVP of zero with the transducer at the level of the right atrium clearly indicates scope for fluid challenge, **but a value of 6 mm Hg or above should be considered high**. An antecubital fossa long line CVP is the safest and least unpleasant route for short term use. This technique is also useful to prevent over-transfusion after caesarean section or haemorrhage, as blood loss is notoriously difficult to assess in these situations.

It is our view that pulmonary artery catheters are only indicated in the presence of pulmonary oedema or renal failure, and are unnecessary in the management of oliguria.

Another important monitor in the prevention of pulmonary oedema is the pulse oximeter. This should be used in all severe preeclamptics. Most cases of pulmonary oedema at SJUH have presented in the first few hours after caesarean section, so pulse oximetry should be used overnight after caesarean section in any degree of preeclampsia, regardless of the anaesthetic technique employed. Basic fluid maintenance after delivery should not exceed 50 ml/hour, plus losses.

MANAGEMENT OF HELLP SYNDROME

Early transfer to a major referral centre is recommended, as in any case of severe preeclampsia. From there, management begins with assessment and stabilization of maternal condition, assessment of foetal status, and a

Table 2.5 Regimen for the treatment of eclampsia and prevention of reconvulsion: magnesium sulphate

Loading dose	4 g (diluted to 20 ml) i.v. over five minutes, followed by 2 g if fits persist
Maintenance	Infuse 1 g per hour i.v. (6 g in 60 ml, 10 ml per hour)
Monitoring	Perform deep tendon reflexes hourly
	Monitor respiratory function with continuous pulse oximetry
	If on oxygen therapy obtain hourly reading in air
	Respiratory rate (rate < 10 or > 25 breaths per minute requires anaesthetic review)
Signs of toxicity	Correct oxygen desaturation with appropriate oxygen therapy
	Discontinue maintenance infusion
	Take blood for Mg^{2+} level
	Consider giving antidote of 1 g calcium gluconate i.v.

Table 2.6 Management of oliguria in preeclampsia

Urine output > 0.4 ml/kg/hour	High osmolarity, no action Low osmolarity, obtain renal consultation (very rare)
Urine output < 0.4 ml/kg/hour	Calculate fluid balance over last 24 hours Correct fluid deficits (e.g. long labour, vomiting etc.)
Urine output still < 0.4 ml/kg/hour	Frusemide 20 mg
Urine output still < 0.4 ml/kg/hour	Site CVP line
CVP below 3 mm Hg	200 ml colloid fluid challenges. Stop if CVP reaches 6 mm Hg
CVP above 3 mm Hg	Choices include cautious fluid challenge, more diuretic, pulmonary artery catheter, mannitol, dopamine, depending on stage of pregnancy, delivery plan, if the patient is postnatal, past medical history etc. **The management of this type of problem should involve consultant level discussion and cannot be safely determined in a fixed protocol.**

Indications for invasive haemodynamic monitoring

- Central venous pressure: oliguria of less than 0.4 ml/kg/hour, despite frusemide to assist fluid management after large blood loss
- Pulmonary artery catheter: pulmonary oedema
  renal failure

---

decision on the need for early delivery. Patients with laboratory evidence of disseminated intravascular coagulation should be delivered promptly, irrespective of gestational age [74, 75]. In the absence of DIC, delivery can be delayed until steroids have been given to increase foetal lung maturity. Prolonged conservative management after the diagnosis of HELLP syndrome exposes the patient to sudden exacerbations of the disease, abruptio placentae, foetal distress, foetal growth retardation and foetal death.

PREECLAMPSIA AND ANAESTHETIC PROCEDURES

The principal anaesthetic concerns in preeclampsia are:

Summary of obstetric management of preeclampsia

- Comprehensive, multidisciplinary antenatal care
- Early referral to day-care unit if hypertension develops
- Early use of antihypertensive agents when diastolic pressure is persistently greater than 100 mm Hg
- Magnesium sulphate to control convulsions/prevent reconvulsions
- Delivery on the best day in the best way
- Careful fluid management
- Counselling

- hypertensive responses to intubation and extubation;
- possible difficult intubation due to airway oedema;
- predisposition to pulmonary oedema;
- precipitous blood pressure fall with regional anaesthesia;
- spinal or epidural techniques in the presence of coagulopathy or thrombocytopenia.

The following discussion of these problems represents the authors' opinions.

HYPERTENSIVE RESPONSES TO INTUBATION AND EXTUBATION

Cerebral haemorrhage in preeclampsia is caused by subjecting a damaged endothelium to high blood pressure, and so the pressor responses to intubation and extubation are moments of potential danger. The prospect of a previously normal patient awaking from her emergency caesarean section with a hemiplegia is not pleasant. So, although there are no data quantifying risks, the pressor responses of anaesthesia should be taken very seriously. In our view, general anaesthesia should only be used if regional techniques are contraindicated. If this condition is satisfied and general anaesthesia is indicated then blood pressure control should be achieved before induction whenever possible, and antihypertensive medication should be continued perioperatively.

Nitroglycerin [76] or labetalol [77, 78] given in increments before induction will reduce the blood pressure, obtund the pressor response to intubation, and do not cause problems with the neonate. Alfentanil is similarly effective and safe at a dose of 10 μg/kg [79], although we have found 15–20 μg/kg to be more effective. Any effect on the neonate is easily antagonized with naloxone, and the maternal effects do not last more than 10 minutes. The ultra short acting-blocker esmolol may cause foetal bradycardia and so is not suitable for intubation in this situation. However, it comes into its own

for preventing the pressor response to extubation [80], when any technique that depresses conscious level or airway reflexes would obviously be inappropriate. A dose of 1.5 mg/kg is effective, lasting only a few minutes.

POSSIBLE DIFFICULT INTUBATION DUE TO AIRWAY OEDEMA

At St James's University Hospital, the failed intubation protocol has been initiated 23 times in 17 years in the maternity unit, and comprehensive data have been collected for all these cases. Airway oedema in preeclampsia does not appear as a prominent risk factor in this series, so it is our conclusion that this problem is overstated.

PREDISPOSITION TO PULMONARY OEDEMA

The reasons for and dangers of pulmonary oedema in preeclampsia have already been discussed. An iatrogenic contribution is common, often in the form of overzealous fluid replacement in the face of haemorrhage or caesarean section. The anaesthetist is often in control of fluid therapy in these circumstances, and the need for extreme caution is sometimes poorly appreciated. Interviewing anaesthetic trainees at the start of their obstetric attachment reveals more concern about renal failure than pulmonary oedema, and a common desire to give generous colloid resuscitation. This view point has sound basis; it is well appreciated by anaesthetists that the reduced circulating volume of non-obstetric hypertensive patients can lead to sudden hypotension and poor organ perfusion during surgery. In these patients, acute tubular necrosis is legitimately the cause of greater concern than pulmonary oedema.

It is therefore necessary to carry out some re-education of anaesthetic trainees when they start obstetrics, and to instil the principles described in the fluid management section of this chapter. Careful assessment of fluid losses at caesarean section and calculation of fasting deficits is naturally important to prevent inadequate fluid therapy, but thereafter a cautious approach is necessary. If in doubt, a long line can be sited quickly and easily. The more generous fluid preload regimens for regional anaesthesia should be avoided because hypervolaemia will occur as the sympathectomy later fades.

PRECIPITOUS BLOOD PRESSURE FALL WITH REGIONAL ANAESTHESIA

It is true of any hypertensive patient that the sympathectomy caused by high spinal and epidural blocks can produce dramatic hypotension. However, patients already vasodilated by antihypertensive agents for long enough to have physiologically compensated for the resultant increase in intravascular space tolerate regional anaesthesia well. If antihypertensive treatment is not well established in preeclamptic patients, but foetal status demands rapid delivery, the danger of sudden hypotension under regional anaesthesia needs to be addressed. There are three common approaches to prevent this phenomenon: the administration of an intravenous fluid preload; ephedrine infusion or boluses; introduction of the sympathetic blockade slowly.

Preloading is seen as an integral part of spinal and epidural anaesthesia for caesarean section by most anaesthetists, although no regimen has been shown to be completely effective. Indeed, one study of normal pregnant women showed no benefit at all and its authors have therefore abandoned the technique [81]. Not only is fluid loading alone of doubtful efficacy, but it is potentially dangerous in preeclampsia. Hypervolaemia before the onset of blockade might provoke pulmonary oedema and fluid tolerated during the block may become excessive as the block recedes. The more generous regimens, involving more than one litre of crystalloid, should not therefore be used in preeclampsia.

It is true that preeclamptic patients are more sensitive to vasoconstrictors, and this causes some practitioners to be concerned about the use of ephedrine during regional anaesthesia. Ephedrine is not dangerous or contraindicated, but simply needs to be given in small increments or by titrated infusion.

The idea of introducing regional blockade gradually in order to avoid sudden hypotension is reasonable, but to contraindicate spinal anaesthesia in preeclampsia would, in our view, be an over-reaction. This approach would condemn preeclamptic patients to receiving the less reliable anaesthesia produced by epidurals for elective caesarean section, and to the dangers of general anaesthesia in the emergency situation. Our approach has therefore been to retain spinal anaesthesia in our armamentarium, but to modify the technique.

At SJUH, the problem of hypotension during regional anaesthesia is managed by combining the three individual methods discussed above. No volume loading is performed prior to regional anaesthesia, but 500 ml of gelatin containing 15 mg ephedrine is attached to the patient's 14G venous cannula. Patients who have been stabilized on antihypertensive regimens receive our usual spinal anaesthetic technique, and the gelatin/ephedrine combination is administered rapidly from the moment the local anaesthetic is injected. If hypotension still occurs, it is treated with boluses of ephedrine in the usual way. If a patient requires an emergency caesarean section before blood pressure control is achieved, we use a combined spinal epidural technique. The spinal is used to produce a block to around T10, which is then gradually topped up with the epidural.

Spinal anaesthesia can be induced with the aid of a spinal catheter. The Food and Drug Administration has banned 32 gauge catheters in the USA because of reports of cauda equina syndrome. These cases involved the use of large doses of 5% lignocaine in 7.5% glucose, which is not licensed for use in the UK. Pooling of hyperbaric solutions is known to occur following intrathecal administration via catheters, so the potential for osmotic damage due to hyperbaric bupivacaine cannot be ignored. To avoid damage to the cauda equina the dose of hyperbaric local anaesthetic should not exceed the normal single shot dose, or isobaric agents should be used. When time permits, a microspinal catheter technique may allow the anaesthetist to produce a slower onset block with some fine tuning of the level.

In summary, we do not see precipitous hypotension as a major problem with regional anaesthesia in preeclampsia. The approach described above is usually effective, and avoids the dangers of excessive fluid administration.

SPINAL OR EPIDURAL TECHNIQUES IN THE PRESENCE OF COAGULOPATHY OR THROMBOCYTOPENIA

This topic is comprehensively covered in Chapter 6, so this section will be restricted to clinical conclusions.

If the platelet count is above $100 \times 10^9/l$, clotting tests are not necessary and all regional techniques can be performed. In the presence of severe coagulopathy with evidence of bleeding, regional anaesthesia is obviously contraindicated. However, between these two extremes there are simply no data available to correlate the risk of an epidural haematoma with any laboratory or clinical tests.

Even if the bleeding times can be reliably and consistently performed, there is very little evidence to support their use as a diagnostic test in individual patients [82, 83]. We have often found thromboelastography to be normal with platelet counts below $100 \times 10^9/l$ and, although this information is reassuring, it still leaves us unable to quantify risks.

One can only conclude that the relative risks of regional and general anaesthesia need to be considered on an individual basis. If it is decided that a regional technique is preferable despite thrombocytopenia or coagulopathy, then we use the small needle techniques of one shot spinal or microspinal catheter.

CONCLUSION

Preeclampsia is a disease which kills previously healthy women, who in most cases are judged to have received substandard care. The condition is complex, but the management strategy need not be. With better awareness of the hazards, improved communication between the relevant professionals, and the adherence to simple management guidelines, there must be room for improvement. It is to be hoped that when a better understanding of the causes and mechanisms of the disease are elucidated, prophylaxis or effective therapy will soon follow.

REFERENCES

1. Department of Health Welsh Office, Scottish Office Home and Health Department, Department of Health and Social Services, Northern Ireland. *Report on Confidential Enquiries into Maternal Deaths in the United Kingdom 1991–1993*, HMSO, London.
2. Saftlas, A.F., Olsen, D.R., Franks, A.L. *et al.* (1990) Epidemiology of preeclampsia and eclampsia in the United States, 1079–1986. *American Journal of Obstetrics and Gynecology*, **163**, 460–5.
3. Mauriceau, F., Desmaladies, D.E.S. and Fennes Grosses, E.T. (1668) *Accouches avec la Bonne et Véritable Méthode*, Cercle du Livre Précieux, Paris.
4. Simpson, J.Y. (1843) Contributions to the pathology and treatment of diseases of the uterus. *Edinburgh Monthly Journal of Medical Sciences*, **3**, 1009.
5. Lever, J.C.W. (1843) Cases of puerperal convulsions with remarks. *Guys Hospital reports*, vol. 1, 2nd series (ed. G.H. Barlow), Samuel Highley, London, p. 495.
6. Vaquez, N. (1897) De la pression artrielle dans l'eclampsia puerparlie. *Bulletin de Medicale Societe de National Hopital, Paris*, **119**, 14.
7. Davey, D.A. and MacGillivray, I. (1988) The classification and definition of hypertensive disorders of pregnancy. *American Journal of Obstetrics and Gynecology*, **158**, 892–8.
8. Perry, I.J., Wilkinson, L.S., Shinton, R.A. and Beavers, D.G. (1991) Conflicting views on the measurement of blood pressure in pregnancy.

British Journal of Obstetrics and Gynaecology, **98**, 241–3.

9. Wichman, K., Ryden, G. and Wichman, M. (1984) The influence of different positions and Korotkoff sounds on the blood pressure measurements in pregnancy. *Acta Obstetricia Gynecologica Scandinavica* [Suppl], **118**, 25–8.

10. The American College of Obstetricians and Gynecologists. Committee on Terminology (1972) in *Obstetric–Gynecologic terminology* (ed. E.C. Hughes), F.A. Davis, Philadelphia, pp. 442–3.

11. Chesley, L.C. (1978) *Hypertensive Disorders in Pregnancy*, Appleton-Century Crofts, New York.

12. MacGillivray, I. (1958) Some observations on the incidence of preeclampsia. *Journal of Obstetrics and Gynaecology of the British Empire*, **65**, 536–40.

13. Jeffcoatte, T.N.A. and Scott, J.S. (1959) Some observations on the placental factor in pregnancy toxaemia. *American Journal of Obstetrics and Gynecology*, **77**, 475–9.

14. Garner, P.R., D'Alton, M.E., Dudley, D.K. *et al.* (1990) Preeclampsia in diabetic pregnancies. *American Journal of Obstetrics and Gynecology*, **163**, 505–8.

15. MacGillivray, I. (1981) Raised blood pressure in pregnancy. Aetiology of preeclampsia. *British Journal of Hospital Medicine*, August, 110–4.

16. Lopez Llera, M. and Hernandez Horta, J.L. (1974) Pregnancy after preeclampsia. *American Journal of Obstetrics and Gynecology*, **119**, 193–8.

17. Sutherland, A., Cooper, D.W., Howie, P.W. *et al.* (1981) Incidence of severe pre-eclampsia amongst mothers and mothers-in-law of pre-eclamptics and controls. *British Journal of Obstetrics and Gynaecology*, **88**, 75–9.

18. Scott, J.R. and Beer, A.A. (1976) Immunological aspects of pre-eclampsia. *American Journal of Obstetrics and Gynecology*, **125**, 418–22.

19. Redman, C.W., Bodmer, J., Bodmer, W.F. *et al.* (1978) HLA antigens in severe pre-eclampsia. *Lancet*, **2**, 397–401.

20. Chen, G., Wilson, R., Cumming, G. *et al.* (1994) Immunological changes in pregnancy-induced hypertension. *European Journal of Obstetrics and Gynaecology and Reproductive Biology*, **53**, 21–5.

21. Chen, G., Wilson, R., Cumming, G. *et al.* (1994) Antioxidants and immunological markers in pregnancy-induced hypertension and essential hypertension in pregnancy. *Journal of Maternal–Fetal Medicine*, **3**, 132–8.

22. Greer, I.A., Dawes, J., Johnston, T.A. and Calder, A.A. (1991) Neutrophil activation is confined to

the maternal circulation in pregnancy-induced hypertension. *Obstetrics and Gynecology*, **78**, 28–32.

23. Greer, I.A., Leak, R., Hudson, B.A. *et al.* (1991) Endothelin, elastase, and endothelial dysfunction in preeclampsia. *Lancet*, **337**, 558.

24. Lyall, F., Greer, I.A., Boswell, F. *et al.* (1994) The cell adhesion molecule, VCAM-1, is selectively elevated in serum in pre-eclampsia: Does this indicate the mechanism of leucocyte activation? *British Journal of Obstetrics and Gynaecology*, **101**, 485–7.

25. Currie, G.A. and Bagshawe, K.D. (1967) The masking of antigens on trophoblastic and cancer cells. *Lancet*, **2**, 708–12.

26. Sheppard, B.L. and Bonnar, J. An ultrastructural study of uteroplacental spiral arteries in hypertensive and normotensive pregnancy and fetal growth retardation. *British Journal of Obstetrics and Gynaecology*, **88**, 695–9.

27. Robertson, W.B., Brosens, I. and Dixon, G. (1975) Uteroplacental vascular pathology. *European Journal of Obstetrics, Gynaecology and Reproductive Biology*, **5**, 47–65.

28. Robertson, W.B., Brosens, I. and Dixon, H.G. (1967) The pathological response of the vessels of the placental bed to hypertensive pregnancy. *Journal of Pathology and Bacteriology*, **93**, 581–92.

29. Kaar, K., Jouppila, P., Kuikka, J. *et al.* (1980) Intervillous blood flow in normal and complicated late pregnancy measured by means of an intravenous 133Xe method. *Acta Obstetricia Gynaecologica Scandinavica*, **59**, 7–10.

30. Ducey, J., Schulman, H. and Farmakides, G. (1987) A classification of pregnancy based on Doppler velocimetry. *American Journal of Obstetrics and Gynecology*, **157**, 860–4.

31. Campbell, S., Pearce, J.M.F., Hackett, G. *et al.* (1986) Qualitative assessment of uteroplacental blood flow: early screening test for high-risk pregnancies. *Obstetrics and Gynecology*, **68**, 649–53.

32. Tominga, T. and Page, E.W. (1996) Accommodation of the human placenta to hypoxia. *American Journal of Obstetrics and Gynecology*, **94**, 679–85.

33. Robbers, D.I.M., Taylor, R.N., Music, T.J. *et al.* (1989) Preeclampsia: An endothelial cell disorder. *American Journal of Obstetrics and Gynecology*, **161**, 1200–4.

34. Zeigler, E.J., McCutchan, J.A., Fierer, J. *et al.* (1982) Treatment of gram-negative bacteraemia and shock with human antiserum to a mutant

Escherichia coli. New England Journal of Medicine, **307**, 1225–30.

35. Friedman, S.A., de Groot, C.J., Taylor, R.N. *et al.* (1994) Plasma cellular fibronectin as a measure of endothelial involvement in preeclampsia and intrauterine growth retardation. *American Journal of Obstetrics and Gynecology*, **170**, 838–41.

36. Roberts, J.M. (1989) Pregnancy related hypertension, in *Maternal Fetal Medicine: Principles and Practice* (eds R.K Creasy and R. Resnik), W.B. Saunders, Philadelphia.

37. Wang, Y., Walsh, S.W., Guo Jingde and Zhang Junyan. (1991) The imbalance between thromboxane and prostacyclin in preeclampsia is associated with an imbalance between lipid peroxides and vitamin E in maternal blood. *American Journal of Obstetrics and Gynecology*, **165**, 1695–700.

38. Speroff, L. (1973) Toxemia of pregnancy: Mechanism and therapeutic management. *American Journal of Cardiology*, **32**, 582–91.

39. Groenendijk, R., Trimbos, M.J. and Wallenburg, H.C.S. (1984) Hemodynamic measurements in preeclampsia: preliminary observations. *American Journal of Obstetrics and Gynecology*, **150**, 232–6.

40. Cotton, D.B., Lee, W.L., Huhta, J.C. and Dorman, K.F. (1988) Hemodynamic profile of severe pregnancy-induced hypertension. *American Journal of Obstetrics and Gynecology*, **158**, 523–9.

41. Mabie, W.C., Ratts, T.E. and Sibai, B.M. (1989) The central hemodynamics of severe preeclampsia. *American Journal of Obstetrics and Gynecology*, **161**, 1443–8.

42. Easterling, T.R. and Benedetti, T.J. (1989) Preeclampsia: A hyperdynamic disease model. *American Journal of Obstetrics and Gynecology*, **160**, 1447–53.

43. Sibai, B.M., Mabie, B.C., Harvey, C.J. and Gonzalez, A.R. (1987) Pulmonary edema in severe preeclampsia–eclampsia: Analysis of thirty-seven consecutive cases. *American Journal of Obstetrics and Gynecology*, **156**, 1174–9.

44. Lindheimer, M.D. and Katz, A.I. (1986) The kidney in pregnancy, in *The Kidney*, 3rd edn (eds B.M. Brenner and F.C. Rector), W.B. Saunders, Philadelphia, pp.1253–95.

45. Clark, S.L., Greenspoon, J.S., Aldahl, D. and Phelan, J.P. (1986) Severe preeclampsia with persistent oliguria: management of hemodynamic subsets. *American Journal of Obstetrics and Gynecology*, **154**, 490–4.

46. Spargo, B.H., McCartney, C. and Winemiller, R. (1959) Glomerular capillary endotheliosis in toxemia of pregnancy. *Archives of Pathology*, **13**, 593–9.

47. Sibai, B.M., Villar, M.A. and Mabie, B.C. (1990) Acute renal failure in hypertensive disorders of pregnancy. Pregnancy outcome and remote prognosis in thirty-one consecutive cases. *American Journal of Obstetrics and Gynecology*, **162**, 777–83.

48. Duley, L. (1992) Maternal mortality associated with hypertensive disorders of pregnancy in Africa, Asia, Latin America, and the Caribbean. *British Journal of Obstetrics and Gynaecology*, **99**, 547–53.

49. Eden, T.W. (1922) Eclampsia: A commentary on the reports presented to the British Congress of Obstetrics and Gynaecology, June 29 1922. *Journal of Obstetrics and Gynaecology of the British Empire*, **29**, 386–401.

50. Medical Research Council Obstetrical Research Committee (1962) Report of eclampsia 1956–1961. *New Zealand Medical Journal*, **59**, 362–3.

51. Hogber, U. and Joelsson, I. (1985) The decline in maternal mortality in Sweden, 1931–80. *Acta Obstetricia Gynaecologica Scandinavica*, **64**, 583–92.

52. Douglas, K.A. and Redman, C.W.G. (1994) Eclampsia in the United Kingdom. *British Medical Journal*, **309**, 1395–400.

53. Sibai, B.M. (1990) The HELLP syndrome (hemolysis, elevated liver enzymes and low platelets): Much ado about nothing? *American Journal of Obstetrics and Gynecology*, **162**, 311–6.

54. Martin, J.N., Blake, P.G., Perry Jr, K.G. *et al.* (1991) The natural history of HELLP syndrome: Patterns of disease progression and regression. *American Journal of Obstetrics and Gynecology*, **163**, 1500–13.

55. Martin Jr, J.N., Blake, P.E., Lowry, S.I. *et al.* (1990) Pregnancy complicated by preeclampsia–eclampsia with the syndrome of hemolysis, elevated liver enzymes, and low platelet count: How rapid is postpartum recovery? *Obstetrics and Gynecology*, **76**, 737–41.

56. Pritchard, J.A., Cunningham, F.G. and Mason, R.A. (1976) Coagulation changes in eclampsia, their frequency and pathogenesis. *American Journal of Obstetrics and Gynecology*, **124**, 855–64.

57. Secher, N.J. and Olsen, S.F. (1990) Fish-oil and pre-eclampsia. *British Journal of Obstetrics and Gynaecology*, **97**, 1077–9.

58. Collaborative Low-dose Aspirin Study in Pregnancy Collaborative Group (1994) CLASP: a randomised trial of low-dose aspirin for the prevention and treatment of pre-eclampsia among 9364 pregnant women. *Lancet*, **343**, 619–29.

59. Sibai, B.M., Taslimi, M., Abdella, T.N. *et al.* (1985) Maternal and perinatal outcome of conservative management of severe preeclampsia in midtrimester. *American Journal of Obstetrics and Gynecology*, **152**, 32–7.

60. Hutton, J.D., James, D.K., Stirrat, G.M *et al.* (1992) Management of severe preeclampsia and eclampsia by UK consultants. *British Journal of Obstetrics and Gynaecology*, **99**, 554–6.

61. Collins, R. and Duley, L. (1994) Any antihypertensive therapy for pregnancy hypertension, Pregnancy and Childbirth Module, in *Cochrane Database of Systematic Reviews* (eds M.W. Enkin, M.J.N.C. Keirse, M.J. Renfrew and J.P. Neilson), Review No. 04426. Update Software, Oxford, Disk Issue 1: 'Cochrane Updates on Disk'.

62. Ahokas, R.A., Mabie, W.C., Sibai, B.M. and Anderson, G.D. (1989) Labetalol does not decrease placental perfusion in the hypertensive term-pregnant rat. *American Journal of Obstetrics and Gynecology*, **160**, 480–4.

63. Ahokas, R.A., Sibai, B.M., Mabie, W.C. and Anderson, G.D. (1988) Nifedipine does not adversely affect uteroplacental blood flow in the hypertensive term-pregnant rat. *American Journal of Obstetrics and Gynecology*, **159**, 1440–5.

64. Redman, C.W., Beilin, L.J.B. and Wilkinson, B.H. (1976) Plasma urate measurements in predicting fetal death in hypertensive pregnancy. *Lancet*, **1**, 1370–4.

65. Walker, J.J., Cameron, A.D., Bjornsson, S. *et al.* (1989) Can platelet volume predict progressive hypertensive disease in pregnancy? *American Journal of Obstetrics and Gynecology*, **161**, 676–9.

66. Sibai, B.M., Gonzalez, A.R., Mabie, W.C. and Moretti, M. (1987) A comparison of labetalol plus hospitalisation versus hospitalisation alone in the management of preeclampsia remote from term. *Obstetrics and Gynecology*, **70**, 323–7.

67. Lucas, M.J., Leveno, K.J. and Cunningham, F.G. (1995) A comparison of magnesium sulphate with phenytoin for the prevention of eclampsia. *New England Journal of Medicine*, **333**, 201–5.

68. Moodley, J. and Moodley, V.V. (1994) Prophylactic anticonvulsant therapy in hypertensive crises of pregnancy – the need for a large, randomised trial. *Hypertension in Pregnancy*, **13**, 245–52.

69. Duley, L., Carroli, G., Belizan, J. *et al.* (1995) Which anticonvulsant for women with eclampsia – evidence from the collaborative eclampsia trial. *Lancet*, **345**, 1455–63.

70. Sibai, B.M. (1990) Magnesium sulphate is the ideal anticonvulsant in preeclampsia–eclampsia. *American Journal of Obstetrics and Gynecology*, **162**, 1141–5.

71. Pritchard, J.A. (1955) The use of the magnesium ion in the management of eclamptogenic toxemias. *Surgery Gynecology and Obstetrics*, **100**, 131–40.

72. Zuspan, F.P. (1966) Treatment of severe preeclampsia and eclampsia. *Clinical Obstetrics and Gynecology*, **9**, 954–72.

73. Sibai, B.M., Graham, J.M. and McCubbin, J.H. (1984) A Comparison of intravenous and intramuscular magnesium sulfate regimens in preeclampsia. *American Journal of Obstetrics and Gynecology*, **150**, 728–33.

74. VanDam, P.A., Renier, M., Baekelandt, T.M. *et al.* (1989) Disseminated intravascular coagulation and the syndrome of hemolysis, elevated liver enzymes, and low platelets in severe preeclampsia. *Obstetrics and Gynecology*, **73**, 97–102.

75. Sibai, B.M., Taslimi, M.M., El-Nazar, A. *et al.* (1986) Maternal–perinatal outcome associated with the syndrome of hemolysis, elevated liver enzymes, and low platelets in severe preeclampsia–eclampsia. *American Journal of Obstetrics and Gynecology*, **155**, 501.

76. Hood, D.D., Dewan, D.M., James, F.M. *et al.* (1985) The use of nitroglycerine in preventing the hypertensive response to tracheal intubation in severe preeclampsia. *Anesthesiology*, **63**, 329–32.

77. Ramanathan, J., Sibai, B.M., Mabie, W.C. *et al.* (1988) The use of labetalol for attenuation of the hypertensive response to endotracheal intubation in preeclampsia. *American Journal of Obstetrics and Gynecology*, **159**, 650–4.

78. Lavies, N.G., Meiklejohn, B.H., May, A.E. *et al.* (1989) Hypertensive and catecholamine response to tracheal intubation in patients with pregnancy-induced hypertension. *British Journal of Anaesthesia*, **63**, 429–34.

79. Dann, W.L., Hutchinson, A. and Cartwright, D.P. (1987) Maternal and neonatal responses to alfentanil administered before induction of general anaesthesia for Caesarean section. *British Journal of Anaesthesia*, **59**, 1392–6.

80. Dyson, A., Isaac, P.A., Pennant, J.H. *et al.* (1990) Esmolol attenuates cardiovascular responses to extubation. *Anesthesia and Analgesia*, **71**, 675–8.

81. Jackson, R., Reid, A. and Thorburn, J. (1995) Volume preloading is not essential to prevent spinal-induced hypotension at caesarean section. *British Journal of Anaesthesia*, **75**, 262–5.

82. Channing-Rogers, R.P. and Levin, J. (1990) A critical review of the bleeding time. *Seminars in Thrombosis and Hemostasis*, **16**, 1–20.

83. Anon. (1991) The bleeding time (editorial). *Lancet*, **337**, 1447–8.

MAJOR HAEMORRHAGE

3

H. Pargger and M. C. Schneider

INTRODUCTION

During the 19th century major haemorrhage was the leading cause of maternal mortality accounting for 44% of all obstetric deaths [1]. One hundred and fifty years later, haemorrhage is still one of the most frequent obstetric catastrophes. After thromboembolism, hypertensive diseases and early pregnancy, haemorrhage is the fourth most important cause of maternal death in the UK (11.6%) [2]. Alarmingly, the number of maternal deaths directly due to haemorrhage has increased during the last decade, and in addition, bleeding has been implicated as a contributory factor in almost as many maternal deaths again, due to other causes. Direct deaths are the result of placenta praevia, placental abruption and postpartum haemorrhage. The authors of this audit found that substandard care was a major factor in 11 out of 15 cases, and amongst these eleven, three were women who had declined blood transfusion [2].

This information suggests that professional education and training in the management of haemorrhage needs to be improved. Excellent communication between obstetricians, anaesthetists, neonatologists, intensivists, midwives and nurses is of paramount importance and allows for a team approach in the care of patients with life-threatening conditions. In 1965, Phillips and Hulka summarized the problem as follows: 'Two common denominators thus account for the contribution of hemorrhage to obstetric mortality, namely, lack of recognition and lack of preparation' [1].

THE PATHOPHYSIOLOGY OF HYPOVOLAEMIA AND HAEMORRHAGIC SHOCK

There are no important differences in the pathophysiological responses to bleeding, hypovolaemia and subsequent haemorrhagic shock between pregnant and non-pregnant women. However, the normal cardiovascular and respiratory changes that occur in late pregnancy imitate some of the early clinical signs of progressive bleeding: dilutional anaemia, tachycardia and hyperventilation [3].

Because blood volume expands by a third during pregnancy, symptoms suggestive of major haemorrhage, such as a rise in pulse rate or a decrease in blood pressure, may not develop until the blood volume has been reduced by 30 to 35%, the equivalent of two litres of blood [4]. The capacity of young and healthy women to compensate for a substantial blood loss without striking changes in baseline cardiovascular parameters can induce

3

Clinical Problems in Obstetric Anaesthesia
Edited by Ian F. Russell and Gordon Lyons. Published in 1997 by Chapman & Hall, London. ISBN 0 412 71600 3.

Table 3.1 Classification of haemorrhage (60 kg gravida, late pregnancy) [5, 6]

Class	Volume lost	Clinical findings

1	≤ 15% of blood volume
	≤ 900 ml
		The clinical symptoms are minimal:
		  mild tachycardia
		  normal blood pressure
		  no change in pulse pressure
		  normal respiration
		  normal urine output

2	15 to 30% of blood volume 1000–1500 ml	Tachycardia (heart rate 110–130) Decreased pulse pressure due to rise in diastolic pressure Mild decrease in urine output (20–30 ml/hour) Moderate tachypnoea Subtle central nervous system changes: anxiety
3	30 to 40% of blood volume 2000 ml	Marked tachycardia (heart rate 120–160) Tachypnoea Decrease in systolic blood pressure Cold, clammy, pallid skin Significant change in mental status
4	≥ 40% of blood volume ≥ 2500 ml	Immediately life-threatening Marked tachycardia Systolic blood pressure below 80 mmHg Peripheral pulses absent Oliguria or anuria Confusion or unconsciousness Circulatory collapse

a false sense of security. Failure to appreciate potential danger may be at its greatest in the presence of an inexperienced attendant and a concealed haemorrhage.

In Table 3.1, a classification of haemorrhage with the expected clinical findings is presented [5, 6]. It is important the clinical state is assessed as a whole because not every parameter will always behave as expected. We emphasize the American College of Surgeons' point of view that 'aggressive fluid resuscitation must be initiated when early signs and symptoms of blood loss are apparent or suspected, not when the blood pressure is falling or absent' [5].

CARDIOVASCULAR RESPONSE TO
HAEMORRHAGE (FIGURE 3.1)

The effect of haemorrhage on the cardiovascular system depends on the amount of loss. With the onset of hypovolaemia, the initial event is a decline in cardiac filling pressures. The reduction in end-diastolic volume is associated with reduced fibre length of the cardiac muscle (preload) and with a consequent decrease in contractility (Starling mechanism). Accordingly, stroke volume and cardiac output decreases which leads to a reduction in pulse pressure (difference between systolic and diastolic blood pressures) and, later, mean arterial pressure. As a consequence, baroreceptor activity is slowed down thereby removing inhibitory, peripheral impulses to the cerebral autonomic control centres. Accordingly, central sympathetic outflow increases and the secretion of adrenaline into the circulation is stimulated. These changes increase myocardial contractility and heart rate and allow for a larger stroke volume at lower filling pressure [7]. Some changes in cardiac parameters due to

Table 3.2 Influence of hypovolaemia on cardiac parameters [7]

Lost blood volume (%)	Preload	Cardiac output	Mean arterial pressure	Contractility	Heart rate
10	↓	0	0	↑	↑
20	↓↓	↓	0	↑↑	↑↑
30	↓↓↓	↓↓	↓	↑↑↑	↑↑↑
40	↓↓↓	↓↓↓	↓↓↓	↑↑↑	↑↑↑

↓ = decrease; ↑ = increase; 0 = no change.

different degrees of blood loss are summarized in Table 3.2.

Sympathetic nervous system stimulation leads to smooth muscle contraction in arterioles and venules, an action elicited by noradrenaline via α-receptors. Normally, the α-effect masks the dilating β2-effect derived from circulating adrenaline. The overall result is an increase in peripheral resistance and a transfer of volume from peripheral to central compartments of the circulation (Figure 3.1) [8].

In addition to these general adaptive mechanisms, local factors have regulatory effects on organ blood flow mediated by metabolic substances, such as CO_2 and lactic acid, hypoxaemia and the endothelium-derived relaxing factor, nitric oxide (NO) [9].

HAEMORRHAGE AND ORGAN PERFUSION

Haemorrhagic shock develops because of a decrease in systemic oxygen transport capacity. Under these conditions, systemic oxygen delivery no longer meets the metabolic needs of the body. Below a critical value for oxygen delivery, supply fails to meet demand,

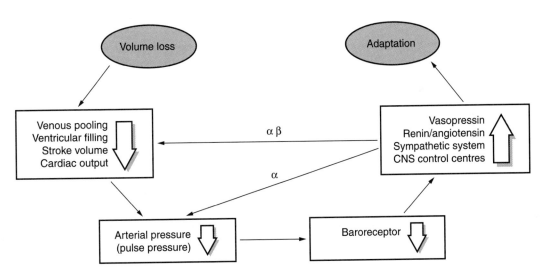

Figure 3.1 Effects of intravascular volume loss on cardiovascular indices and adaptive mechanisms. The stimulation of the sympathetic system by noradrenergic nerve fibres via α_1- receptors results in vasoconstriction and, therefore, in an increase of the diastolic blood pressure, whereas the systolic blood pressure is maintained up to a volume loss of 30%. This explains why a decrease in pulse pressure (systolic minus diastolic blood pressure) often is the only sign of a haemorrhage class 2 (Table 3.1). The increase of circulating adrenaline and the stimulation of cardiac sympathetic fibres via β_1-stimulation leads to an increase of contractility and heart rate.

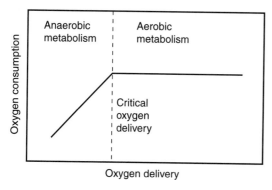

Figure 3.2 Relationship between oxygen delivery and oxygen consumption. Under normal conditions the amount of oxygen transported to the organs is far above the needs of these organs. As long as the delivery of oxygen to the organs exceeds the demand, oxygen consumption remains constant irrespective of the amount of oxygen delivered. The entire metabolism is aerobic. Below a critical oxygen delivery the amount of transported oxygen no longer meets the demands of the tissue. With a further decrease in oxygen delivery, oxygen consumption also decreases and results in partially anaerobic metabolism.

and metabolism becomes anaerobic (Figure 3.2) [8].

In response to hypovolaemia, cardiovascular shut down is selective. Oxygen delivery to the gut, kidneys, skin and skeletal muscle is decreased, while flow to the heart, liver and brain is increased [10]. This selective vasoconstriction is responsible for the development of relative ischaemia in these organs. If this state is not corrected, a progressive acidosis can occur which may lead to multiple organ failure [11].

THE PRINCIPLES OF MANAGEMENT

The principal goal of management is successful maternal resuscitation, and all foetal issues are secondary to this. Successful resuscitation is dependent on achieving adequate oxygen delivery to all organs, including the uteroplacental unit. Major principles in the management of major haemorrhage are set out below.

- Define the source and/or the cause of the haemorrhage.
- Define the degree of the haemorrhage.
- Have guidelines and a written protocol for the management of massive haemorrhage [2].
- Monitor the patient.
- Assess the effectiveness of resuscitative therapy and revise whenever appropriate.
- Plan postoperative intensive care as early as possible.

Identifying the aetiology of the bleeding is necessary to direct therapy. It is not possible to stop surgical bleeding or haemorrhage from an atonic uterus by replacing coagulation factors alone; nor does it make sense to manage haemorrhage from vaginal lacerations solely by surgery, when the picture is complicated by dilutional coagulopathy.

By classifying the degree of haemorrhage, the magnitude and the urgency of the problem can be defined. Organ function may be adversely affected by inadequate oxygen delivery, and should be assessed, as this has a major impact on postoperative or postresuscitation outcome.

In the hectic atmosphere of emergency resuscitation it becomes extremely difficult to analyse the efficiency of decisions and procedures. The way to improve efficacy is to be fully prepared. Policies for the management of obstetric haemorrhage should include raising the alarm, the allocation of the responsibilities and an algorithm for clinical management. The infrastructure requires access to a blood bank and specialized laboratory facilities 24 hours a day. Policies must be adapted to local circumstances because of differences in the infrastructure and availability of special expertise. Figure 3.3 is one suggestion for successful management. All participating disciplines – the obstetricians, anaesthetists, midwives, operating theatre personnel and laboratory personnel – should understand the policy and their role in it.

Monitoring of the patient is the only way of evaluating the effectiveness of the treatment.

Call immediately: anaesthetist and obstetrician

Patient history and assessment

antepartum, postpartum, foetus, complications during pregnancy
personal history: allergies, medication, previous operations and hospitalizations
class of haemorrhage (Table 31)
source of bleeding
ultrasound

Initial resuscitation

★ **i.v.-Access** two large-bore, peripheral catheters (7F, 14G)
external and/or internal jugular vein, femoral vein, venous cutdown

★ **Laboratory Testing** blood group, blood for cross-matching
haemoglobin, haematocrit, platelets, leucocytes
sodium, potassium, creatinine
coagulation screening

★ **Fluid Administration** Ringer's lactate, hydroxyethyl starch

★ **Oxygen**

★ **Urinary Catheter and Urimeter**

★ **Obstetric Measures** oxytocin, uterus massage, tamponade

Organization and preparation

★ **Order** 10 units packed red cells, type-specific or O Rh neg uncross-matched

★ **Call** consultant

★ **Inform** anaesthesia team (if possible, get more personnel)
preparations: Drugs: ketamine, suxamethonium, etomidate, vasoactive drugs
Intubation material
Monitoring: ECG, non-invasive blood pressure, pulse oximeter
capnograph, temperature, invasive blood pressure
Fluids: warmed
Ringer's lactate, hydroxyethyl starch, packed red cells
Special: rapid infusion device
cell saver

Decision

Emergency Operation?

Operation

★ **Treat Hypovolaemia/Shock** packed red cells, hydroxyethyl starch, Ringer's lactate

★ **Check Equipment and Drugs**

★ **Patient Ready?** positioning, disinfection, diathermy

★ **Team Ready?** anaesthesia team, obstetricians, surgeons, nurses

★ **Start General Anaesthesia** rapid sequence induction, reduced dosage

★ **Start Operation**

Stabilization

continue fluid resuscitation
intravenous anaesthetics if necessary
ventilation with high inspired oxygen concentration

Source of Bleeding Found?
Bleeding Stopped?

Call blood bank: supply   **Consider** arterial line   **Order** more blood
intensive care unit   central venous line   fresh frozen plasma
gastric tonometer   platelets
vasoactive drugs   cryoprecipitate
fresh frozen plasma
aprotinin
calcium

Reassessment

★ **Laboratory Testing** arterial blood gases, haemoglobin, haematocrit, platelets, sodium potassium
clotting profile, lactate ionized calcium

★ **Arterial Pressure Curve Form and Heart Rate** volume status

★ **Urimeter** renal perfusion

★ **Pulse oximetry/Skin** oxygenation, peripheral perfusion

★ **Capnography** cardiac output, metabolism global organ perfusion

★ **Intramucosal pH** gastro-intestinal perfusion

★ **Temperature**

★ **Pupils and Need for Sedation** cerebral perfusion

Complications

coagulopathy (dilutional coagulopathy, disseminated intravascular coagulation, thrombocytopenia), renal
failure, gastro-intestinal ischaemia, hypothermia, capillary leak, cerebral damage

Postoperative therapy

★ **Intensive Care Unit**

★ **Postoperative Ventilation**

★ **Tertiary Referral**

Figure 3.3 Treatment protocol for major obstetric haemorrhage.

Reassessment is the key word. On the receipt of clinical and laboratory-based information, the clinician should be prepared to revise, change and amend the strategy as appropriate.

Even when resuscitation appears to achieve its goal, single or multiple organ failure cannot be ruled out. Renal, respiratory, haematological and cardiovascular support may be required for some time after the initial insult, and intensive continuing therapy is necessary for the best outcome.

PRACTICAL MANAGEMENT

This section summarizes the important points in the practical treatment of a major haemorrhage. The order reflects our opinion as to the importance of each single issue for the anaesthetist. However, we would like to emphasize that for a successful resuscitation most of the actions have to take place more or less in parallel rather than in series.

ORGANIZATION

It is impossible for one person to treat a major haemorrhage without support. As bleeding may be unnoticed and the degree of haemorrhage underestimated, matters may suddenly become life-threatening. Effective therapy must be instituted immediately and the alarm sounded. The anaesthetist should become involved as soon as there is any suspicion of maternal bleeding, and if severe, senior and additional help should be summoned without delay.

INTRAVENOUS ACCESS

As soon as obstetric haemorrhage is recognized, at least two large-bore intravenous infusions should be established. Simultaneously blood should be taken for cross-matching and baseline laboratory investigations before starting fluid resuscitation. The cannulae should be short and fat because the flow increases as a function of the fourth power of the diameter

and decreases proportionally with length [12]. The best peripheral sites for intravenous access are the forearms and the antecubital fossae. Under some circumstances the saphenous vein or the external jugular vein may be used for rapid intravenous cannulation. Central venous access will come later. Hypovolaemia often results in peripheral venous vasoconstriction and intravenous access may be difficult or impossible. Under these conditions, options include a rapid infusion device which allows the replacement of an 18 gauge catheter by a 7 French cannula utilizing the Seldinger technique. In profound hypovolaemic shock, central venous lines can be set up by way of the internal jugular, subclavian or the femoral vein, although this is not for the inexperienced. According to the American College of Surgeons' Committee on Trauma, a venous cutdown represents the most appropriate approach after two failed percutaneous punctures in shocked patients [5]. We believe that either approach is good as long as the person performing the procedure has practical experience, the equipment is readily available and the venous access is established within five minutes.

Adequate venous access is the first important step of anaesthetic management. The second step consists of rapid infusion of warmed fluids. Most of the commercially available warming devices are not efficient enough for rapid infusions. A warming bath will work, but immediate infusion is impossible and there is a delay in temperature equilibration. The best device for achieving rapid infusion of warmed fluids utilizes an air compressor and a highly effective countercurrent warming system [12]. It is essential to bear in mind that volume resuscitation keeps several staff members busy, and by using this device, fewer personnel are occupied.

FLUID THERAPY

The controversy surrounding crystalloid versus colloid resuscitation and, more recently, on small-volume resuscitation with hypertonic sodium chloride solutions is unresolved. Although clinical studies have failed to show improved mortality or morbidity with one fluid regimen compared to another, fluid regimens used for the resuscitation of patients in haemorrhagic shock have both advantages and limitations.

Crystalloid

Under most circumstances a balanced crystalloid solution will be adequate for the primary resuscitation. Balanced crystalloids such as 0.9% sodium chloride or Ringer's lactate remain within the extracellular compartment of the body. Hypotonic or dextrose containing solutions are unsuitable or even dangerous when fast intravascular replacement is the goal of fluid therapy as only a fraction will remain in the circulation.

When replacing blood loss by crystalloid, at least three times the lost volume has to be administered to counterbalance the distribution of much of the administered solution to the extravascular compartment. Oedema formation is the potential consequence of this treatment. It is unclear if and when extravascular fluid sequestration becomes a problem for the patient. It is also unclear if avoiding this problem with colloid therapy improves the outcome [13]. Crystalloid has no capacity for oxygen carriage and will dilute clotting factors, but as the first step in fluid resuscitation it has a useful role.

Colloids

The important advantage of colloids over crystalloids is that colloids remain, at least initially, almost entirely within the intravascular compartment. Therefore, restoration of blood flow is faster following administration of colloids compared with crystalloids. In addition, the effect of colloids on intravascular volume is likely to be longer lasting.

The synthetic colloid of choice in our institution is hydroxyethyl starch (HES). Up to a daily dosage of 2 g/kg body weight is recommended. The dose limit, which is a matter of constant discussion [13], depends on the molecular weight, the substitution degree and the concentration of the solution. It is part of our routine management of haemorrhagic shock to use 1 to 1.5 litres of 6% HES with a mean molecular weight of 70 000 and a substitution degree of 0.5. The administration of all colloid solutions in any volume is likely to dilute clotting factors, while at the same time, the process of haemorrhage removes them. When large volumes are infused, dilutional coagulopathy should be anticipated [13].

Dextrans are not used to replace blood loss due to haemorrhage. They tend to reduce platelet stickiness and have a negative effect on coagulation [14].

When gelatins which have a molecular weight in the region of 30 000 are used, the volume effect and its duration are less pronounced than with HES. Therefore, twice the effective volume loss has to be replaced in order to restore normovolaemia [14]. We believe that gelatin has no advantage compared with Ringer's lactate.

For 20 years the potential benefit of using pasteurized human albumin solutions in various concentrations (5 to 25%) over synthetic colloids or Ringer's lactate for volume replacement has been subject to debate. In our opinion, there is now enough data showing that albumin solutions are not superior to HES in terms of efficacy during volume therapy, outcome and rate of complications [13]. Albumin solutions are about five to six times more expensive than a comparable HES solution and we feel that albumin should no longer be used to correct acute blood loss or hypovolaemia.

With all colloid solutions, including human albumin, there is a risk of severe anaphylactic or anaphylactoid reaction. Modern methods of preparation have tended to reduce this risk.

Small-volume resuscitation

The principle of small-volume resuscitation is based on the infusion of a small volume of hypertonic (7.5%) sodium chloride. Due to the osmotic effect of a high intravascular concentration of sodium, there is a flux of free water from the intracellular and the interstitial compartment into the vessels. Obviously, this effect lasts only as long as there is an effective osmotic gradient; eventually sodium leaves the vessels and the flux of water reverses [15]. Small-volume resuscitation has never been used under controlled conditions for obstetric haemorrhage, and the effects of a high sodium concentration and the osmotic pressure gradients on the foetus are unclear. Therefore, we consider the use of hypertonic sodium chloride solutions in the management of major obstetric bleeding as experimental.

BLOOD COMPONENT THERAPY

When massive loss of red cells occurs oxygen delivery becomes impaired. When this happens, coagulation is also likely to suffer as clotting factors are also lost. Blood component therapy is based on the principle of restoring a measured loss of function, according to assessments using appropriate serial haematological tests. Falling haematocrit will point to red cell replacement, and abnormal coagulation screen or thromboelastograph will point to replacement with clotting factors. The availability of different blood products differs from region to region and it may be important that the local protocol for obtaining various blood products is understood.

For many years, our blood bank has provided us with blood components. Instead of whole blood or fresh blood we use components such as packed red cells, fresh frozen plasma, platelet concentrates, fibrinogen and cryoprecipitate. Even platelets are available within one hour's notice 24 hours a day. We find that the availability of components is a highly effective way to give the patient exactly what is needed and makes efficient use of donated blood.

In addition to blood component therapy, we consider the use of a cell saver in every case of a major haemorrhage. This device allows the continuous salvaging of blood from the operating field. The salvaged fluid is washed, centrifuged, and the erythrocytes are suspended in isotonic sodium chloride without plasma proteins, clotting factors or platelets. The cell saver is a highly effective device which reduces the need for stored red cells, although it does require an additional person to run the machine.

Blood group

Occasionally blood loss is so massive that transfusion has to be started before the cross-match is completed. In such an emergency, group O rhesus negative red blood cells should be used until cross-matched blood becomes available. Blood banks in large hospitals usually have a supply of two to ten units of O negative packed red cells. Untested O negative blood may result in haemolytic reactions due to small amounts of anti-A or anti-B antibodies.

Often the woman's blood group is known, or there may be time to group from a fresh sample before transfusion. In this event, we prefer to use type-specific, uncross-matched blood. It takes only five to 10 minutes to determine the blood group of the recipient. The group-matched red cells have an excellent safety record [16].

Although blood subjected to complete cross-match has the lowest incidence of transfusion reactions, it is often not possible to wait 60 minutes to two hours in emergency situations for a complete cross-match. Under these circumstances type- or group-specific blood is a good and safe choice.

Packed red cells

Packed red cells are prepared by centrifugation of a unit of whole blood. After removing the plasma, a preservative solution, which extends the storage period to 42 days, is added. It is possible to reduce the white blood cell number by filtration. Such 'buffy-poor' red cells decrease the number and severity of febrile reactions due to blood transfusion [16].

Fresh frozen plasma

Plasma separated from whole blood and cooled within six hours to −18°C is called fresh frozen plasma. This product contains all clotting factors in almost normal concentrations, including factors V and VIII, which are labile at room or refrigerator temperature.

Fresh frozen plasma should not be used for volume replacement but only to treat an impaired coagulation system. There is a clear relationship between the amount of blood loss and the severity of coagulation disorders. As a rule of thumb, two units fresh frozen plasma may be given for every five units packed red cells [17]. An exchange transfusion without replenishing lost clotting factors risks dilutional coagulopathy [18].

Factor concentrates and cryoprecipitate

Several different products are likely to be available from the transfusion service. Obstetric-related haemorrhage may be associated with a degree of fibrinogen depletion, and infusion of cryoprecipitate which contains fibrinogen and factor VIII should be considered early [17].

Platelet concentrate

Because 'fresh blood' is no longer used, the need for platelets for resuscitation during major haemorrhage has increased. Such a treatment should be considered as soon as the platelet count falls below 100 000/µl in the presence of a clinically detectable problem. Serial platelet counts should be performed alongside coagulation screening during massive transfusion. When the count is below 50 000/µl and there is profuse bleeding, we order platelets.

Each unit contains platelets from six donors and when administered increases the platelet count by about 30 000/µl. We try to give platelets towards the end of the operation, when hopefully, surgical sources of haemorrhage have been dealt with.

Hypocalcaemia

A rapid infusion of large amounts of blood and protein-containing solutions may result in a decrease of ionized calcium. Calcium is adsorbed by excess citrate which is used as an anticoagulant in stored blood. In hypothermia and with liver failure, the conversion of citrate to bicarbonate is impaired resulting in a further decrease of ionized calcium [19]. Ideally, the ionized calcium should be measured to guide the treatment. If ionized calcium levels cannot be monitored, the prolongation of the QT interval on the electrocardiogram may be used as an indication for the presence of hypocalcaemia [20].

Because abrupt decreases in ionized calcium are associated with hypotension and increased left ventricular end-diastolic pressure [20], we routinely administer calcium chloride during massive transfusion accompanied by hypotension. If a bolus of 8 mg $CaCl_2$/kg body weight (1 ml 10% $CaCl_2$ = 2.8 mmol Ca^{2+} = 56 mg Ca^{2+}) results in an immediate increase in blood pressure, hypocalcaemia is very likely. In order not to overtreat and cause hypercalcaemia, ionized calcium plasma levels should be monitored.

Aprotinin

Aprotinin is a serine protease inhibitor derived from bovine lungs. It is used to reduce blood loss in cardiac surgery [21], liver transplantation [22] and orthopaedic procedures [23]. Aprotinin reduces blood loss during haemorrhage, including postpartum haemorrhage [24], blood loss related to elective surgery, and has beneficial and potential life-saving effects in situations of dilutional coagulopathy after massive transfusions. It should be considered when diffuse bleeding persists after massive transfusion despite attempts to correct coagulopathy by administration of fresh frozen plasma, cryoprecipitate and platelets.

Two hundred thousand to 2 000 000 units followed by an infusion of 50 000 to 500 000 units/hour have been effective in reducing blood loss [24]. Recent reports demonstrate, however, that, at least in elective surgery, such high doses of aprotinin do not appear to offer additional benefits [22]. Therefore, we recommend an initial dose of 500 000 units followed by an infusion of 150 000 units/hour for about 12 hours.

VASOACTIVE DRUGS

During haemorrhagic shock, there is reduced perfusion of all organs [13]. The gastrointestinal tract appears to be particularly susceptible to ischaemic damage as evidenced by translocation of bacteria from the gut in an experimental model [25]. Persistent gastrointestinal ischaemia, ultimately, leads to multiple organ failure, the major cause of death in intensive care units [26, 27].

Successful resuscitatation in haemorrhagic shock is by aggressive volume therapy. However, there is evidence that, despite volume resuscitation, low flow may persist in the splanchnic organs [13] and that dopamine may improve gut ischaemia [28, 29]. Dopamine also has beneficial effects on urine production in surgical patients after resuscitation [30]. The potential role of other vasoactive drugs like noradrenaline or adrenaline following resuscitation from haemorrhagic shock is not yet established. Persistent hypotension after volume resuscitation requires treatment. An appropriate vasopressor may improve the cerebral, cardiovascular and gastrointestinal perfusion pressures without changing flow, and therefore can be beneficial [31].

Based on these considerations, the threshold for using vasoactive drugs in the treatment of haemorrhagic shock is low. As a first line, dopamine infusion can be started when volume resuscitation is ongoing. As soon as bleeding has been stopped and normovolaemia is re-established, a noradrenaline infusion may be given to patients remaining hypotensive without pre-existing or ischaemia-related acute cardiac disease. To evaluate the cardiac situation, we prefer to perform a transoesophageal echocardiography rather than insert a pulmonary artery catheter. Some authorities would choose the appropriate drug according to measurements of systemic vascular resistance, and right and left cardiac function, and tailor the dose to achieve desirable changes in these parameters.

OBSTETRIC MANAGEMENT

The obstetric management of a major haemorrhage in a pregnant patient before or after delivery depends on the origin of the bleeding. We will not discuss special obstetric treatment options for placenta praevia, placenta accreta, abruptio placentae or uterine rupture but, rather, describe general guidelines.

When called to see a patient who is profusely bleeding, it is important to determine rapidly the aetiology and assess the severity of the haemorrhage. In the case of antepartum haemorrhage, physical examination should include measurement of foetal heart rate and diagnostic ultrasound [6, 32]. In this manner a definitive diagnosis of placental abruption, placenta praevia or uterine rupture can be made. In patients with postpartum haemorrhage, lacerations along the birth canal, uterine atony and retained placenta are among the most common aetiologies [33]. In the case of intra-abdominal haemorrhage, transabdominal ultrasound may be helpful in establishing the diagnosis. Whereas abdominal or vaginal delivery represents the ultimate therapy for antepartum haemorrhage, management of postpartum haemorrhage is based on the administration of drugs that enhance uterine contraction after delivery such as oxytocin, ergonorine or methylergometrine and prostaglandin $PGF_{2\alpha}$. Any of these drugs can be administered intravenously or injected intramyometrially by the obstetrician.

MONITORING

Monitoring should be sophisticated and extended to as many useful parameters as possible. It will allow performance to be assessed and treatment strategies revised whenever necessary. It will also give the clinician an opportunity to identify complications of treatment.

CARDIOVASCULAR MONITORING

Direct measurement of arterial pressure via an arterial cannula offers a number of advantages, especially in the haemodynamically unstable patient. The beat-to-beat reading allows the early recognition of hypotension. Visual analysis of the pressure curve gives some information about cardiac contractility, stroke volume, systemic vascular resistance, and blood volume [34]. Arterial cannulation for blood pressure monitoring should never delay more important resuscitative measures, but should be introduced at the earliest opportunity.

During the initial phase there is no need for a central venous catheter, except when it is impossible to insert a peripheral large-bore catheter. As soon as haemodynamic stability is restored, central venous pressure monitoring should be instituted. In addition to the fine tuning of volume replacement, it permits administration of vasoactive drugs [34].

In our view, there are very few indications for a pulmonary artery catheter in patients with major obstetric haemorrhage, because most of these individuals are relatively young and healthy. We believe the best indication is an additional primary cardiac problem. Pulmonary artery catheterization may have major complications [34], especially in patients with coagulopathy, and no study has ever demonstrated a reproducible, beneficial effect. Nevertheless, many intensive care units use pulmonary artery catheters routinely, and some would consider them essential when monitoring the effects of inotropic infusions.

Transoesophageal echocardiography is an alternative for a pulmonary artery catheter. It is a safe, semi-invasive method [35] that can distinguish between cardiogenic and hypovolaemic shock, and guide volume therapy in patients with cardiac disease. If the equipment and a well-trained investigator are available, in our hands, this method is superior to pulmonary artery catheterization.

CAPNOGRAPHY

Capnography is part of the minimal monitoring required for the safe administration of general anaesthesia in our and many other institutions. It is the only device that permits immediate recognition of oesophageal intubation and, therefore carries a recommendation for routine use in obstetric practice [2]. Failed tracheal intubation occurs once in 300 to 750 general anaesthetics for caesarean delivery [36]. This frequency is eight-fold higher than that in a general surgical population. There may be other reasons for advocating the use of the capnograph; it can be used as a crude monitor of cardiac output, and as a diagnostic tool. An increase in the arterial to end-expiratory carbon dioxide tension might indicate cardiopulmonary disease [37].

PULSE OXIMETRY

The pulse oximeter measures the oxygen saturation of haemoglobin, and provides a beat-to-beat measurement of the important variables determining oxygen transport. However, without an intact peripheral circulation, the monitor fails. During severe hypovolaemia and hypothermia, peripheral vasoconstriction impedes reliable reading of peripheral oxygen saturation. Once intravascular volume has been restored and hypothermia corrected, the pulse oximeter can be reimplemented. Readings can be used as an indication of adequate perfusion of the periphery and give some insight into the perfusion of other organs [38].

MONITORING THE KIDNEYS AND THE GASTROINTESTINAL SYSTEM

During emergency resuscitation the only way to monitor kidney function is by assessing urine output. During the acute phase of resuscitation, we may assume kidney perfusion to be sufficient as long as urine output exceeds 0.5 ml/hour/kg body weight. Because the kidneys are very sensitive to hypoperfusion careful observation of the urimeter is recommended; this provides important information on the effectiveness of resuscitation.

The gut is prone to early injury during shock. For several years, it has been possible to assess the adequacy of gastrointestinal perfusion by using a silicone balloon at the tip of a nasogastric tube filled with saline [39, 40]. Carbon dioxide freely diffuses from the gastric mucosa into the silicone balloon. After an equilibration time of 20 to 60 minutes, the saline is aspirated for the determination of carbon dioxide tension. Using the Henderson–Hasselbalch equation and assuming that the mucosal bicarbonate content is the same as in arterial blood, it is possible to calculate the intramucosal pH. Given some limitations, intramucosal pH is still a useful measure of stomach perfusion [41] and, therefore, can be used as a guide for volume resuscitation in hypovolaemic shock.

LABORATORY INVESTIGATIONS

Laboratory tests are important markers for the efficacy of resuscitation. Ideally, with the insertion of the first peripheral catheter, the anaesthetist should take blood for crossmatching as well as chemistry, haematology and coagulation baseline values. With the insertion of an arterial line, the laboratory profile is completed with an arterial blood gas analysis.

It is difficult to give exact recommendations for the intervals between different tests, because they depend on the patient and the course of the treatment. Haemoglobin, platelets, sodium, potassium, coagulation screen and an arterial blood gas analysis have to be repeated frequently, at least hourly.

ANAESTHETIC CONSIDERATIONS

In a situation of major antepartum or postpartum haemorrhage the chances are high that the patient will immediately need general anaesthesia for a life-saving surgical procedure. A regional method (spinal or epidural) would be deleterious because of the sympathetic blockade and, therefore, should not be used in these patients.

The recommendations for general anaesthesia are the same for all patients in hypovolaemic shock. The fact that a viable foetus may still be present should not change the procedure, because the foetus will only survive if the mother survives.

Before induction of anaesthesia it is crucial to improve the volume status of the patient. At least two large-bore (7 French, 12 or 14 gauge) peripheral catheters have to be used for maximum speed volume resuscitation. If available, there should be one person responsible for every line, knowing exactly which fluid bag has to be infused next. Before induction of anaesthesia all materials, monitors, machines and drugs have to be checked.

For induction of patients in hypovolaemic shock we recommend a reduced dose of ketamine (0.4 to 1 mg/kg i.v.) and suxamethonium (1 mg/kg i.v.) for muscle relaxation. As an alternative, a reduced dose of etomidate (0.1 to 0.2 mg/kg i.v.) may be administered. The anaesthetist should expect cardiovascular deterioration after administration of any anaesthetic. After endotracheal intubation the patient's lungs are ventilated with a high oxygen concentration [42, 43].

As long as the patient remains in shock, we do not use nitrous oxide or inhalational agents.

Anaesthesia may be maintained, if necessary, with small doses of ketamine. Once the patient has reached haemodynamic stability, a mean arterial pressure above 50 mm Hg, and the bleeding has stopped, anaesthesia can be maintained according to personal preferences. The dosage of all drugs, however, should still be adjusted to the patient's condition.

REFERENCES

1. Phillips, O.C. and Hulka, J.F. (1965) Obstetric mortality. *Anesthesiology*, **26**, 435–46.
2. Department of Health, Welsh Office, Scottish Office Home and Health Department of Health and Social Security, Northern Ireland (1996) *Report on Confidential Enquiries into Maternal Deaths in the United Kingdom 1991–1993*, HMSO, London.
3. McMorland, G.H. (1995) Cardiovascular and respiratory changes in late pregnancy, in *Common Problems in Obstetric Anesthesia*, 2nd edn (ed. S. Datta), Mosby-Year Book, St Louis, pp. 1–5.
4. Marx, G.F. (1965) Shock in the obstetric patient. *Anesthesiology*, **26**, 423–34.
5. Subcommittee on Advanced Trauma Life Support of the American College of Surgeons Committee on Trauma 1988–1992 (1993) *Advanced Trauma Life Support* The American College of Surgeons, Chicago.
6. Goldberg, S. and Norris, M.C. (1993) Obstetric hemorrhage, in *Obstetric Anesthesia* (ed. M.C. Norris), J.B. Lippincott Company, Philadelphia, pp. 579–98.
7. Traber, D.L., Meyer, J. and Traber, L.D. (1995) Cardiac function during hypovolemia, in *Pathophysiology of Shock, Sepsis, and Organ Failure* (eds G. Schlag and H. Redl), Springer-Verlag, Berlin, Heidelberg, pp. 194–99.
8. Gutierrez, G. and Brown, S.D. (1995) Response of the macrocirculation, in *Pathophysiology of Shock, Sepsis, and Organ Failure* (eds G. Schlag and H. Redl), Springer-Verlag, Berlin, Heidelberg, pp. 215–29.
9. Palmer, R.M.J., Ferrige, A.G. and Moncada, S. (1987) Nitric oxide release accounts for the biological activity of endothelium-derived relaxing factor. *Nature (London)*, **327**, 524–526.
10. Crystal, G.J. and Salem, M.R. (1989) Myocardial and systemic responses to arterial hypoxemia during cardiac tamponade. *American Journal of Physiology*, **257**, H726–33.
11. Fiddian-Green, R.G. (1988) Splanchnic ischaemia and multiple organ failure in the critical ill. *Annals of the Royal College of Surgeons of England*, **70**, 128–34.
12. Stene, J.K., Grande, C.M. and Giesecke, A. (1991) Shock resuscitation in *Trauma Anesthesia* (eds J.K. Stene and C.M. Grande), Williams & Wilkins, Baltimore, pp. 100–32.
13. Engelhardt, W. (1995) Gibt es gesicherte Indikationen für Humanalbumin in der Anästhesiologie und Intensivmedizin? *Anaesthesiologie Intensivmedizin*, **36**, 120–27.
14. Larsen, R. (1994) *Anästhesie*, Urban und Schwarzenberg, München.
15. Mattar, J.R. (1989) Hypertonic and hyperoncotic solutions in patients. *Critical Care Medicine*, **17**, 297–8.
16. Edelman, B. and Heyman, M.R. (1991) Blood component therapy for trauma patients, in *Trauma Anesthesia* (eds J.K. Stene and C.M. Grande), Williams & Wilkins, Baltimore, pp. 133–76.
17. Schneider, J.M. (1995) Hemorrhage: Related obstetric and medical disorders, in *Principles and Practice of Obstetric Analgesia and Anesthesia* (eds J.J. Bonica and J.S. McDonald), Williams & Wilkins, Baltimore, pp. 865–917.
18. Murray, D.J., Pennell, B.J., Weinstein, S.L. *et al.* (1995) Packed red cells in acute blood loss: dilutional coagulopathy as a cause of surgical bleeding. *Anesthesia and Analgesia*, **80**, 336–42.
19. Stoelting, R.K. (1987) *Pharmacology and Physiology in Anesthetic Practice*, J.B. Lippincott Company, Philadelphia.
20. Scheidegger, D. and Drop, L.J. (1979) The relationship between duration of Q–T interval and plasma ionized calcium concentration. *Anesthesiology*, **51**, 143–8.
21. Alvarez, J.M., Quiney, N.F., McMillan, D. *et al.* (1995) The use of ultra-low-dose aprotinin to reduce blood loss in cardiac surgery. *Journal of Cardiothoracic and Vascular Anesthesia*, **9**, 29–33.
22. Soilleux, H., Gillon, M.-C., Mirand, A. *et al.* (1995) Comparative effects of small and large aprotinin doses on bleeding during orthotopic liver transplantation. *Anesthesia and Analgesia*, **80**, 349–52.
23. Murkin, J.M., Shannon, N.A., Bourne, R.B. *et al.* (1995) Aprotinin decreases blood loss in patients undergoing revision or bilateral total hip arthroplasty. *Anesthesia and Analgesia*, **80**, 343–8.

24. Valentine, S., Williamson, P. and Sutton, D. (1993) Reduction of acute haemorrhage with aprotinin. *Anaesthesia*, **48**, 405–6.
25. Koziol, J.M., Rush, B.F., Smith, S.M. *et al.* (1988) Occurrence of bacteremia during and after hemorrhagic shock. *Journal of Trauma*, **28**, 10–6.
26. Border, J.R. (1992) Multiple systems organ failure (editorial). *Annals of Surgery*, **216**, 111–6.
27. Deitch, E.A. (1992) Multiple organ failure: pathophysiology and potential future therapy. *Annals of Surgery*, **216**, 117–34.
28. Segal, J.M., Phang, P.T. and Walley, K.R. (1992) Low-dose dopamine hastens onset of gut ischemia in a porcine model of hemorrhagic shock. *Journal of Applied Physiology*, **73**, 1159–64.
29. Nordin, A., Mäkisalo, H. and Höckerstedt, K. (1994) Dopamine infusion during resuscitation of experimental hemorrhagic shock. *Critical Care Medicine*, **22**, 151–6.
30. Flancbaum, L., Choban, P.S. and Dasta, J.F. (1994) Quantitative effects of low-dose dopamine on urine output in oliguric surgical intensive care unit patients. *Critical Care Medicine*, **22**, 61–6.
31. Breslow, M.J., Miller, C.F., Parker, S.D. *et al.* (1987) Effect of vasopressors on organ blood flow during endotoxin shock in pigs. *American Journal of Physiology*, **252**, H291–H300.
32. Biehl, D.R. (1987) Antepartum and postpartum hemorrhage in *Anesthesia for Obstetrics* (eds S.M. Shnider and J.L. Levinson), Williams & Wilkins, Baltimore, pp. 281–9.
33. Winikur, L.J. (1991) Treatment of postpartum hemorrhage in *Anesthesiology Review* (ed. R.J. Faust), Churchill Livingstone, New York, p. 402.
34. Hug, C.C. (1986) Monitoring, in *Anesthesia* (ed. R.D. Miller), Churchill Livingstone, New York, pp. 411–64.
35. Rafferty, T., LaMantia, K.R., Davis, E. *et al.* (1993) Quality assurance for intraoperative transesophageal echocardiography monitoring: A report of 846 procedures. *Anesthesia and Analgesia*, **76**, 228–32.
36. Lussos, S.A. (1995) Anesthesia for cesarean delivery, in *Common Problems in Obstetric Anesthesia* (ed. S. Datta), Mosby-Year Book, St Louis, pp. 203–28.
37. Hatle, L. and Rokseth, R. (1974) The arterial to end-expiratory carbon dioxide tension gradient in acute pulmonary embolism and other cardiopulmonary diseases. *Chest*, **66**, 352–7.
38. Moller, J.T., Pedersen, T., Rasmussen, L.S. *et al.* (1993) Randomized evaluation of pulse oximetry in 20,802 patients: I and II. *Anesthesiology*, **78**, 436–53.
39. Grum, C.M, Fiddian-Green, R.G., Pittenger, G.L. *et al* (1984) Adequacy of tissue oxygenation in intact dog intestine. *Journal of Applied Physiology*, **56**, 1065–69.
40. Antonsson, J.B., Boyle, C.C and, Kruithoff, K.L. (1990) Validation of tonometric measurement of gut intramural pH during endotoxemia and mesenteric occlusion in pigs. *American Journal of Physiology*, **259**, G519–23.
41. Fiddian-Green, R.G. (1995) Gastric intramucosal pH, tissue oxygenation and acid–base balance. *British Journal of Anaesthesia*, **74**, 591–606.
42. Schneider, M.C. (1995) Antepartum hemorrhage in *Common Problems in Obstetric Anesthesia* (ed. S. Datta), Mosby-Year Book, St Louis, pp. 271–86.
43. Weiskopf, R.B. (1987) Anesthesia for major trauma, in *Review Course Lectures*, International Anesthesia Research Society, Ohio, pp. 73–9.

PERIPARTUM ANAESTHESIA

4

M.C. Schneider and K.F. Hampl

INTRODUCTION

Within the last few decades, there has been an increasing trend towards delivery by caesarean section. Rates have soared worldwide reaching a high of 30% in some industrialized countries such as the USA [1]. Recourse to abdominal delivery is being challenged as pressure from public and professional sources puts greater emphasis on the advantages that vaginal delivery has in terms of maternal and foetal outcome [2]. Trials of labour in pursuit of a vaginal delivery after a previous caesarean section have become common practice in many obstetric units. Certainly, such a policy requires that, in the event of maternal or foetal emergencies, skilled anaesthetic support is immediately available. Such support should be managed by a team prepared to administer anaesthesia within a reasonably short response time [3, 4]. In the future, demands for peripartum anaesthesia are likely to increase in parallel to the implementation of wait-and-see policies in obstetric practice in order to reduce the incidence of surgical deliveries.

In this chapter we consider some aspects of the organization and delivery of an obstetric anaesthetic service. Some indications for anaesthetic involvement are regular occurrences, while others represent rare events. The examples quoted are intended to serve as a blueprint for both common and rare situations.

HAZARDS OF EMERGENCY AND UNPLANNED ANAESTHESIA

Peripartum anaesthesia is frequently synonymous with anaesthesia for women requiring unplanned or emergency surgical intervention. Risk is higher in women undergoing emergency procedures compared with those presenting electively. One contributing factor is the lack of time for adequate pre-anaesthetic preparation and emergency anaesthesia is known to make maternal morbidity and death more likely [5].

Furthermore, ignorance of the special condition called pregnancy and its implication for anaesthetic practice in so-called 'healthy' patients has also made its contribution [5–7]. The role of the preoperative visit to women who require peripartum anaesthesia is to raise standards and improve safety (Table 4.1). It should form an essential part of any policy intended to make childbirth uneventful and improve maternal satisfaction.

Clinical Problems in Obstetric Anaesthesia
Edited by Ian F. Russell and Gordon Lyons. Published in 1997 by Chapman & Hall, London. ISBN 0 412 71600 3.

Table 4.1 Pregnant women who should have an antenatal assessment by the anaesthetist

Maternal request for epidural analgesia
High-risk pregnancy and/or delivery:
• pre-existing maternal disease (cardiovascular, pulmonary, renal, endocrine, neurologic, immunologic, haematologic disorders)
• pregnancy-induced maternal disease (preeclampsia, thromboembolic disease)
• obstetrical history (vaginal birth after caesarean section)
• problems related to labour and delivery (intra-uterine growth retardation, preterm labour, abnormal foetal presentation, multiple gestation, trial of labour)
High-risk anaesthesia:
• difficult airway (morbid obesity, preeclampsia, anatomic abnormalities)
• severe preeclampsia, significant maternal disease (American Society of Anesthesiology physical status ≥ III)
• drug addiction

PHYSIOLOGICAL CHANGES AND IMPLICATIONS FOR THE ANAESTHETIST

Pregnancy is associated with important changes in anatomy, and physiological functions are adapted to meet increased metabolic and respiratory demands [8, 9]. Most of these alterations have direct bearing on the management of general as well as regional anaesthesia. On one hand, the increase in both total blood volume and extravascular fluid volume effectively protects against hypovolaemia due to blood loss at delivery. On the other hand, about 20% of cardiac output flows through the vascular bed of the gravid uterus at term, which corresponds to 500 ml per minute. This explains why uterine atony and/or lacerations may result in massive haemorrhage. Other important circulatory changes which occur in late pregnancy are associated with the supine position. The gravid uterus puts pressure on both major intra-abdominal vessels, the aorta and inferior vena cava, thus reducing venous return, stroke volume, cardiac output and uteroplacental perfusion, resulting in acute hypotension and foetal distress [10].

Respiratory function is significantly influenced by the expanding uterus which displaces the diaphragm cephalad. While functional residual capacity progressively decreases, closing volume increases so that airway closure occurs within the normal tidal volume in about 50% of pregnant women [8]. Anatomical changes may contribute to an eight-fold increase in the frequency of difficult orotracheal intubations in pregnant as compared with non-pregnant women [11]. Moreover, the soft tissues lining the oral, nasal and pharyngeal cavities are prone to bleeding and swelling following mechanical manipulation, which can impair visualization of the larynx.

Although controversial, it is wise to assume that gastric emptying may be unpredictably prolonged in pregnant patients, and the presence of a full stomach should always be anticipated irrespective of the time between the last meal and the onset of labour [12]. Placental gastrin adds to the likelihood that large volumes of low pH gastric juices are produced [12]. In addition, intra-abdominal pressure and cephalad displacement of the stomach may reduce the effectiveness of gastro-oesophageal sphincter function.

PREANAESTHETIC ASSESSMENT AND MEDICATION

The ideal time to conduct an anaesthetic assessment is before labour has started. Such a visit is necessary to achieve high standards, but in practice, ideal timing is often hard to achieve. A team approach to management in the presence of increased obstetrical risk should include

Table 4.2 Measures aimed at preventing the risks of aspiration of gastric contents in parturients deemed candidates for peripartum anaesthesia

Dietary policies concerning oral intake during labour:
- Only clear liquids or ice chips allowed

Pharmacologic acid aspiration prophylaxis:
- non-particulate antacid:
  0.3 M sodium citrate, 30 ml orally
  H_2 receptor antagonist: ranitidine, 50 mg i.v. or 150 mg orally
  cimetidine, 200 mg i.v. or 400 mg orally as effervescent (cimetidine/sodium citrate)
- metoclopramide, 10 mg i.v. or orally (central antidopaminergic and intestinal cholinergic action)
- proton pump inhibitor:
  omeprazole, 40 mg i.v. or orally
- antimuscarinic agents:
  atropine, hyoscine (placental transfer)
  glycopyrrolate (almost no placental transfer)

early warning. Multidisciplinary cooperation may help to ameliorate the stress that may accompany unexpected and sometimes dire peripartum situations. Failure to communicate at an early stage may hamper task co-ordination and impinge negatively on the performance of team members, resulting in both maternal and foetal morbidity or mortality [13].

Obstetric risk (Table 4.1) may be related to significant pre-existing or pregnancy-related disease, breech and other abnormal presentations. Some maternal conditions may be associated with particular anaesthetic hazards, for example morbid obesity, the difficult airway, preeclampsia and drug addiction. During the course of an adequate preoperative meeting, the options for anaesthetic management can be thoroughly overhauled. A supportive relationship should be established with the woman which should serve to reduce her anxiety and stress. However, experience tells us that unforeseen problems will continue to arise in obstetric practice, and that rapid intervention in unprepared women will continue to be a feature. A calm and reassuring manner is necessary to win confidence, allay anxiety, and win co-operation whilst simultaneously preparing for anaesthesia.

The presence of pre-existing or pregnancy-induced disease should be carefully evaluated. When conditions such as coagulation dis-orders, maternal sepsis, active central nervous system disease or absolute refusal, preclude the administration of regional anaesthesia, the patient's upper airway must be examined carefully in order to assess the relative risk of difficult tracheal intubation [14]. If difficult intubation is expected, the possibility of an awake and/or fibre optic intubation should be discussed with the patient.

While candidates for a general anaesthetic (Table 4.1) should not be allowed to eat solid food during labour, drinking of clear liquids may be permissible (Table 4.2) [15]. Precise timing of childbirth is impossible, and a preoperative fasting period of at least four hours may be wishful thinking [16]. The prophylactic administration of 0.3 M sodium citrate (20–30 ml), a non-particulate oral antacid, immediately before induction, is compulsory. When administered with H_2-receptor antagonists, like cimetidine or rantidine, the combination is beneficial and has been shown to be effective in reducing the volume of gastric contents and the acidity of gastric secretion [17]. In this context, use of the dopaminergic antagonist metoclopramide as the third component is recommended both to shorten gastric emptying time and to increase the lower oesophageal sphincter pressure by an intestinal cholinergic action [18]. Sedatives for reducing apprehension are not routinely prescribed. In the emergency situation the onset time is often too long, central nervous depression is undesirable, and when relevant, so too is foetal transmission.

GUIDELINES, POLICIES AND STANDARDS

Institutions which care for women in labour should define guidelines for the management of foetal as well as maternal complications. Minimum standards have been proposed by the Obstetric Anaesthetists' Association [3] and by the American Society of Anesthesiologists [4]. These guidelines not only define the availability of anaesthetic personnel and their professional qualifications but they also define infrastructural requirements which might include facilities for immediate surgical intervention or access to specialized neonatal care units.

In the *Report on Confidential Enquiries into Maternal Deaths 1991–1993* [5], pulse oximetry is recommended for perioperative and early postoperative routine monitoring in addition to standard monitoring which includes a CO_2 analyser, intermittent blood pressure and continuous electrocardiographic recording.

FOETAL INDICATIONS

SHOULDER DYSTOCIA, HEAD ENTRAPMENT, UMBILICAL CORD COMPRESSION AND PROLAPSE

Severe foetal distress as a result of shoulder dystocia in the vertex position or head entrapment during vaginal breech deliveries or delivery of the second twin, umbilical cord compression or, occasionally, by cord prolapse has always been a challenge in obstetric practice. Additional to the usual hazards associated with emergency anaesthesia, there may also be a request for general anaesthesia in the lithotomy or other position. The traditional teaching has been that it is impossible to practice to the required standard under this restriction,

and that maternal interests should outweigh obstetric and foetal distress. A particular concern has been the inability to turn a woman who regurgitates. Where effective regional blockade is in place this dilemma should not arise. Goals of anaesthetic care include pain relief and relaxation of the pelvic floor without interfering with the mother's ability to push effectively. If an epidural catheter is in place, immediate uterine relaxation can be achieved by increments of 100–200 µg intravenous nitroglycerine [19]. However, often a general anaesthetic may be necessary. In such a case, a rapid sequence induction using thiopentone or propofol and suxamethonium is recommended following four deep breaths of 100% oxygen for denitrogenation [20]. Cricoid pressure should be applied until correct endotracheal tube position is confirmed. Any potent volatile anaesthetic may be used in concentrations high enough to achieve cervical relaxation. Neonatal depression will result from asphyxia rather than exposure to anaesthetics. Expert neonatal resuscitation may be crucial in determining long-term outcome.

MATERNAL INDICATIONS FOR PERIPARTUM ANAESTHESIA

Maternal indications are given below.

- Antepartum:
  cervical suture
- Intrapartum:
  forceps delivery
  inversion of the uterus
- Postpartum:
  haemorrhage
  manual removal of the placenta
  perineal tears
  evacuation of vulvar haematoma
  exploration of wound
  tubal ligation

When bulging membranes are associated with prematurity, a cervical suture may be inserted as an emergency procedure. Kielland's forceps requires either emergency regional or general anaesthesia, and where there is a well-established epidural analgesia service, additional intervention is a rare event. Postpartum haemorrhage is defined as a blood loss in excess of 500 ml caused by injury of the perineum, lacerations within the birth canal or originating within the uterine cavity. A vulvar haematoma may require evacuation, and there is a tendency to underestimate blood loss from this source. Occasionally following caesarean delivery, especially when coagulation is for diagnosis and therapy, there is often the need for analgesia or anaesthesia, and while principles of management are common to all, some of these conditions carry individual cautions.

Minor lesions involving the perineum or the distal vagina may be repaired under submucosal infiltration anaesthesia. For more extensive perineal exploration or repair, a bilateral pudendal nerve block can provide perineal pain relief. Spinal or epidural anaesthesia (if an epidural catheter is already in place) are valuable alternatives assuming that hypovolaemia is corrected. Vaginal or uterine explorations, including removal of retained placenta, may be performed without further analgesic medication. Sometimes, however, manual removal of the placenta may only be accomplished following relaxation of the cervix by intravenous nitroglycerine in dosages as low as 50–100 µg [19] or as a sublingual aerosol spray delivering 0.8 mg [21]. For patients without epidural labour analgesia, spinal anaesthesia can be recommended as a method that avoids the risks of a general anaesthetic under less than perfect conditions. Both bupivacaine and lignocaine are appropriate. For general anaesthesia, any potent inhalational anaesthetic in a concentration above 0.5 of the minimum anaesthetic concentration (MAC) may be used in order to relax the contracted uterus [22]. It is important to note that concentrations in excess of 2 MAC may diminish the uterine response to oxytocin infusion [23]. Once the placenta is removed, the inhalational agent should be discontinued immediately and an oxytocin infusion should be started.

Inversion of the uterus is a rare but life-threatening complication [24]. The cause of uterine inversion is often strong traction of the umbilical cord while vigorous fundal pressure is applied at the other end. As exsanguination may rapidly occur, prompt therapy is of crucial importance. Fluid resuscitation via large-bore intravenous lines must be started immediately while manual repositioning of the uterus should be attempted. However, uterine inversion may occur without significant blood loss, but a form of neurogenic shock with hypotension may be confused with haemorrhagic shock. The temptation to correct neurogenic hypotension with large volumes of fluid should be resisted. Failure to reverse this condition may be due to cervical contraction. Uterine relaxation may then be achieved by intravenous administration of nitroglycerine [25], tocolytics such as terbutaline, ritodrine or magnesium sulphate, or by inhalational anaesthesia. However, as a consequence of hypovolaemia, deep inhalational anaesthesia may result in hypotension. As soon as the uterus is repositioned, uterine relaxation should be stopped by administration of uterotonic agents to prevent further haemorrhage. If these measures fail to be effective, prompt laparotomy under general anaesthesia is required.

ANAESTHESIA FOR POSTPARTUM TUBAL LIGATION

Postpartum tubal ligation offers many advantages over interval laparoscopic sterilisation. First, only single hospitalization is required as a matter of convenience and cost savings. Second, surgical and postpartum recovery are combined. Third, childbirth may be the one and only occasion that many women come into contact with the health care system. Therefore, elective tubal ligation at this time appears to be an ideal option.

The risk of pulmonary aspiration of gastric contents is reduced after delivery, but nevertheless, some of the anatomical and physiological changes of pregnancy persist for a while. As the results of studies on gastro-intestinal function for this period conflict [26–28], anaesthetic management of postpartum tubal ligation should include the same precautionary measures to protect against the aspiration of gastric contents as in the pre and intrapartum periods. In addition, the patient should be fasted for at least eight hours before elective postpartum surgery. For the same reasons, a regional anaesthetic technique is highly preferable to general anaesthesia for this procedure. General anaesthesia should only be performed when regional anaesthetic techniques are contraindicated or refused by the patient. A rapid sequence induction (as described above) should always be performed. Because these procedures tend to be short, a reduced dosage of short-acting non-depolarizing muscle relaxants or a suxamethonium drip may be used to maintain muscle relaxation. Before extubation, recovery from neuromuscular block should be detected by using a peripheral nerve stimulator and clinical signs. If necessary, pharmacologic reversal agents should be given.

When an epidural catheter is in place, epidural anaesthesia may be reinstated. The local anaesthetic requirement may be considerably increased compared with the prepartum period [29]. If there are doubts about epidural efficacy, elective spinal anaesthesia is an excellent choice. It avoids the embarrassment of unsatisfactory epidural anaesthesia and rescue with a general anaesthetic. Spinal anaesthesia has many advantages over epidural anaesthesia for postpartum tubal ligation. The former is simple to perform, has a rapid onset and provides excellent anaesthesia with a minimal risk of local anaesthetic toxicity. For years, the only objection against spinal anaesthesia in young patients was an unacceptably high incidence of post-dural puncture headache. This problem has been largely resolved by the introduction of small pencil-point spinal needles into clinical practice [30]. Spinal puncture is performed at the L2/3 or L3/4 interspace after prehydration with Ringer's solution. For adequate anaesthe-

sia, a sensory level of T4 is required. This may be achieved by administration of either plain or hyperbaric solutions of lignocaine or bupivacaine.

ACKNOWLEDGEMENT

We wish to thank Mrs Joan Etlinger for her excellent secretarial work.

REFERENCES

1. Lussos, S.A. and Datta, S. (1992) Anesthesia for cesarean delivery. Part 1: General considerations and spinal anesthesia. *International Journal of Obstetric Anaesthesia*, **1**, 79–91.
2. Myers, S.A. and Gleicher, N. (1988) A successful program to lower cesarean-section rates (special article). *New England Journal of Medicine*, **319**, 1511–6.
3. Obstetric Anaesthetists' Association (1995) Recommended minimum standards for obstetric anaesthesia services (Guidelines). *International Journal of Obstetric Anaesthesia*, **4**, 125–8.
4. American Society of Anesthesiologists (1995) Guidelines for regional anesthesia in obstetrics. *International Journal of Obstetric Anaesthesia* **4**, 129–30.
5. Hibbard, B.M., Anderson, M.M., Drife, J.O. *et al.* (eds) (1994) *Report on Confidential Enquiries into Maternal Deaths in the United Kingdom 1991–1993*. HMSO, London, pp. 87–102.
6. Morgan, M. (1987) Anaesthetic contribution to maternal mortality. *British Journal of Anaesthesia*, **59**, 842–55.
7. Sachs, B.J., Oriol, N.E., Ostheimer, G.W. *et al.* (1989) Anesthetic-related maternal mortality, 1954 to 1985. *Journal of Clinical Anesthesia*, **1**, 333–8.
8. Moir, D.D. (1980) Physiology of pregnancy and labour, in *Obstetric Anaesthesia and Analgesia*. Baillière Tindall, London, pp. 8–37.
9. Camaan, W.R. and Ostheimer, G.W. (1990) Physiological adaptations during pregnancy. *International Anesthesiology Clinics*, **28**, 2–10.
10. Eckstein, K.-L. and Marx, G.F. (1974) Aortocaval compression and uterine displacement. *Anesthesiology*, **40**, 92–6.
11. Samsoon, G.L.T. and Young, J.R.B. (1987) Difficult tracheal intubation: a retrospective study. *Anaesthesia*, **42**, 487–90.

12. Roberts, R.B. and Shirley, M.A. (1974) Reducing the risk of acid aspiration during cesarean section. *Anesthesia and Analgesia*, **53**, 859–68.

13. McDonald, J.S. and Jacoby, J. (1995) Complications of general anesthesia, in *Principles and Practice of Obstetric Analgesia and Anesthesia*, 2nd edn (eds J.J. Bonica and J.S. McDonald), Williams and Wilkins Company, Baltimore, pp. 672–711.

14. Rocke, D.A., Murray, W.B., Rout, C.C. and Gouws, E. (1992) Relative risk analysis of factors associated with difficult intubation in obstetric anaesthesia. *Anesthesiology*, **77**, 67–73.

15. Elkington, K.W. (1991) At the water's edge: where obstetrics and anesthesia meet (clinical commentary). *Obstetrics and Gynecology*, **77**, 304–8.

16. Lewis, M. and Crawford, J.S. (1987) Can one risk fasting the obstetric patient for less than 4 hours? *British Journal of Anaesthesia*, **59**, 312–4.

17. Okasha, A.S., Motaweh, M.M. and Bali, A. (1983) Cimetide–antacid combination as premedication for elective Caesarean section. *Canadian Anaesthetists' Society Journal*, **30**, 593–7.

18. Hey, V.M.F. and Ostick, D.G. (1978) Metoclopramide and the gastro-oesophageal sphincter. A study in pregnant women with heartburn. *Anaesthesia*, **33**, 462–5.

19. DeSimone, C.A., Norris, M.C. and Leighton, B.L. (1990) Intravenous nitroglycerin aids manual extraction of a retained placenta. *Anesthesiology*, **73**, 787.

20. Norris, M.C., Kirkland, M.R., Torjman, M.C. and Goldberg, M.E. (1989) Denitrogenation in pregnancy. *Canadian Journal of Anaesthesia*, **36**, 523–5.

21. Redick, L.F. and Livingstone, E. (1995) A new preparation of nitroglycerin for uterine relaxation. *International Journal of Obstetric Anaesthesia*, **4**, 14–6.

22. Warren, T.M., Datta, S., Ostheimer, G.W. *et al.* (1983) Comparison of the maternal and neonatal effects of halothane, enflurane, and isoflurane for cesarean delivery. *Anesthesia and Analgesia*, **62**, 516–20.

23. Naftalin, N.J., McKay, D.M., Phear, W.P.C. and Goldberg, A.H. (1977) The effect of halothane on pregnant and non-pregnant human myometrium. *Anesthesiology*, **46**, 15–9.

24. Shah-Hosseini, R. and Evrard, J.R. (1989) Puerperal uterine inversion. *Obstetrics and Gynecology*, **73**, 567–70.

25. Altabef, K.M., Spencer, J.T. and Zinberg, S. (1992) Intravenous nitroglycerin for uterine relaxation of an inverted uterus. *American Journal of Obstetrics and Gynecology*, **166**, 1237–8.

26. Blouw, R., Scatliff, J., Craig, D.B. and Palahniuk, R.J. (1976) Gastric volume and pH in postpartum patients. *Anesthesiology*, **45**, 456–7.

27. James, C.F., Gibbs, C.P. and Banner, T. (1984) Postpartum perioperative risk of aspiration pneumonia. *Anesthesiology*, **61**, 756–9.

28. O'Sullivan, G.M., Sutton, A.J., Thompson, S.A. *et al.* (1987) Noninvasive measurement of gastric emptying in obstetric patients. *Anesthesia and Analgesia*, **66**, 505–11.

29. Abouleish, E.I. (1986) Postpartum tubal ligation requires more bupivacaine for spinal anesthesia than does cesarean section. *Anesthesia and Analgesia*, **65**, 897–900.

30. Halpern, S. and Preston, R. (1994) Postdural puncture headache and spinal needle design. Metaanalyses. *Anesthesiology*, **81**, 1376–83.

D. Thorin, D. Bracco and Y. Vial

INTRODUCTION

During the second half of pregnancy many conditions can result in maternal and/or foetal damage. Many antepartum emergencies present as antepartum haemorrhage, but some conditions (ruptured gravid uterus, placental abruption, foetal hypoxia, etc.) can lead to serious foetal and/or maternal morbidity without brisk haemorrhage. Antepartum haemorrhage continues to be reported as the second largest cause of maternal mortality in the USA (following preeclampsia/eclampsia), contributing to 10.8–16% of all direct maternal deaths [1, 2]. Among the 22 deaths from antepartum and postpartum haemorrhage reported in the *Triennial Report on Confidential Enquiries into Maternal Deaths in the United Kingdom 1988–1990*, five deaths were due to abruptio placentae, five to placenta praevia and one to coagulopathy following intra-uterine death. Haemorrhage is a major direct cause of maternal death and frequently complicates the treatment of the sick obstetric patient. In the UK, the number of deaths directly due to haemorrhage rose from 10 to 22 per triennium between 1985 and 1990. Every year there are five deaths due to obstetric haemorrhage [3]. The first two pathologies (abruptio placentae and placenta praevia) account for more than half of all vaginal bleeding after 20 weeks' gestation [4]. Other less clinically important causes

of antepartum haemorrhages are also briefly considered: placenta accreta/increta, ruptured gravid uterus, vasa praevia, velamentous cord insertion and trauma (Table 5.1).

Clinical assessment of the volume of blood loss during the second and third trimesters may be extremely difficult. Management of these women is often complex. A multidisciplinary approach which includes obstetricians, anaesthetists and neonatologists is necessary for effective care. Basic rules must be established as guidelines for the management of massive antepartum vaginal bleeding. These will include clinical evaluation of mother and foetus, gradation of the severity of the vaginal haemorrhage and determination of obstetric and anaesthetic strategies.

ABRUPTIO PLACENTAE

Abruptio placentae is defined as the premature separation of a normally inserted placenta from the uterus prior to the third stage of labour. Commonly, the bleeding of placental abruption is apparent through the cervix, and this is termed external haemorrhage. In some cases, haemorrhage is invisible within the uterine cavity, and this is called a concealed haemorrhage. The likelihood of inappropriate appraisal of maternal blood loss and coagulopathy is greater in abruptio placentae with concealed haemorrhage. Abruptio placentae is

Clinical Problems in Obstetric Anaesthesia
Edited by Ian F. Russell and Gordon Lyons. Published in 1997 by Chapman & Hall, London. ISBN 0 412 71600 3.

Table 5.1 Causes of antepartum emergencies

Pathologies	Incidence	Maternal morbidity	Foetal morbidity
Functional abnormalities of the placenta			
Preeclampsia, eclampsia	1:15 to 1:20	++	++
Pregnancy-induced hypertension	1:10 to 1:15	++	+
Anatomical abnormalities of the placenta			
Placenta praevia	1:200	++	++
Abruptio placentae	1:40 to 1:500	+	+++
Placenta accreta, increta, percreta	1:2500 to 1:7000	+++	+
Abnormalities of the uterus and membranes			
Uterine rupture	1:1500 to 1:3000	++	+++
Rupture of membranes	1:10	−	+
Abnormalities of the foetus			
Malpositions	1:15	−	−
Breech head retention	rare	+	+++
Retention of a dead foetus	rare	+	
Abnormalities of the cord			
Cord prolapse	1:300	−	+++
Vasa praevia	1:100	−	+++
Velamentous insertion of the umbilical cord	1:100	−	+++

classified according to the blood loss (from less than 100 ml to more than 500 ml), maternal condition, uterine tone and foetal heart rate, into mild (65%) moderate (23%) and severe (12%) categories [5]. Reported incidences vary widely, ranging from 0.2 to 2.4% of deliveries [4]. In subsequent pregnancies, the risk of recurrence is estimated to be 5 to 15%[6]. The overall maternal mortality is less than 5% and represents 15% of all perinatal deaths, even when the severe forms associated with coagulopathy and renal failure are taken into account [7]. Foetal mortality, mainly due to prematurity and anoxia, is influenced by the degree of placental separation [6]. The factors most frequently associated with abruptio placentae are age, high parity, hypertension, trauma, uterine abnormalities, previous abruptio placentae and premature rupture of membranes (Table 5.2). Treatment with low-dose aspirin could be a risk factor [8].

The signs and symptoms depend on the clinical category of abruptio placentae. Common manifestations include vaginal bleeding and/or abnormal hypertonic uterine contractions and/or abdominal pain and/or foetal distress. The association of maternal hypotension with tachycardia out of proportion to the external blood loss, lower abdominal pain and a tense uterus suggests the diagnosis of abruptio placentae with concealed haemorrhage. Often marginal placental abruption leads to massive vaginal bleeding without interfering too greatly with placental gas exchange, whereas central placental abruption leads to delayed haemorrhage with severe placental surface abruption and foetal distress (Figure 5.1).

Ultrasonography is helpful in the diagnosis of placenta praevia, but cannot rule out an abruptio placentae if negative [9]. The most helpful laboratory tests include a full blood

Table 5.2 Antepartum emergencies and their risk factors

Risk factors	Pathologies			
	Abruptio placentae	Placenta previa	Placenta accreta	Uterine rupture
Maternal age	Yes	Yes		
High parity	Yes	Yes	Yes	Yes
Multiple pregnancy				Yes
Smoking		Yes		
Previous caesarean section		Yes	Yes	Yes
Previous uterine surgery		Yes	Yes	Yes
Previous abortion		Yes	Yes	
Oxytocin use				Yes
Hypertension	Yes			

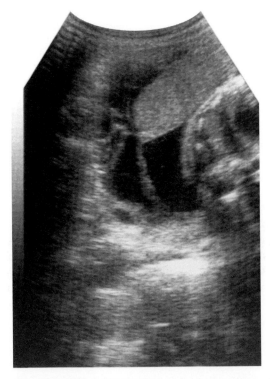

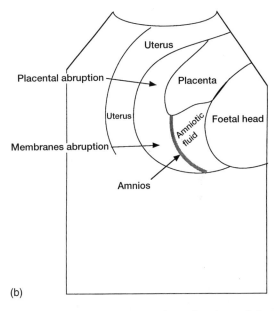

(b)

Figure 5.1 Placental abruption: (a) ultrasound and (b) marginal placental abruption at 22 weeks of pregnancy by transabdominal ultrasound. Ultrasound by Y. Vial.

and platelet count, a serial evaluation of the plasma concentration of fibrinogen and fibrin split products. A sudden fall in fibrinogen concentration associated with an elevation of fibrin split products and progressive thrombocytopenia indicates a life-threatening coagulopathy [5]. It should not be forgotten that foetomaternal bleeding also occurs in these situations and Rh immune globulin should be given if indicated (single dose of anti-D 200 mg intramuscularly).

MANAGEMENT

Immediate hospitalization is required if abruptio placentae is suspected. Half of the related perinatal deaths occur before hospital admittance and 20% between admittance and delivery.

Immediate management of placental abruption involves

- immediate and continuous foetal assessment if the foetus is alive;
- oxygen administration by face mask;
- fluid management by one or two large-bore intravenous lines as indicated by the maternal haemodynamic state;
- cross-match, haematocrit and coagulation profile;
- hourly assessment of urine output.

The obstetric management depends on foetomaternal condition and the clinical category of abruptio placentae. When abruption is mild in the presence of foetal prematurity, conservative management with steroid therapy to hasten foetal lung maturation is indicated. Prompt delivery is recommended when abruption is moderate to severe.

Maternal morbidity seems to be lower with vaginal rather than abdominal delivery, particularly when there is severe coagulopathy [10]. Perioperative bleeding from surgical incision of the uterine wall or placental bed can result in hysterectomy [10]. Vaginal delivery is recommended after foetal death, in the hope that morbidity related to caesarean delivery can be avoided.

ANAESTHETIC CONSIDERATIONS

Anaesthetic management is dictated by the clinical state of the patient. Regional analgesia for labour and vaginal delivery, and anaesthesia for cesarean section should be considered in

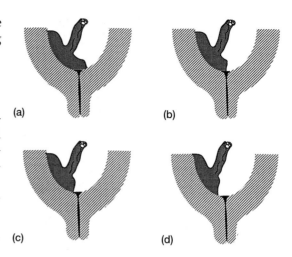

Figure 5.2 Classification of placenta praevia. (a) Total or complete placenta praevia: internal os totally covered by placenta; (b) partial placenta praevia: internal os partially covered by placenta; (c) marginal placenta praevia: placenta is proximate to the internal os; (d) low-lying placenta praevia; implantation in the lower uterine segment.

the presence of normovolaemia, and in the absence of coagulopathy and foetal distress. A low platelet count, an abnormal bleeding time, prothrombin (PT), activated partial thromboplastin time (APTT) or thromboelastogram, and/or a fibrinogen below 1 g/l associated with increased fibrin split products contraindicate regional anaesthesia.

Haemorrhage, hypovolaemia, acute foetal distress or severe coagulopathy indicate general anaesthesia with a rapid-sequence induction. Although ketamine is frequently used as the induction agent, it has the potential to increase the uterine tone and aggravate an abruption [11].

PLACENTA PRAEVIA

Placenta praevia is defined as an implantation of the placenta over or near the internal os of the uterus. The types of placenta praevia are summarized in Figure 5.2 and an example is shown in Figure 5.3. The incidence of placenta praevia is approximately 0.5% of deliveries [12]. The

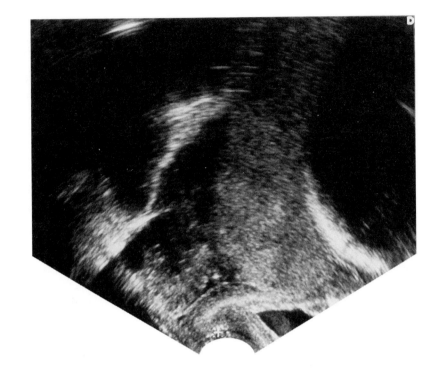

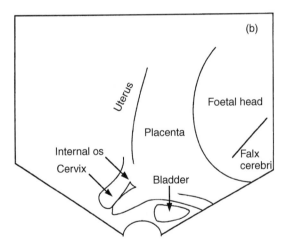

Figure 5.3 Placenta praevia: (a) ultrasound and (b) illustration of total placenta praevia by endovaginal ultrasound at 34 weeks of pregnancy. Ultrasound by Y. Vial.

risk factors are outlined in Table 5.2. In the UK, one fifth of all maternal deaths due to haemorrhage are due to placenta praevia [3].

Placenta accreta may be responsible for up to 15% of significant revealed haemorrhages contributing to maternal morbidity and mortality. Factors influencing perinatal mortality include significant haemorrhage, placental insufficiency and prematurity. Its incidence reaches 10% when bleeding occurs during the third trimester [13].

Painless haemorrhage is the main manifestation of placenta praevia, occurring in more than 90%. Thirty per cent of placenta praevia bleed before 30 weeks' gestation and 30% after 36 weeks' gestation [12].

Diagnosis of placenta praevia is usually made by ultrasonography. A spontaneous resolution rate as high as 90% may be expected when the diagnosis is made during the second trimester. Placental migration explains this very high resolution rate and the success of conservative care. The growth of the lower

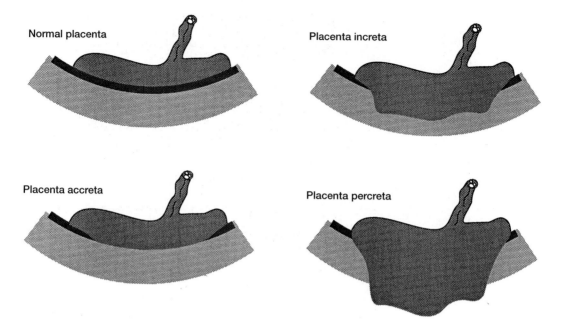

Figure 5.4 Degrees of myometrial invasion in placenta accreta, increta and percreta.

segment means that a low placenta in the second trimester may be found in the fundus near term.

Full blood and platelet count, coagulation profile and ABO/Rh antibody status should be obtained. Foetomaternal bleeding may occur and Rh immune globulin should be given if indicated.

MANAGEMENT

The aim of a conservative approach is to reduce perinatal mortality and morbidity associated with prematurity by extending foetal maturation for as long as possible [14]. Bed rest, and monitoring the haemorrhage, the maternal vital signs and the foetal heart rate fails in approximately 2:10 women, and a more aggressive approach is needed [5].

Emergency caesarean section is considered as the delivery of choice, particularly when the foetus is viable and distressed, or if the woman is actively bleeding. In the case of marginal or low-lying placenta, vaginal delivery may be

considered but the possibility of haemorrhage carries risks for mother and foetus. A high standard of care is required.

ANAESTHETIC CONSIDERATIONS

Both epidural and general anaesthesia may be appropriate techniques for a caesarean section in the context of placenta praevia. Maternal hypovolaemia or clotting abnormalities and acute foetal distress contraindicate regional anaesthesia. Combined spinal–epidural anaesthesia may be considered if a more complex surgical procedure such as hysterectomy is anticipated.

Precautions for regional and general anaesthesia for placenta praevia are similar to those in elective situations, provided there is normovolaemia and haemodynamic stability. Epidural techniques are as safe as general anaesthesia in term of perioperative blood loss and foetomaternal outcome [15]. However, anaesthetists should be aware that profuse bleeding can result when a placenta implanted

Table 5.3 Vertical and lower segment uterine rupture

	Vertical segment rupture	*Lower segment rupture*
Incidence	2.2%	0.5%
Maternal mortality	5%	0%
Foetal mortality	73%	12.5%
Time of rupture	Before labour	During labour
Severity of symptoms	Brisk collapse	+/− symptoms

over the anterior lower uterine segment becomes part of a surgical incision. If the surgeon cannot quickly identify the edge of the placenta and enter the amniotic sac, he/she should proceed promptly through the placenta. Whatever anaesthetic technique is chosen, two large-bore intravenous lines should be established before any surgical procedure.

PLACENTA ACCRETA, INCRETA AND PERCRETA

A defective formation of the decidua, with direct contact between chorionic villi and myometrium in such a way that placental separation cannot occur, characterizes placenta accreta. Placenta acquires the suffix accreta, increta or percreta according to the depth of uterine invasion by the placenta (Figure 5.4). Removal of the placenta may be difficult or impossible and massive blood loss (more than 1000 ml) can accompany attempts at placental separation. The incidence of placenta accreta is approximately 1:2500 pregnancies [16]. The diagnosis is made when several attempts to remove the placenta fail. Total abdominal hysterectomy may be life-saving in controlling massive haemorrhage. Women presenting with a known placenta praevia and a uterine scar from a prior caesarean section must be suspected of placenta accreta and the increased risk of caesarean hysterectomy [17].

Massive bleeding associated with an unsuspected placenta accreta during vaginal or abdominal delivery may be life-threatening, irrespective of the anaesthetic technique.

Prompt resusitation, which involves obstetricians and anaesthetists, is of paramount importance if a successful outcome is to be achieved.

RUPTURED GRAVID UTERUS

The incidence of ruptured gravid uterus is estimated to be between 1:1500 to 1:3000 births [18]. The particular risk occurs with vaginal delivery when the uterus is scarred by a previous caesarean section. There has been considerable debate regarding the risks and benefits of vaginal delivery after a caesarean section. At the present time there is a consensus that maternal and foetal benefits outweigh the risk of a routine repeat caesarean section, and trial of labour is associated with an 80% rate of success [19]. The incidence of emergency caesarean section in women during trial of labour is comparable to that in the general labouring population [20, 21]. Uterine rupture following caesarean section greatly depends upon the kind of uterine incision performed. Rupture of the uterine body through the scar of a classical vertical incision has a different clinical presentation from lower segment rupture [23, 24] (Table 5.3).

Although uterine rupture is associated with a scarred uterus, it is frequently not the case. As many as 70% of ruptures occur in unscarred uteri. A few of them may be related to external trauma, but a large part of uterine ruptures cannot be related to classical factors. Two risk factors identified are grand parity (risk is 20 times higher in women parity seven or higher), and excessive or inappropriate

Table 5.4 Complete versus partial uterine rupture

Complete rupture	Partial rupture (dehiscence)
Full thickness ruptured	Partial thickness rupture
Uterine content extrusion	No uterine content extrusion
Abdominal pain	Less abdominal pain
Peritoneum ruptured	Peritoneum intact
Hypovolaemic shock	Lower blood loss
Higher maternal and foetal mortality	Lower maternal and foetal mortality
More often in the myometrium	More often in the lower segment

oxytocin use. Uterine rupture encompasses a spectrum of problems, from the physiologic rupture of some fibres during labour, through incomplete rupture (dehiscence) to complete rupture with extrusion of the uterine content (Table 5.4).

In some circumstances, uterine rupture occurs without any symptoms. Manifestations are protean and a high index of suspicion is necessary. Major clinical signs are abdominal pain (up to 75% of patients), foetal distress (50 to 70%) and vaginal bleeding (17 to 67%). Later

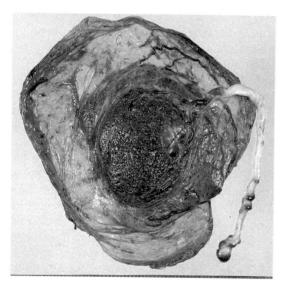

Figure 5.5 Velamentous cord insertion. The vessels travel from the placenta to the foetus in an umbilical cord without Wharton's jelly. The risk of trauma is evident. Courtesy of Professor R. Laurini, Department of Pedopathology, Institute of Pathology, University Hospital, Lausanne, Switzerland.

signs include recession of the presenting part (25 to 50%) and shock (50%) [18]. Maternal and foetal prognosis largely depends upon the rapidity of the surgical intervention. There is no place for expectant or medical management.

ANAESTHETIC CONSIDERATIONS

It is well recognized that epidural analgesia during labour does not mask the clinical signs and symptoms of uterine rupture. Abdominal pain, hypertension, tachycardia or foetal demise, related to a peritoneal tear or soiling by blood or amniotic fluid, point to uterine rupture [24–26]. Obstetricians who monitor scar tenderness as an indication of impending uterine rupture may be dismayed by epidural analgesia [27]. This has not been subjected to scientific evaluation. Moreover, epidural analgesia does not increase the risk of repeat caesarean section during trial of labour [25].

Appropriate foetal and maternal monitoring must be instituted and the weakest but effective epidural mixture must be used. In such conditions, bupivacaine 0.0625 or 0.125% in combination with fentanyl 2.5 to 5.0 µg/ml, injected to obtain a symmetrical sensitive block at or below Th10, can be safely administrated.

Anaesthetic management in uterine rupture includes rapid haemodynamic resuscitation and prompt caesarean section. Uterine bleeding may be massive and an unequivocal obstetric strategy must be followed. Surgery must not be delayed because it is the only way to control the arterial bleeding and to remove uterine contents.

VARIOUS ANTEPARTUM EMERGENCIES

VASA PRAEVIA AND VELAMENTOUS CORD INSERTION

Umbilical vessels usually travel from the placenta to the foetus through Wharton's jelly, which has a protective cushioning effect. Velamentous insertion of the vessels describes an abnormality of the vessels travelling through the thin amniotic sac. Without Wharton's jelly, these vessels are fragile and prone to compression and trauma (Figure 5.5). Vasa praevia are vessels inserted on the placenta in front of the presenting part of the foetus.

Vasa praevia complicates 1% of pregnancies and velamentous insertion of the umbilical cord 0.5 to 1% of pregnancies [28]. The usual clinical presentation is the palpation of a pulsate mass during labour before membrane rupture, or brisk bleeding and foetal distress after rupture of the membranes. Foetal mortality is very high due to rapid exsanguination, reaching 75 to 100%. Foetal survival requires a high index of suspicion and immediate caesarean delivery.

FOETAL HAEMORRHAGE

Foetal haemorrhage is a rare condition (1:800 births), which, in exceptional circumstances, can cause disturbance to the mother. At term, the foetus and the placenta have a blood volume of approximately 300 ml. A loss of 30 to 50 ml produces foetal distress and more than 100 ml may be life-threatening for the foetus. Causes of foetal haemorrhage are related to obstetrical trauma (scalp blood sampling, forceps, umbilical cord trauma), abnormal umbilical cord (vasa praevia, velamentous insertion of the cord) or to medical conditions such as foetal haemophilia or thrombocytopenia. Umbilical cord trauma, in particular

during instrumental deliveries, can lead to rapid foetal exsanguination.

Frequently, a foetal haemorrhage is accompanied by bleeding into the amniotic fluid, the retroamniotic space or the maternal circulation. The success of neonatal resuscitation depends on the delay between the diagnosis of foetal haemorrhage and the delivery.

FOETAL BLOOD SAMPLING

Foetal blood sampling is a procedure which is increasingly being performed for diagnostic and therapeutic purposes in high-risk pregnancies. Quoted incidences of foetal loss during cordocentesis range from less than 1 to 2.5% [29–32]. Foetal loss is related to trauma or haematoma of the umbilical cord by impeding blood flow between the placenta and the foetus, and also by exsanguination into the amniotic fluid. Five cases of lethal foetal exsanguination have been reported in association with alloimmune thrombocytopenia [33]. For successful outcome, potential complications must be carefully eliminated, and if necessary, the foetus must be delivered by emergency caesarean section.

EXTERNAL CEPHALIC VERSION

External cephalic version is an efficient therapeutic option for breech presentation in late pregnancy. The overall success rate is approximately 65%, and the procedure can also be safely performed in women with a previous low transverse caesarean section scar [34, 35]. There is a traditional fear of uterine rupture during this procedure, though the risk cannot be quantified. Currently recommendations are that version should be performed in women who have fasted six hours, under tocolysis, with foetal monitoring and anti-D immune globulin for rhesus negative patients. As many as 40% are associated with foetal heart rate changes; foetal asystole and unexplained foetal deaths are reported [36, 37]. Foetal heart rate monitoring and immediate surgical facilities might prevent these problems, though foetal heart rate variations are usually harmless and resolve spontaneously. Foetomaternal bleeding, amniotic fluid embolism, placental abruption or premature rupture of membranes have been reported, and foetal distress requiring emergency caesarean delivery should be anticipated. [38].

CORD PROLAPSE

Cord prolapse is a rare complication occurring once in every 300 deliveries and it may have disastrous neonatal effects. Pregnancies at risk include small infants (lighter than 2500 g), premature labour and breech presentation [39]. Umbilical cord prolapse associated with cord compression requires immediate delivery (= 25%). If cord compression can be alleviated (= 75%), delivery by emergency caesarean section is still required, but without the dire urgency of the former. The prolapse is intravaginal in 75%, extravaginal in 5% and occult in 20% of the cases [40]. If the foetus is still alive, one management protocol recommends intravenous tocolysis, a rapid infusion of 500 to 750 ml of normal saline into the bladder to lift the presenting part and alleviate cord compression. Simultaneously, the mother must be prepared for emergency caesarean section.

RETENTION OF A DEAD FOETUS

Foetal death during the third trimester is relatively rare, occurring in 0.8% of pregnancies. The main cause is placental abruption, but foetal or cord abnormalities account for some foetal deaths. Usually, spontaneous labour begins within 10 to 15 days after the foetal death. If the dead foetus remains in the uterine cavity for more than four to six weeks, coagulation disorders can be expected in approximately 25%. Thromboplastin released from necrotic foetal tissues may activate the maternal coagulation cascade. A decrease of fibrinogen concentration lower than non-pregnant values, an increase of fibrin degradation prod-

ucts and a progressive decrease in platelet count are common. Thrombocytopenia is a late sign and seldom severe. In the case of multiple pregnancies with one foetus still alive, consumptive coagulopathy may affect the living twin worse than the mother. Treatment includes low doses of intravenous heparin and replacement of clotting factors with fresh frozen plasma if defibrinogenation is severe [41, 42]. Necrotic tissues within the uterus are very prone to infection and conditions such as premature rupture of membranes will lead to chorioamnionitis within a few hours. Any evidence of sepsis or chorioamnionitis requires urgent evacuation of uterine contents.

To avoid caesarean section during the second trimester, before the development of the lower segment, per vaginam evacuation is recommended. Induction of labour is performed by intracervical and retroamniotic prostaglandins. In the absence of infection and coagulopathy, an epidural can be left in place for maternal comfort and uterine cavity revision if necessary. Bupivacaine 0.0625 or 0.125% with fentanyl 2.5 μg/ml, at a perfusion rate of 10 ml/h or controlled by the patient, is the preferred solution. At follow-up, infection and coagulopathy should be excluded. Like the intravenous formulations, intracervical and retroamniotic prostaglandin administration may have systemic effects, which include fever, rash, dizziness, hyperemesis, fatigue, nausea, vomiting and diarrhoea. Usually these symptoms respond to supportive care and antiemetics. Oxytocin may be sufficient to induce labour for a dead foetus near term, but before 34 weeks' gestation its efficiency is low. Intra-amniotic hypertonic saline is not recommended, given that amniotic fluid volume is reduced because of its potential for systemic toxicity.

REFERENCES

1. Kaunitz, A., Hughes, J., Grimes, D. *et al.* (1985) Causes of maternal mortality in the United States. *Obstet. Gynec.* **65**, 605–12.

2. Rochat, R., Koonin, L., Atrash, H. and Jewell, J. (1988) Maternal mortality in the United States: report from the maternal Maternity Collaborative. *Obstet. Gynec.*, **72**, 91–7.

3. *Report on the Confidential Enquiries into Maternal Deaths in the United Kingdom 1988–1990*, HMSO London, 1994; p. 34–42.

4. Beihl, D. (1987) Antepartum and postpartum haemorrhage, in *Anaesthesia for Obstetrics*, 2nd edn (eds S. Shnider and J. Levinson), Williams & Wilkins, Baltimore, pp. 281–9.

5. King, J. (1993) Antepartum bleeding in advanced pregnancy, in *Clinical Manual of Obstetrics*, 2nd edn (eds D. Shaver, S. Phelan, C. Beckman and F. Ling) McGraw-Hill, New York, pp. 329–39.

6. Abdella, T., Sibai, B., Hays, J. J. and Anderson, G. (1984) relationship of hypertensive disease to abruptio placentae. *Obstet. Gynec.*, **63**, 365–70.

7. Iyasu, S., Saftlas, A. K., Rowley, D. L. *et al.* (1993) The epidemiology of placenta previa in the United States, 1979 through 1987. *Am. J. Obstet. Gynecol.*, **168**, 1424–9.

8. Sibai, B., Caritis, S., Thorn, E. *et al.* (1993) Prevention of preeclampsia with low-dose aspirin in healthy, nulliparous pregnant women. *N. Engl. J. Med.*, **329**, 1213–8.

9. Hurd, W., Miodovnik, M., Hertzberg, V. and Lavin, J. (1983) Selective management of abruptio placentae: a prospective study. *Obstet. Gynec.*, **61**, 467–73.

10. Stanco, L., Schrimmer, D., Paul, R. and Mishell, D. (1993) Emergency peropartum hysterectomy and associated risk factors. *Am. J. Obstet. Gynecol.*, **168**, 879–83.

11. Gatt, S. (1986) Anaesthetic management of the obstetric patient with antepartum or intrapartum haemorrhage. *Clin. Anaesthesiol.*, **4**, 373–88.

12. Clark, S., Koonings, P. and Phelan, J. (1985) Placenta previa/accreta and prior cesarean section. *Obstet. Gynec.*, **66**, 89–92.

13. Chantigian, R. (1987) Antepartum haemorrhage, in *Common Problems in Obstetric Anaesthesia*, 2nd edn (eds. S. Datta and G. Ostheimer), Year Book Medical Publishers, Chicago, pp. 236–48.

14. Mouer, J. R. (1994) Placenta previa: antepartum conservative management, inpatient versus outpatient. *Am. J. Obstet. Gynecol.*, **170**, 1683–5.

15. Chestnut, D., Dewan, D., Redick, L. *et al.* (1989) Anaesthetic management for obstetric hysterectomy: a multi-institutional study. *Anesthesiology*, **70**, 607–10.

16. Read, J., Cotton, D. and Miller, F. (1980) Placenta accreta: changing clinical aspects and outcome. *Obstet. Gynec.*, **56**, 31–4.

17. Sibai, M. H., Rahman, J., Rahman, M. S. and Butalack, F. (1987) Emergency hysterectomy in obstetrics – a review of 117 cases. *Aust. NZ. J. Obstet. Gynaecol.*, **27**, 180–4.

18. Elkady, A. A., Bayomy, H. M., Bekhiet, M. T. *et al.* (1993) A review of 126 cases of ruptured gravid uterus. *Int. Surg.*, **78**, 231–5.

19. Bedoya, C., Bartha, J. L., Rodriguez, I. *et al.* (1992) A trial of labour after cesarean section in patients with or without a prior vaginal delivery. *Int. J. Gynaecol. Obstet.*, **39**, 285–9.

20. Flamm, B. L., Goings, J. R., Liu, Y. and Wolde, T. G. (1994) Elective repeat cesarean delivery versus trial of labour: a prospective multicenter study. *Obstet. Gynec.*, **83**, 927–32.

21. Cowan, R. K., Kinch, R. A., Ellis, B. and Anderson, R. (1994) Trial of labour following cesarean section delivery. *Obstet Gynec.*, **83**, 933–6.

22. Nordin, A. J. and Richardson, J. A. (1993) Lower segment uterine scar rupture during induction of labour with vaginal prostaglandin E2 (letter). *Postgrad. Med. J.*, **69**, 592.

23. Razinger, M., Fuentes, A. and Smyk, L. V. (1994) Spontaneous rupture of a low transverse cesarean scar. *South. Med. J.*, **87**, 1001–2.

24. Guedj, P. and Eldor, J. (1992) Prerupture of unscarred uterus masked by an epidural analgesia (letter). *Int. J. Gynaecol. Obstet.*, **38**, 50–1.

25. Rowbottom, S. J. and Tabrizian, I. (1994) Epidural analgesia and uterine rupture during labour. *Anaesth. Intensive Care*, **22**, 79–80.

26. Abraham, R. and Sadovsky, E. (1992) Delay in the diagnosis of rupture of the uterus due to epidural anaesthesia in labour. *Gynaecol. Obstet. Invest.*, **33**, 239–40.

27. Burmucic, R. and Hofmann, P. (1992) Is palpation of the healed section scar after previous Cesarean section with subsequent vaginal delivery necessary? *Gynakol. Geburtshilfliche Rundsch.*, **32**, 76–7.

28. Dougall, A. and Baird, C. H. (1987) Vasa praevia–report of three cases and review of literature. *Br. J. Obstet. Gynaecol.*, **94**, 712–5.

29. Sanzeni, W., Vial, Y., Hohlfeld, P. *et al.* (1994) Cordocentèse: Analyse des indications et des complications sur une série de 478 cas (Abstract). *Arch. Gynaecol. Obstet.*, **255**, 417.

30. Hohlfeld, P., Forestier, F., Kaplan, C. *et al.* (1994) Fetal thrombocytopenia: A retrospective survey of 5194 fetal blood sampling. *Blood*, **84**, 1851–6.

31. Ghidini, A., Sepulveda, W., Lockwood, C. and Romero, R. (1993) Complications of fetal blood sampling. *Am. J. Obstet. Gynecol.*, **168**, 1339–44.

32. Wilson, R., Farquharson, D., Wittman, B. and Shaw, D. (1994) Cordocentesis: overall pregnancy loss rate as important as procedure loss rate. *Fetal. Diag. & Therapy*, **9**, 142–8.

33. Paidas, M., Berkowitz, R., Lynch, L. *et al.* (1995) Alloimmune thrombocytopenia: fetal and neonatal losses related to cordocentesis. *Am. J. Obstet. Gynecol.*, **172**, 475–9.

34. Zhang, J., Bowes, W. and Fortney, J. (1993) Efficacy of external cephalic version: A review. *Obste. Gynec.*, **82**, 306–12.

35. Flamm, B., Fried, M., Lonky, N. and Giles, W. (1991) External cephalic version after previous cesarean section. *Am. J. Obstet. Gynecol.*, **165**, 370–2.

36. Phelan, J., Stine, L., Müller, E. *et al.* (1984) Observation of fetal heart rate characteristics related to external cephalic version and tocolysis. *Am. J. Obstet. Gynecol.*, **149**, 658–61.

37. Kurup, A., Arulkumaran, S., Montan, S. and Ratnam, S. (1993) Need for fetal assessment prior to and during external cephalic version. Occurrence of transient cardiac asystole. *Acta Obstet. Gynaecol. Scand.*, **72**, 60–2.

38. Stine, L., Phelan, J., Wallace, R. *et al.* (1985) Update on external cephalic version performed at term. *Obstet. Gynec.*, **65**, 642–6.

39. Critchlow, C., Leet, T., Benedetti, T. and Daling, J. (1994) Risk factors and infants outcomes associated with umbilical cord prolapse: a population based case-control study among birth in Washington state. *Am. J. Obstet. Gynecol.*, **170**, 613–6.

40. Katz, Z., Shoham, Z., Lancet, M. *et al.* (1988) Management of labour with umbilical cord prolapse: 1 5-year study. *Obstet. and Gynec.*, **72**, 278–81.

41. Wheeler, A. and Rubenstein, E. (1994) Current management of disseminated intravascular coagulation. *Oncology*, **8**, 69–73.

42. Hasbu, J., Munoz, H., von Muhlenbrock, R. *et al.* (1992) The successful prolongation of a twin preterm pregnancy complicated by a dead fetus and disseminated intravascular coagulation. *Revista Chilena de Obstetrica y Gynecologica*, **57**, 293–6.

HAEMATOLOGICAL DISORDERS IN PREGNANCY

6

L. Hawthorne

'Birth is bloody, sometimes fatally so'
M.H. Plumer

INTRODUCTION

In the most recent confidential enquiry into maternal deaths [1] maternal haemorrhage was cited as a major cause of maternal mortality. Obstetric haemorrhage may be catastrophic, is often unpredictable and can occur in patients with normal haematological systems. Patients with haematological disorders, congenital or acquired, may be more susceptible to haemorrhage, or as a consequence of their coagulopathy, influence our anaesthetic technique. This chapter deals with the physiological and pathological changes in the haematological system that may be encountered during pregnancy and discusses the anaesthetic management of these patients while highlighting the potential obstetric problems.

PHYSIOLOGICAL CHANGES IN COAGULATION AND FIBRINOLYSIS IN NORMAL PREGNANCY

Plasma volume increases steadily from the sixth week of gestation and tends to plateau around the 24th week at some 50% over non-pregnant values. Although there is an increase of 20% in absolute red cell volume (RCV), the mean RCV per kg body weight remains constant [2]. This results in the 'physiological' anaemia of pregnancy with a haemoglobin concentration of 11 g/dl considered to be the lower limit of normal for pregnancy [3].

Despite the large increase in plasma volume, a 'hypercoagulable state' develops during pregnancy [4]. Procoagulants tend to increase while anticoagulants tend to decrease. These changes are a physiological adaptation to protect the parturient from life-threatening bleeding during delivery. Many of these changes are also found in women taking oral contraceptives [5] and so are, at least in part, hormonally induced.

Hypercoagulation may be due to:

- increased platelet aggregation;
- increased concentration of coagulation factors;
- decreased levels of coagulation inhibitors;
- decreased fibrinolytic capacity.

The changes in coagulation, anticoagulant and fibrinolytic proteins are summarized in Table 6.1.

Clinical Problems in Obstetric Anaesthesia
Edited by Ian F. Russell and Gordon Lyons. Published in 1997 by Chapman & Hall, London. ISBN 0 412 71600 3.

Table 6.1 The changes in coagulation, anticoagulant and fibrinolytic proteins in pregnancy

Protein	Change in pregnancy
Procoagulant	
Fibrinogen	↑↑
II	↑
VII	↑
VIII	↑
X	↑
XI	↑
V	No change
IX	No change
Prekallikrein	No change
HMWK	No change
XI	↓
XII	↓
Anticoagulant	
ATIII	No change
Protein C	No change
Protein S	↓
Fibrinolytic	
tPA	↓
PAI-1	↑
PAI-2	↑
FDPs*	↑

*Products of fibrinolysis, but also have anticoagulant properties.

LABORATORY AND BEDSIDE TESTS

PROTHROMBIN TIME (PT)

This test was first described 60 years ago by Quick [6]. It measures the plasma coagulation time in the presence of added tissue factor and calcium. The PT provides an assessment of the **extrinsic** and **common** pathways, and is affected by changes in factors II, V, VII and fibrinogen. As such, alterations in three of the four factors affected by warfarin (II, VII, IX, X), will be detected by the PT [7].

The PT will be prolonged if factors V, VII or X are reduced by 50% or more, factor II by 70%, or if the fibrinogen concentration is less than 1 g/l [8]. The commonest causes of a prolonged PT are:

- oral anticoagulants;
- liver disease, especially obstruction;
- vitamin K deficiency;
- disseminated intravascular coagulation (DIC);
- deficiency of factors II, V, VII, X or fibrinogen.

ACTIVATED PARTIAL THROMBOPLASTIN TIME (APTT)

This test, also known as the kaolin clotting time (KCCT), is sensitive to changes in the **intrinsic** and **common** pathways. It is used to measure heparin therapy.

Deficiencies of any factor except VII may cause a prolonged result [9], but it is most sensitive to reductions in factors VIII and IX. The APTT becomes prolonged once these factors are 25–30% below normal [8]. Isolated prolongation of the APTT may be due to circulating inhibitors [7]. Correction of the APTT by mixing the test plasma in a 50:50 volume with normal plasma implies factor deficiency rather than the presence of inhibitors [9]. The main causes of a prolonged APTT are:

- DIC;
- liver disease;
- massive transfusion with stored blood;
- heparin;
- circulating anticoagulant;
- deficiency of any factor other than VII.

THROMBIN TIME (TT)

This test, which determines the time plasma takes to clot after the addition of a standard solution of buffered thrombin, is abnormal if longer than 18 s [10]. The concentration of thrombin solution is adjusted to clot normal plasma in 15 s. Prolongation of the thrombin time may result from:

- heparin;
- circulating anticoagulants;
- fibrinogen deficiency;
- fibrin degradation products;
- dysfibrinogenaemia.

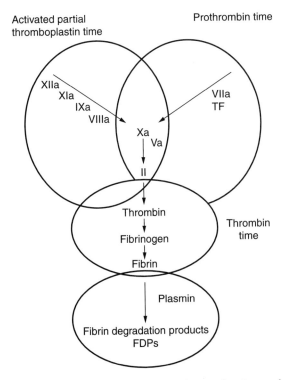

Figure 6. 1 Diagram indicating the mechanisms of blood coagulation examined by common laboratory tests (TF, tissue factor). Adapted from reference [10]; published by Blackwell Scientific, 1989.

FIBRIN DEGRADATION PRODUCTS (FDPs)

Plasmin degrades both fibrinogen and fibrin to form fragments X, Y, D and E. These are commonly measured by their ability to agglutinate latex beads coated with antibody. A more accurate test for the proteolytic products of plasmin cleavage is the D-dimer test [8]. FDPs, as determined by standard tests, are elevated in:

- liver disease;
- impaired renal function;
- pregnancy.

The mechanism of blood coagulation examined by common tests is summarized in Figure 6.1.

BLEEDING TIME (BT)

The bleeding time (BT) has been suggested as an *in vivo* test of platelet function [11] but, despite modifications, the validity of the test has not been improved [12]: there is high interobserver variation and there is no evidence that the BT correctly predicts the risk of epidural haematoma.

THROMBOELASTOGRAPHY

The use of thromboelastography was first described by Hartert in 1948 [13]. Until recently it was mainly used as a research tool, but it is now gaining popularity in clinical practice in cardiac surgery, liver transplantation and the obstetric unit. Not only does the thromboelastogram (TEG) allow global assessment of haemostatic function but information regarding all aspects of clotting is available within 20 to 30 minutes. Subsequent clot stability and fibrinolysis can be evaluated over the next 60 minutes [8].

While routine laboratory tests are measured in plasma, the TEG uses whole blood and thus assesses the interaction between platelets, the coagulation cascade and fibrinogen. In addition the TEG provides information about clot stability and fibrinolysis [13]. Figure 6.2 shows a schematic drawing of a TEG trace: it is

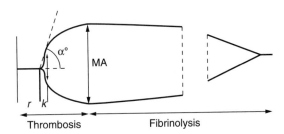

Figure 6.2 Schematic representation of the thromboelastogram. TEG parameters measured from the trace include *r* time (reaction time or time to initial fibrin formation); *k* time (clot formation time); alpha angle which denotes the speed at which the clot forms; MA (maximum amplitude) which is a measure of maximum clot strength.

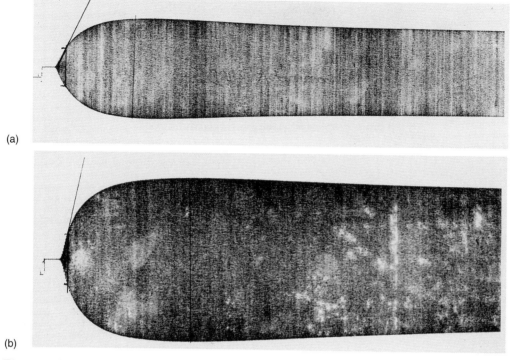

Figure 6.3 (a) TEG of non-pregnant woman, MA = 64°; (b) TEG of pregnant woman showing hypercoagulable trace, MA = 77°.

the maximum amplitude which is the most appropriate TEG measurement for the assessment of platelet function. In pregnancy a more hypercoagulable trace is seen (Figure 6.3). The TEG has also been shown to be of greater value than the routine tests for predicting the safe practice of regional anaesthesia [14].

As will be noted later in this chapter many studies use the bleeding time as an indication of platelet function. While it may be true that bleeding time, assessed by an experienced technician, is useful, acquiring such expertise in an acute clinical situation is rarely possible. For this reason the TEG is regaining popularity among clinicians and is viewed by some as providing a rapid and simple way of assessing coagulation in the clinical setting. Indeed, in difficult cases within our unit, the TEG is the preferred method of assessing coagulation prior to regional anaesthesia.

ANAEMIAS

THALASSAEMIA

The thalassaemia syndromes are due to inherited defects in the synthesis of one or more of the polypeptide chains making up the haemoglobin tetramer. The syndromes are classified according to the decreased production in affected α- or β-chains. The disease is prevalent in people from Mediterranean, Asian and African countries and in areas where malaria is endemic [15].

α-Thalassaemia

This is more prevalent in South East Asia and comprises four subtypes:

- $\alpha°$-thalassaemia (Barts hydrops);
- haemoglobin H disease;

- α-thalassaemia trait;
- silent carrier.

In Barts hydrops there are no functioning genes and death *in utero* usually occurs. Mothers carrying infants with α°-thalassaemia haemoglobinopathy have an increased incidence of anaemia, pregnancy-induced hypertension (PIH), antepartum and postpartum haemorrhage, and retained placenta. In haemoglobin H disease haemolytic anaemia, splenomegaly and fatigue may occur, but hospitalization is rarely required and patients have a normal life span [16]. Silent carriers and those with α-thalassaemia trait are asymptomatic and are not at increased risk of complications during pregnancy or surgery.

β-Thalassaemia

There are three subtypes according to the severity of the disease:

- thalassaemia major – homozygous (Cooley's anaemia);
- thalassaemia intermedia – two mutations, one severe and one mild;
- thalassaemia minor – heterozygous.

Thalassaemia major

Patients afflicted by homozygous β-thalassaemia suffer from severe anaemia and hypersplenism and are dependent on blood transfusions. The consequent hypoxia and massive tissue iron deposition lead to cardiac, hepatic and endocrine failure [17] but, due to improved paediatric and haematological management, patients with thalassaemia major are now surviving into the third and fourth decades. Despite the increased incidence of spontaneous abortion and intrauterine death, Jensen [18] has reported 16 successful conceptions, which resulted in 13 live births, in 11 women with β-thalassaemia major.

Pregnancy results in increased metabolic demands, higher transfusion requirements and worsening heart failure. During this time it is essential to maintain the haemoglobin concentration above 10 g/dl. Diabetes mellitus and cardiomyopathy are not uncommon in these patients [18], the latter often preventing the achievement of a full-term pregnancy.

While obstetric management is directed towards a trial of labour, the characteristically small maternal stature often results in cephalopelvic disproportion [18] and caesarean section is common in this group. Splenomegaly may result in thrombocytopenia, so platelet counts should be checked before regional anaesthesia. Most patients undergo splenectomy at a young age, and have platelet counts in excess of $500 \times 10^9/l$. This, coupled with the hypercoagulable state normally found in pregnancy, predisposes women to venous thrombosis, hence deep venous thrombosis prophylaxis must be ensured. Because these patients are susceptible to significant cardiac compromise epidural anaesthesia may be preferable to spinal for caesarean section. While epidural block may be technically difficult due to skeletal abnormalities one should not forget that difficult intubation secondary to hypertrophy of the maxilla has been reported [19].

Thalassaemia intermedia and minor

Thalassaemia intermedia has variable clinical manifestations but usually only requires the administration of folic acid supplements. Thalassaemia minor has a benign clinical course and does not affect anaesthetic management.

SICKLE CELL DISEASE

Sickle cell disease results from polymerization of haemoglobin S. The geographical distribution of sickle cell disease mirrors that of plasmodium falciparum malaria and it is common in Africa, Asia, the Arabian peninsula, Southern Europe and the Americas but the disease tends to be milder in Asians compared to Africans. The clinical features are related to haemolytic anaemia and vascular occlusion [15]. Diagnosis is confirmed by anaemia (haemoglobin 6–8 g/dl), high reticulocyte count, sickle cells in the peripheral blood film and haemoglobin electrophoresis.

Crises may be precipitated by infection, dehydration, hypoxia and acidosis and may manifest in three forms [16]:

- infarctive, secondary to vasoocclusion;
- aplastic, secondary to reduced erythropoiesis due to infection;
- sequestration, due to pooling of erythrocytes in the spleen.

In pregnancy the complications of sickle cell disease are exacerbated, vasoocclusion being the most common. Maternal mortality may be as high as 1% [20]; this is usually secondary to pulmonary embolism or infection. Placental infarction may result in spontaneous abortion or intra-uterine growth retardation with 20% foetal and 5% neonatal death rates. The incidences of preterm labour, abruption, placenta praevia and preeclampsia are also increased [21].

Using blood transfusions, management goals are aimed at maintaining a haemoglobin concentration of greater than 8 g/dl with haemoglobin A comprising more than 40% of the total haemoglobin. Prophylactic partial exchange transfusion has been advocated by some [22] but, until the results of trials with contemporary controls are reported, it would seem wise to continue individualized therapy [23].

Anaesthetic management is directed towards the provision of good analgesia in labour, usually by epidural. Operative delivery is accomplished under general or regional anaesthesia but attention should be paid to the following:

- warming of fluids, gases and the general environment;
- provision of supplemental oxygen and the avoidance of hypoventilation;
- maintenance of adequate red blood cell numbers to maintain oxygen delivery;

- prevention of venous stasis.

Adequate preloading with a gradual onset of blockade is advisable. It is essential to avoid the risks of sudden marked hypotension and the consequent use of vasopressors. As such, an incremental regional anaesthesia technique may be preferable to a 'one-shot' spinal technique.

Sickle cell trait is usually asymptomatic but factors which precipitate a crisis should be avoided.

HAEMOLYTIC AND APLASTIC ANAEMIA

These conditions, which may coexist in pregnant women, are relatively rare. Their management and clinical course is beyond the scope of this chapter but, needless to say, treatment should be individualized and a haematological opinion sought.

PERNICIOUS ANAEMIA

Although pernicious anaemia usually occurs in older age groups, it can present in pregnancy and may be a coincidental finding on routine blood testing. B_{12} and folate deficiency may result in congenital malformations, pre or postpartum haemorrhage, placental abruption and prematurity [24]. It is important to exclude any neuropathy before instituting regional blockade.

CONGENITAL COAGULOPATHIES

VON WILLEBRAND'S DISEASE

Von Willebrand's disease is the commonest congenital coagulopathy affecting women and, in most cases, has an autosomal dominant inheritance. It is a disorder involving the von Willebrand portion of the factor VIII complex; factor VIII comprises a procoagulant factor (VIII Act) and von Willebrand factor (vWF). The disease can be classified as type I, with a quantitative defect in vWF, or type II, with a qualitative defect.

Type I

This is usually a mild condition and represents 80% of cases of von Willebrand's disease. It is characterized by reduced levels of both factor VIII Act and vWF activity [25] and the bleeding time may be normal or prolonged. During pregnancy factor VIII complex levels normally rise and most patients with type I von Wille-brand's disease attain normal levels of vWF and diminished bleeding problems. Provided that the bleeding time is normal and factor VIII Act levels are >50 i.u./dl, uncomplicated vaginal delivery is possible [26]. In those with reduced factor VIII complex levels, infusion of 1-deamino-8-*p*-arginine vasopressin (DDAVP) has been used in the puerperium and for oper-ative delivery [27]. If the patient is unrespon-sive to this form of treatment, fresh frozen plasma (FFP) or cryoprecipitate will be required (FFP contains more vWF than cryo-precipitate).

As far as regional anaesthesia is concerned, it is said that there is no contraindication pro-vided factor VIII complex levels are normal and the bleeding time is not prolonged [27]. Since the mild form of von Willebrand's disease is likely to cause more postpartum than intrapartum problems [27], it is prudent to remove the epidural catheter as soon as possible after delivery since factor VIII complex levels decrease to prepregnant levels very quickly once the uterus is empty [27].

Type II

This disease is characterized by a severe bleed-ing disorder, a prolonged bleeding time and low vWF activity. These patients can also develop thrombocytopenia (type IIb). Obstet-ric management should be individualized, but in those with severe disease, elective caesarean section is recommended. These patients with type II disease are unresponsive to DDAVP

Table 6.2 Suggested levels of factor VIII complex required for various stages of the delivery process

Stage in pregnancy	Factor VIII level (% of normal)
During labour	50
Caesarean section	80
Postpartum	25

and clotting does not improve during preg-nancy. An elective caesarean section allows the planned administration of blood products con-taining vWF to control bleeding in the mother. Furthermore, since the severity of the disease in the neonate may be unknown an elective section is recommended to prevent bleeding complications in the neonate [25]. Suggested levels of factor VIII complex for various stages of the delivery process are summarized in Table 6.2.

Regional blockade in this group should be approached with caution. In patients receiving replacement therapy it is safe to administer a conduction block if laboratory and *in vivo* tests are normal. However, if the procedure is bloody or technically difficult then persistent attempts should be abandoned.

HAEMOPHILIA

Haemophilia A (reduced factor VIII Act) and haemophilia B (reduced factor IX, Christmas disease) are X-linked recessive disorders and, as such, usually afflict the male population. The prevalences of haemophilia A and B in the UK population are 90 per 1 000 000 and 20 per 1 000 000, respectively [28]. Although women are normally only carriers of the gene, 'full blown' haemophilia can occur by mutation. Although carriers would be expected to have factor levels reduced by around 50% of normal, in fact a wide range of functional activity has been reported, and one in ten carrier women will have excessive bleeding [26]. The diseases are usually classified according to the circulat-ing concentration of the respective factor: severe (0%), moderate (1–4%) or mild (5–25%)

[29]. The diagnosis of haemophilia A is suggested by the past history, a prolonged APTT, normal PT and low factor VIII Act activity.

Trial of labour and vaginal delivery is recommended for heterozygous carriers, but vacuum extraction should be avoided as it can cause cephalic haematoma in the neonate [29]. Since half the infants of a heterozygous carrier may be affected, in the absence of a prenatal foetal diagnosis, foetal scalp blood sampling or the use of forceps should be carefully considered before they are attempted. Factor VIII Act activity of 30% is generally sufficient for haemostasis. If levels are low, factor supplements or plasma exchange with FFP or cryoprecipitate are needed before or during delivery [30]. If surgery is planned, factor levels should be normalized to 100%. Postpartum, factor VIII levels drop dramatically and haemorrhage can occur. Close monitoring of levels is necessary and DDAVP may be useful [31].

ACQUIRED COAGULOPATHIES

DISSEMINATED INTRAVASCULAR COAGULATION

The paradox of simultaneous thrombosis and haemorrhage, the marked variation in severity, and the wide spectrum of diseases associated with disseminated intravascular coagulation (DIC) have resulted in confusion and misunderstanding. DIC is never a primary event but is always a secondary phenomenon triggered by the release of procoagulant material into the circulation or by damage to the vascular endothelium. Manifestations of DIC range from a chronic, compensated state to acute life-threatening haemorrhage. Diagnosis of fulminant DIC is usually made on clinical grounds, with bleeding from wound and venepuncture sites, and profound hypotension secondary to haemorrhage and vasoactive substances. Laboratory diagnosis is confirmed by:

- decreased platelets;
- increased PT (increases before APTT);
- increased APTT;
- decreased fibrinogen;
- increased FDPs.

As indicated above the bleeding time is unreliable and subjective unless performed by experienced personnel but the thromboelastogram may be useful in this situation and is our preferred method.

In obstetric practice the most common triggering events for DIC are:

- placental abruption;
- dead foetus;
- amniotic fluid embolism;
- sepsis;
- PIH.

Placental abruption

This is the commonest cause of DIC in the parturient. It occurs in 0.5–1.3% of deliveries and of these, 10–30% have some coagulation disturbance [3]. Blood loss is always underestimated as bleeding may be largely retroplacental [28]. The mainstay of treatment is correction of hypovolaemia and expeditious delivery. Once the foetus and placenta are delivered, myometrial contraction will reduce or stop placental bleeding. It is important to ensure that the uterus remains well contracted and oxytocics may be required.

Retained dead foetus

Today, with induction of labour and early delivery of the foetus this is now a rare occurrence. Coagulopathy is usually not apparent until the foetus has been *in utero* for three to four weeks. A coagulation defect may be seen in the case of a dead twin or selective foeticide where the dead foetus may remain *in utero* for several weeks alongside its live sibling [28].

Amniotic fluid embolism

Amniotic fluid embolism is a rare complication of pregnancy resulting in cardiovascular collapse, cyanosis and bleeding from venepuncture sites and the genital tract. It bears a high maternal mortality and can present during or shortly after labour, or at caesarean section, but typically it occurs when a patient has just completed a strenuous labour with an intact amniotic sac. The management of this fulminant type of DIC is discussed below.

Sepsis

Gram-negative septicaemia is often responsible for a subacute form of DIC in which haemorrhage is uncommon. Some other organisms however, particularly meningococci, *Strep. pyogenes* and *Staph. aureus*, may produce a more fulminant haemorrhagic condition [32].

Pregnancy-induced hypertension

PIH is associated with a chronic low-grade DIC but laboratory tests are often normal and excessive bleeding is rarely a problem. Thrombocytopenia is more common however, occurring in up to 20% of patients [4].

MANAGEMENT OF FULMINANT DIC

Maternal mortality is high with death due to the underlying cause (embolism), haemorrhage or end-organ failure (ARDS, renal failure). Treatment should be prompt and aggressive (Table 6.3).

If general anaesthesia is required for caesarean section, reduced doses of induction and volatile agents may be necessary in order to prevent further hypotension. Invasive monitoring, including an arterial line and pulmonary artery catheter, will be required for the critically ill. Fulminant DIC is a contraindication to regional anaesthesia but insertion of an epidural catheter may have preceded the event. This should not be removed until the platelet count is $> 50 \times 10^9/l$ and coagulation tests have normalized.

Table 6.3 Management of fulminant DIC

Prepare for immediate delivery
Large-bore cannulae
Fluids/blood (avoid dextrans)
Left lateral tilt
Inotropes/vasopressors
O_2–IPPV if any airway problems or altered consciousness
FFP as source of fibrinogen (plasma level ↑ 10–20 mg with each unit)
Cryoprecipitate if volume overload
Platelets (aim for count $> 50 \times 10^9/l$)
Cardiopulmonary resuscitation may be required

Alternative treatment

The use of heparin and antifibrinolytic drugs is controversial [33]. Clinical studies have yet to prove the benefits of these treatments in the obstetric setting and the successful use of these agents is, to date, anecdotal.

MASSIVE BLOOD TRANSFUSION

Obstetric haemorrhage is still one of the leading causes of maternal mortality [1] and necessitates the rapid replacement of large volumes of blood. Storage of blood results in considerable loss of functional platelets and the labile coagulation factors V and VIII. Blood replacement with packed cells and plasma expanders compounds the deleterious effects of haemorrhage on haemostasis. Massive blood transfusion is often associated with a multifactorial clotting disorder due to:

- dilutional platelet 'washout';
- procoagulant factor V and VIII dilution;
- acute haemolytic transfusion reactions (less than 0.7% are of this type);
- platelet-specific antibodies;
- depletion of adenosine triphosphate (ATP) stores (required for platelet aggregation) [31].

It can be difficult to differentiate the coagulopathy seen following massive transfusion from that during DIC. In fact the two may coexist, as DIC may be attributed to the under-lying pathology necessitating transfusion.

Management

Like most other clinical problems, 'prevention is better than cure'. The bleeding diathesis caused by massive transfusion may be pre-vented by the administration of FFP (one unit) with every five units of stored transfused blood. Occasionally platelet transfusion (5–6 units) will also be required if platelet levels fall to $20 \times 10^9/l$ and bleeding persists. Treatment, guided by consideration of the patient's clini-cal condition and the results of coagulation tests, is two-fold: stemming the bleeding from anatomical lesions and modifying the under-lying disease [32].

LIVER DISEASE

Liver impairment in late pregnancy is not uncommon. Although cardiac output is 50% more than the prepregnant value, hepatic blood flow remains unchanged. This results in the percentage of cardiac output passing through the liver being decreased by 35%. As well as 'normal' patient exposure to viral hepatitis, alcoholic liver disease and drug hypersensitivities, pregnancy is specifically associated with a number of liver disorders:

- acute fatty liver of pregnancy;
- cholestasis;
- hepatic rupture secondary to preeclampsia;
- HELLP syndrome (haemolysis, elevated liver enzymes, low platelets).

Significant coagulopathy does not occur until severe liver disease is present with bleed-ing being secondary to a combination of factors:

- deficiency of procoagulant factors II, V, VII, IX and X;
- DIC;
- hypofibrinogenaemia;
- thrombocytopenia.

Table 6.4 Platelet disorders in pregnancy

Immune (idiopathic) thrombocytopenic purpura
Gestational (incidental) thrombocytopenia
Preeclampsia/HELLP
Thrombotic thrombocytopenic purpura/
    haemolytic uraemic syndrome
Systemic lupus erythematosus
Drug-induced thrombocytopenia
Hereditary thrombocytopenia (May–Hegglin
    anomaly)

As many of these patients have a severe coagulopathy, regional anaesthetic techniques are probably contraindicated. However, general anaesthesia in any patient with fulmi-nant liver disease is a hazardous undertaking and should involve experienced personnel.

THROMBOCYTOPENIAS

Thrombocytopenia in pregnant individuals may result from physiological or pathological processes. Reduced platelet numbers are secondary to decreased production or acceler-ated destruction of platelets. The latter is responsible for most cases of thrombocytope-nia seen in pregnancy. Important conditions that may be associated with platelet disorders during pregnancy are listed in Table 6.4.

IMMUNE THROMBOCYTOPENIC PURPURA

Immune thrombocytopenic purpura (ITP) is relatively common during pregnancy, occur-ring once or twice in every 1000 deliveries [34]. The disease is characterized by a decreased platelet count, due to their destruction by platelet autoantibodies directed against platelet surface antigens. The course of ITP is not affected by pregnancy but the disease may influence pregnancy outcome significantly. The main risk to the mother is haemorrhage during and after childbirth. The platelet autoantibodies, usually immunoglobulin G (IgG), may enter the foetal circulation and cause immune destruction of foetal platelets

[35]. An affected foetus may be born with dangerously low platelet counts and be susceptible to intracranial haemorrhage.

Diagnosis of ITP is often one of exclusion. A patient with isolated thrombocytopenia, normal or mildly enlarged platelets on the peripheral blood film, and bone marrow with normal or increased numbers of megakaryocytes is presumed to have ITP [36]. Routine laboratory coagulation tests are normal (PT, APTT) and although the platelet count is less than $100 \times 10^9/l$, the bleeding time is usually normal or even shortened. This is due to increased numbers of young platelets, which are haemostatically more competent, in the circulation [4].

Maternal management

The goal of therapy is a haematologically asymptomatic patient and not necessarily a normal platelet count [37]. Factors that aggravate ITP should be avoided; these include aspirin, alcohol, infection, vaccinations.

Corticosteroids form the mainstay of treatment with the aim being to maintain the platelet count above $50 \times 10^9/l$. Splenectomy is rarely indicated in pregnancy and immunosuppressive agents are not suitable because of their potential teratogenicity [35]. Intravenous IgG can result in a rapid reversal of thrombocytopenia in ITP and has been used successfully in pregnancy. Intravenous IgG may also be useful in situations of acute haemorrhage or in preparation for splenectomy [35,37]. Platelet transfusions are not indicated unless there is life-threatening haemorrhage or a very low platelet count in patients undergoing surgery [31]. Unnecessary transfusion of platelets in the absence of haemostatic failure may stimulate more antibodies and worsen maternal thrombocytopenia [35].

Foetal considerations

Thrombocytopenia in infants born to mothers with ITP is relatively common [34, 38] and the risk of neonatal bleeding is inversely proportional to the platelet count [39]. Attempts have been made to identify those infants at greatest risk, but no maternal characteristic has been found to accurately predict the neonatal platelet count [40]. There is said to be a risk of bleeding associated with foetal sampling procedures but recent evidence suggests that neonatal outcome is unaffected by them [41]. Bleeding complications are rare with maternal platelet counts greater than $50 \times 10^9/l$ [39, 40] and therefore this is the arbitrary level considered safe for vaginal delivery. Vaginal delivery has never been proven to be the cause of intracranial haemorrhage [39], and no association between route of delivery and neonatal bleeding complications was found in 474 infants of mothers with ITP [40]. Thus current recommendations are to perform delivery by caesarean section for obstetric indications only without determining the foetal platelet count.

GESTATIONAL THROMBOCYTOPENIA

Incidental thrombocytopenia of pregnancy (GTP) describes a common (up to 5% of pregnant women), mild to moderate, asymptomatic thrombocytopenia (but usually $> 80 \times 10^9/l$) [34, 39]. GTP, which probably represents an acceleration of the physiological pattern of increased platelet destruction during pregnancy, accounts for more than 70% of cases of thrombocytopenia in pregnant women. GTP is not easily distinguishable from ITP but, compared to ITP, there is no antenatal history of thrombocytopenia and foetal thrombocytopenia is not a risk factor [36, 39, 42]. No specific treatment is required.

PREGNANCY-INDUCED HYPERTENSION

PIH is a common disorder occurring in 3–12% of all pregnancies. Approximately 20% of these parturients will demonstrate evidence of a consumptive thrombocytopenia with an additional defect in platelet function [4]. The management of this type of thrombocytopenia is essentially that of preeclampsia. An extreme variant of preeclampsia is the HELLP syndrome. Thrombocytopenia is a prominent feature of this disorder, and may be severe with platelet counts less than $50 \times 10^9/l$. Inadequate haemostasis or excessive bleeding are common and blood/FFP/platelet transfusions are often required [43].

THROMBOTIC THROMBOCYTOPENIC PURPURA AND HAEMOLYTIC URAEMIC SYNDROME

Thrombotic thrombocytopenic purpura (TTP) is a rare condition but its progression is often rapid and fatal [35]. It is characterized by a pentad of findings: thrombocytopenia, haemolytic anaemia, neurological dysfunction, renal failure and fever. The pathological process consists primarily of widespread thrombotic occlusion of arterioles and capillaries, involving multiple organs [36]. Pregnancy may be a predisposing factor. It is often difficult to differentiate TTP from severe PIH or HELLP syndrome [44] but TTP usually presents in the second trimester whereas PET and HELLP present most commonly after 36 weeks' gestation [36].

A major breakthrough in the treatment of TTP is the use of exchange transfusion or plasmapheresis with FFP. Antiplatelet drugs (aspirin, dipyridamole) have also been used and high-dose prednisolone may be effective in mild cases without central nervous system involvement [32]. A combination of plasma exchange and steroids can result in a dramatic improvement [37]. There is no evidence that prompt delivery influences the course of TTP and, as the syndrome usually occurs in the second trimester, this may not be a therapeutic option [35, 36]. Emergency delivery by caesarean section should be considered if renal failure, hypertension or refractory anaemia intervene [37].

Haemolytic uraemic syndrome (HUS) is a similar condition to TTP, usually occurring in the postpartum period with primary patho-

Table 6.5 Common drugs affecting platelet number or function

Thrombocytopenia:
- heparin
- quinine
- penicillins
- thiazides
- hydralazine
- H$_2$-receptor antagonists
- digoxin
- cocaine

Impaired platelet function:
- non-steroidal anti-inflammatory drugs
- dextran
- alcohol (in high concentration)

logical changes largely confined to the kidneys [35].

SYSTEMIC LUPUS ERYTHEMATOSUS

Thrombocytopenia can occur in up to one third of patients with systemic lupus erythematosus (SLE). It is particularly common in SLE patients with antiphospholipid antibody. Interestingly, intravascular thrombosis is a greater problem than haemorrhage [35]. This will be discussed in a later section of this chapter.

DRUG-INDUCED THROMBOCYTOPENIA

Thrombocytopenia may occur secondary to many drugs (Table 6.5) and this cause needs to be excluded in all cases. Drugs may produce thrombocytopenia by direct depression of platelet production (thiazides), or more commonly, by increased platelet destruction due to immune mechanisms or direct toxic effects [35]. In most instances bleeding manifestations develop within 24 hours of drug exposure and disappear over a period of three to four days following drug withdrawal. Occasionally the problem is severe and steroids, IgG or platelet transfusion is necessary [31].

Some drug-induced syndromes are relatively unique to pregnancy. Cocaine ingestion has been associated with acute onset thrombocytopenia occurring within hours of drug exposure. Platelet counts can decrease dramatically over the ensuing week, without further re-exposure to the drug. Screening for thrombocytopenia may be advisable if there is a risk of cocaine use [45]. Thiazide diuretics or hydralazine administered to the mother may cause a neonatal thrombocytopenia.

HEREDITARY THROMBOCYTOPENIA

The May–Hegglin anomaly is a rare autosomal dominant platelet disorder. Patients are usually asymptomatic but serious bleeding can occur and platelet infusions may be required at delivery [35].

ANAESTHETIC MANAGEMENT OF PATIENTS WITH THROMBOCYTOPENIA

The main dilemma facing the obstetric anaesthetist is whether regional anaesthesia is safe in the thrombocytopenic patient. The decision to perform a conduction block depends on the degree of thrombocytopenia and its aetiology. Determining the cause involves a thorough history (bleeding problems, drugs), examination (petechiae, ecchymoses, oedema, abdominal or neurological signs) and a review of appropriate laboratory tests (blood film, electrolytes, liver function).

In our unit we consider the following points in deciding whether regional anaesthesia is appropriate.

- If the platelet count is below $50 \times 10^9/l$ regional anaesthesia is contraindicated.
- If the platelet count is above $100 \times 10^9/l$ regional anaesthesia may be safely performed.
- Platelet counts between 50 and $100 \times 10^9/l$ create the most concern and are considered on an individual basis.

As regards the safe lower limit of platelet count deemed necessary for regional blockade, opinions are changing. Provided platelet function is normal, as it is in gestational thrombocytopenia and ITP, then a platelet count of $50 \times 10^9/l$ is considered safe [4, 36]. However, if platelet function is impaired (e.g. PIH) then tests of platelet function will be required. We have found the thromboelastogram to be an invaluable tool in this situation and, in fact, have demonstrated normal TEGs in patients with platelet counts less than $50 \times 10^9/l$ although we do not yet advocate regional blockade in this group. An important exception to the above guidelines is the patient with a rapidly falling platelet count (e.g. HELLP syndrome). In this situation, despite the platelet count being above $50 \times 10^9/l$, their number can decrease rapidly with development of a bleeding diathesis before regional anaesthesia can be instituted

In such high-risk cases intrathecal analgesia using local anaesthetic and/or opioids may be considered if the benefits of regional analgesia far outweigh the risks. This should only be performed by experienced personnel. For caesarean section general anaesthesia, or subarachnoid block in exceptional circumstances, is indicated.

HYPERCOAGULABLE STATES

Normal pregnancy tends to induce a hypercoagulable state, but there are pathological conditions which heighten this propensity and may require the use of anticoagulant drugs.

SYSTEMIC LUPUS ERYTHEMATOSUS

The pathophysiology of SLE and the antiphospholipid syndrome are discussed in Chapter 8. Leucopenia, lymphopenia and thrombocytopenia are common in active SLE but clotting defects, although they have been reported, are uncommon [46]. Antiphospholipid antibodies, namely lupus anticoagulant (LA) and anticardiolipin antibody (ACL), may be found in SLE [47] and both are associated with venous and arterial thrombosis [48]. LA is of particular interest to the anaesthetist because of its effect on the coagulation screen. There is a prolongation of the APTT (and rarely the PT), but these are *in vitro* phenomena and there is no *in vivo* bleeding tendency: isolated elevation of APTT does not confer a bleeding tendency [46]. The presence of inhibitors is confirmed, as neither APTT nor PT is correctable by a 50/50 mixture of the patient's plasma with normal plasma.

Treatment of SLE usually includes the administration of high-dose steroids and low-dose aspirin [48]. Anaesthetic options encompass all types of anaesthesia but must take into account the multisystem nature of the disease, the severity of organ involvement and the drugs used in treatment. When considering regional anaesthesia in the lupus patient, the presence of peripheral neuropathies must be appreciated and documented [46]. Since both platelet number and function are affected by SLE a coagulation screen which includes platelet count and tests of platelet function (e.g. TEG) should be done on all patients. In general, a normal TEG or bleeding time is reassuring but therapy with aspirin may confound the picture.

Some confusion may reside over the differentiation between SLE and the antiphospholipid syndrome. The antiphospholipid syndrome is considered a distinct entity from SLE and is characterized by the presence of antiphospholipid antibodies (LA and ACL), but patients do not have features of SLE or any other well-defined autoimmune disease [47,49].

ANTITHROMBIN III DEFICIENCY

Antithrombin III (ATIII) deficiency occurs in 1 in 5000 people and can be quantitative (type I) or qualitative (type II) [16]. In untreated patients, the risk of thrombosis in pregnancy is 55–68%. The mainstay of treatment is anticoagulation with heparin, both during pregnancy and in the postpartum period. Warfarin is occasionally used in the second trimester. Adjuvant ATIII concentrates may be required in the peripartum period [16, 50].

PROTEIN C AND PROTEIN S DEFICIENCY

Protein C acts by inhibiting factors V and VIII and a deficiency occurs in 1 in 15 000 individuals [16]. Thrombosis occurs in 25% of pregnant patients unless anticoagulant treatment is given. Anticoagulation is with heparin in the first and third trimesters, and either heparin or warfarin in the second trimester and post partum.

Protein S acts as a cofactor for protein C and the treatment for protein S deficiency is as above.

ANTICOAGULANT THERAPY

Thromboembolic disease remains a major cause of maternal death in the UK [1] and the use of anticoagulant drugs, either therapeutically or prophylactically, to modify this disease creates considerable dilemmas for the obstetric anaesthetist. The risk of haematoma within the spinal canal, which may be associated with substantial or permanent neurological damage, is the main concern. Such a haematoma after central nervous blockade (CNB) is very rare: 61 cases of epidural and/or subdural haematomata were found between 1906 and 1994 (only five of these were pregnant and no details are given) [51]. The most constant factor in this series was the presence of an anticoagulant drug or clotting disorder. Although baseline figures are unknown, epidural anaesthesia accounted for 45 of the haematomata and spinal anaesthesia for 15, figures which tend to support the view that subarachnoid block is less traumatic than epidural. Interestingly, bleeding into the spinal canal occurred immediately after removal of the epidural catheter in almost half the patients [51].

In acute thrombotic disease therapeutic anticoagulation with heparin or warfarin is required. It is generally agreed that regional blockade is contraindicated in this group until the coagulation profile is normal [31, 52, 53]. However, the situation with low-dose heparin or low-molecular-weight heparin as thrombo-prophylaxis is more controversial.

LOW-DOSE HEPARIN AND LOW-MOLECULAR-WEIGHT HEPARIN

Spinal haematoma after epidural or spinal insertion or epidural catheter removal has not been reported in association with low-dose heparin (LDH) [54]. In theory the new low-molecular-weight heparins (LMWH) may be even safer as they have less effect on platelet activity and have a more predictable bioavailability [51]. In controlled studies at least 10 000 patients have received the combination of LMWH and regional blockade without complication [55]. The risk of fatal pulmonary thromboembolism because of omitted thromboprophylactic treatment probably exceeds the risk of spinal haemorrhage with the combination of LDH or LMWH and regional blockade. As such, the institution of regional anaesthesia in these patients is safe provided the following precautions are borne in mind [51, 53]:

- site block/remove catheter before first dose or four to six hours after the last dose of LDH;
- site block/remove catheter before first dose or 12 hours after the last dose of LMWH;
- experienced anaesthetist should perform block in order to minimize vessel trauma;
- consider platelet count in patients on long-term LDH therapy.

ASPIRIN

The use of aspirin in the obstetric population is not uncommon (PIH, SLE) and consequently these patients present for regional anaesthetic procedures [56]. Low-dose aspirin therapy results in a prolonged bleeding time due to irreversible inhibition of platelet aggregation [51]. For affected platelets this inhibition of aggregation lasts up to seven to ten days after the last administration of drug (i.e. the entire lifetime of the affected platelets) [51]. Despite this well-known influence on platelet function, there is no evidence that low-dose aspirin increases the risk of spinal haemorrhage following regional blockade [54]. More than 3000 women received uncomplicated epidural anaesthesia for labour and delivery while being treated with low-dose aspirin for the prevention and treatment of PIH [57, 58]. Provided there is no underlying pathology affecting the coagulation process which merits investigation (e.g. PIH), and no other clinical or laboratory indications of a bleeding diathesis, it is regarded as safe practice to undertake regional anaesthesia in patients receiving aspirin therapy [56].

CONCLUSION

In summary, the patient with a bleeding diathesis poses a dilemma for the obstetric anaesthetist – the benefits of regional anaesthesia for labour and delivery on the one hand versus the potential risk of spinal canal haematoma caused by instrumentation on the other. Regional blockade is said to be contraindicated in patients with severe coagulopathies (e.g. DIC or HELLP syndrome) or in those receiving therapeutic anticoagulants. But since it is not known which coagulation screening tests are relevant for predicting the occurrence of spinal canal haematomata and spontaneous haematomata occur in the absence of any spinal instrumentation, the risk of haematoma formation is difficult, if not impossible, to predict for the majority of patients. Despite the widespread use of regional techniques in obstetric anaesthetic practice, haematomata of the spinal canal are very rare but it is not known if this rarity is due to vigilance on the part of the obstetric anaesthetist or if the risk of spinal canal haematomata is much less than we are led to believe.

REFERENCES

1. Department of Health Welsh Office, Scottish Office Home Health Department, Department

of Health and Social Security Report on Health and Social Subjects (1994) *Report on Confidential Enquiries into Maternal Deaths in the United Kingdom 1988–1990*, HMSO, London.

2. Lund, C.J. and Donovan, J.C. (1967) Blood volume during pregnancy. *American Journal of Obstetrics and Gynecology*, **98**, 393–403.

3. Kelton, J.G. and Cruickshank, M. (1988) Hematologic disorders of pregnancy, in *Medical Complications During Pregnancy* (eds G.N. Burrow and T.F. Ferris), W.B. Saunders, Philadelphia, pp. 65–94.

4. Douglas, J.M. (1991) Coagulation abnormalities and obstetric anaesthesia. *Canadian Journal of Anaesthesia*, **38**, R17–R21.

5. Poller, L. (1978) Oral contraceptives, blood clotting and thrombosis. *British Medical Bulletin*, **34**, 151–156.

6. Thomenson, J.A. and Thomson, J.M. (1985) Standardisation of the prothrombin time, in *Blood Coagulation and Haemostasis* (ed. J.M. Thomson), Churchill Livingstone, Edinburgh, pp. 370–409.

7. Laffan, M.A. and Bradshaw, A.E. (1995) Investigation of haemostasis, in *Practical Haematology* (eds J.V. Dacie and S.M. Lewis), Churchill Livingstone, Edinburgh, pp. 297–315.

8. Orlikowski, C.E.P. and Rocke, D.A. (1994) Coagulation monitoring in the obstetric patient. *International Anaesthesiology Clinics*, **32**, 173–91.

9. Kay, L.A. (1988) The coagulation laboratory, in *Essentials of Haemostasis and Thrombosis* (ed. L.A. Kay), Churchill Livingstone, Edinburgh, pp. 228–76.

10. (1989) Coagulation disorders, in *de Gruchy's Clinical Haematology in Medical Practice* (eds F. Firkin, C. Chesterman, D. Pennington and B. Rush), Blackwell Scientific, Oxford, pp. 406–53.

11. Macdonald, R. (1991) Aspirin and extradural blocks. *British Journal of Anaesthesia*, **66**, 1–3.

12. Rodgers, R.P.C. and Levin, J. (1990) A critical appraisal of the bleeding time. *Seminars in Thrombosis and Hemostasis*, **16**, 1–20.

13. Mallett, S.V. and Cox, D.J.A. (1992) Thromboelastography. *British Journal of Anaesthesia*, **69**, 307–13.

14. Bigeleisen, P.E. and Kang, Y. (1991) Thromboelastography as an aid to regional anaesthesia. *Regional Anaesthesia*, **16**, 59–61.

15. Sivakumaran, M. and Wood, J.K. (1994) The red cell, in *Anaesthesia* (eds W.S. Nimmo, D.J. Rowbotham and G. Smith), Blackwell Scientific, Oxford, pp. 325–35.

16. Lechner, R.B. (1994) Haematologic and coagulation disorders, in *Obstetric Anesthesia* (ed. D.H. Chestnut), Mosby, St Louis, pp. 815–32.

17. Mordel, N., Birkenfeld, A., Goldfarb, A.N. and Rachmilewitz, E.A. (1989) Successful full-term pregnancy in homozygous b-thalassemia major: Case report and review of the literature. *Obstetrics and Gynecology*, **73**, 837–40.

18. Jensen, C.E., Tuck, S.M. and Wonke, B. (1995) Fertility in b-thalassaemia major: a report of 16 pregnancies, preconceptual evaluation and a review of the literature. *British Journal of Obstetrics and Gynaecology*, **102**, 625–9.

19. Orr, D. (1967) Difficult intubation; A hazard in thalassaemia. *British Journal of Anaesthesia*, **39**, 585–6.

20. Poddar, D., Maude, G.H., Plant, P.J. *et al.* (1986) Pregnancy in Jamaican women with homozygous sickle cell disease. Fetal and maternal outcome. *British Journal of Obstetrics and Gynaecology*, **93**, 727–32.

21. Koshy, M., Burd, L., Wallace, D. (1988) *et al.* Prophylactic red-cell transfusions in pregnant patients with sickle cell disease. *New England Journal of Medicine*, **319**, 1447–52.

22. Morrison, J.C. and Wiser, W.L. (1976) The use of prophylactic partial exchange transfusion in pregnancies associated with sickle cell hemoglobinopathies. *Obstetrics and Gynecology*, **48**, 516.

23. Charache, S., Scott, J., Niebyl, J. and Bonds, D. (1980) Management of sickle cell disease in pregnant patients. *Obstetrics and Gynecology*, **55**, 407–10.

24. Hoffbrand, A.V. (1987) Megaloblastic anaemia and miscellaneous deficiency anaemias, in *Oxford Textbook of Medicine* (eds D.J. Weatherall, J.G.G. Ledingham and D.A. Warrel), Oxford Medical Publications, Oxford, pp. 19.93–19.108.

25. Chediak, J.R., Alban, G.M. and Maxey, B. (1986) von Willebrand's disease and pregnancy: Management during delivery and outcome of offspring. *American Journal of Obstetrics and Gynecology*, **155**, 618–24.

26. Greer, I.A., Lowe, G.D.O., Walker, J.J. and Forbes, C.D. (1991) Haemorrhagic problems in obstetrics and gynaecology in patients with congenital coagulopathies. *British Journal of Obstetrics and Gynaecology*, **98**, 909–18.

27. Milaskiewicz, R.M., Holdcroft, A. and Letsky, E. (1990) Epidural anaesthesia and von Willebrand's disease. *Anaesthesia*, **45**, 462–4.

28. Walker, I.D., Walker, J.J., Colvin, B.T. *et al.* (1994) Investigation and management of haemorrhagic disorders in pregnancy. *Journal of Clinical Pathology*, **47**, 100–8.

29. Ljung, R., Lindgren, A., Petrini, P. and Tengborn, L. (1994) Normal vaginal delivery is to be recommended for haemophilia carrier gravidae. *Acta Paediatrica*, 609–11.

30. Seeds, J.W., Cefalo, R.C., Miller, D.T. and Blatt, P.M. (1983) Obstetric care of the affected carrier of hemophilia B. *Obstetrics and Gynecology*, **62**, 23S–25S.

31. Gatt, S. (1990) Haematological disorders responsible for maternal bleeding in late pregnancy. *Anaesthesia and Intensive Care*, **18**, 335–47.

32. Chesterman, C.N. and Chong, B.H. (1995) Acquired haemostatic failure. *Medicine*, **23**, 518–30.

33. Wollman, L. (1995) Disseminated intravascular coagulation, in *Obstetric Anaesthesia* (ed. S. Datta), Mosby, St Louis, pp. 363–71.

34. Burrows, R.F. and Kelton, J.G. (1990) Thrombocytopenia at delivery: A prospective survey of 6715 deliveries. *American Journal of Obstetrics and Gynecology*, **162**, 731–4.

35. Biswas, A., Arulkumaran, S. and Ratnam, S.S. (1994) Disorders of platelets in pregnancy. *Obstetrical and Gynecological Survey*, **49**, 585–93.

36. McCrae, K.R., Samuels, P. and Schreiber, A.D. (19) Pregnancy-associated thrombocytopenia: Pathogenesis and management. *Blood*, **80**, 2697–714.

37. Kitay, D.Z. (19) Thrombocytopenia: The ITP and TTP syndromes, in *Management of High-risk Pregnancy* (ed. J.T. Queenan), Blackwell Scientific, Boston, pp. 212–23.

38. Garmel, S.H., Craigo, S.D. and Morin, L.M. *et al.* (1995) The role of percutaneous umbilical blood sampling in the management of immune thrombocytopenic purpura. *Prenatal Diagnosis*, **15**, 439–45.

39. Silver, R.M., Branch, D.W. and Scott, J.R. (1995) Maternal thrombocytopenia in pregnancy: Time for a reassessment. *American Journal of Obstetrics and Gynecology*, **173**, 479–82.

40. Cook, R.L., Miller, R.C., Katz, V.L. and Cefalo, R.C. (1991) Immune thrombocytopenic purpura in pregnancy: A reappraisal of management. *Obstetrics and Gynecology*, **78**, 578–83.

41. Burrows, R.F. and Kelton, J.G. (1995) Pregnancy in patients with idiopathic thrombocytopenia purpura: assessing the risks for the infant at delivery. *Obstetrical and Gynecological Survey*, **48**, 781–8.

42. Burrows, R.F. and Kelton, J.G. (1993) Fetal thrombocytopenia and its relation to maternal thrombocytopenia. *New England Journal of Medicine*, **329**, 1463–6.

43. Crosby, E.T. (1991) Obstetrical anaesthesia for patients with the syndrome of haemolysis, elevated liver enzymes and low platelets. *Canadian Journal of Anaesthesia*, **38**, 227–33.

44. Hsu, H.W., Belfort, M.A., Vernino, S. *et al.* (1995) Postpartum thrombotic thrombocytopenic purpura complicated by Budd–Chiari syndrome. *Obstetrics and Gynecology*, **85**, 839–43.

45. Kain, Z.N., Mayes, L.C. and Pakes, J. (19) Thrombocytopenia in pregnant women who use cocaine. *American Journal of Obstetrics and Gynecology*, **173**, 885–90.

46. Davies, S.R. (1996) Systemic lupus erythematosus and the obstetrical patient – implications for the anaesthetist. *Canadian Journal of Anaesthesia*, **38**, 790–6.

47. Reid, R.W. and Chestnut, D.H. (1994) Autoimmune disorders, in *Obstetric Anesthesia* (ed. D.H. Chestnut), Mosby, St Louis, pp. 735–45.

48. Resnik, R. (1994) Systemic lupus erythematosus, in *Management of High-risk Pregnancy* (ed. J.T. Queenan), Blackwell Scientific, Boston, pp. 298–301.

49. Fabregues, F., Ingelmo, M. and Vanrell, J.A. (1993) Low-dose aspirin for prevention of pregnancy losses in women with primary antiphospholipid syndrome. *Human Reproduction*, **8**, 2234–9.

50. Neerhof, M.G., Krewson, D.P., Haut, M. and Librizzi, R.J. (1993) Heparin therapy for congenital antithrombin III deficiency in pregnancy. *American Journal of Perinatology*, **10**, 311–2.

51. Vandermeulen, E.P., Van Aken, H. and Vermylen, J. (1994) Anticoagulants and spinal–epidural anaesthesia. *Anaesthesia and Analgesia*, **79**, 1165–77.

52. Bullingham, A. and Strunin, L. (1995) Prevention of postoperative venous thromboembolism. *British Journal of Anaesthesia*, **75**, 622–30.

53. Wildsmith, J.A.W. and McClure, J.H. (1991) Anticoagulant drugs and central nerve blockade. *Anaesthesia*, **46**, 613–4.

54. Sage, D.J. (1990) Epidurals, spinals and bleeding disorders in pregnancy: A review. *Anaesthesia and Intensive Care*, **18**, 319–26.

55. Bergqvist, D., Lindblad, B. (1992) and Matzsch, T. Low molecular weight heparin for thrombo-

prophylaxis and epidural/spinal anaesthesia – is there a risk? *Acta Anaesthesiologica Scandinavica*, **36**, 605–9.

56. Orlikowski, C.E.P., Payne, A.J., Moodley, J. and Rocke, D.A. (1992) Thrombelastography after aspirin ingestion in pregnant and non-pregnant subjects. *British Journal of Anaesthesia*, **69**, 159–61.

57. Collaborative Low-dose Aspirin Study in Pregnancy Collaborative Group (1994) CLASP: a randomised trial of low dose aspirin for the prevention and treatment of pre-eclampsia among 9364 pregnant women. *Lancet*, **343**, 619–29.

58. Horlocker, T.T., Wedel, D.J., Offord, K.F. *et al.* (1994) Preoperative antiplatelet drugs do not increase the risk of spinal hematoma associated with regional anaesthesia. *Regional Anaesthesia*, **19**, 8.

CARDIAC DISEASE AND RESUSCITATION

7

B. M. Gray

INTRODUCTION

Pregnancy places considerable stress on the cardiovascular system but the apparent ease with which most women tolerate this should not mask the risks to women with pre-existing cardiac disease. The combination of improved medical care enabling more women with serious cardiac pathology to attain reproductive age and a rising consumer expectation that pregnancy, with a healthy infant at the end, is a right leads to increasing numbers of women with the potential for cardiovascular instability presenting with an established pregnancy. Ideally, while every female with cardiac disease should be made aware of the consequences of pregnancy on her well-being before she becomes pregnant problems can arise with regard to who should take the lead in such counselling. Women first achieving pregnancy at an older age when ischaemic heart disease is already present may have no knowledge of their disease, or young teenagers with complex congenital cardiac problems may never have had the issue of pregnancy raised by the paediatric cardiologist. The first time many of these women realize the risk is when they are pregnant.

PHYSIOLOGICAL CHANGES DURING NORMAL PREGNANCY, LABOUR AND THE PUERPERIUM

By term, plasma volume rises to approximately 150% of prepregnancy values, with the most rapid increase occurring early in pregnancy: approximately half the increase occurs by 10 weeks' gestation and some 80% of the rise is complete by 20 weeks. The red cell mass increases by only some 25% in a more linear fashion over the whole pregnancy. The discrepancy between these changes in red cell mass and plasma volume leads to a reduced haemoglobin concentration: the 'physiological anaemia of pregnancy' [1, 2].

There is a definite rise in pulse rate during pregnancy, mostly occurring by eight weeks' gestation, but ultimately reaching a value of 10 to 20 beats per minute faster at term: stroke volume has been shown to increase and decrease but is usually unchanged [3]. Overall, during pregnancy, cardiac output rises by 40%, with the greatest rise in the second trimester. Cardiac output peaks by about 32 weeks and remains at this level until delivery. The changes in cardiac output occur in response to the increased oxygen consumption of pregnancy. Previous reports of a fall in cardiac output towards term are now thought to be the result of aortocaval compression and reduced venous return leading to a reduced stroke

Clinical Problems in Obstetric Anaesthesia
Edited by Ian F. Russell and Gordon Lyons. Published in 1997 by Chapman & Hall, London. ISBN 0 412 71600 3.

volume. Using data from pulmonary artery catheters inserted into 10 healthy pregnant women at term and again at 12 weeks postpartum Clark *et al.* [4] were able to confirm a decrease in cardiac output in the supine position. This fall could be obtunded by using either the right or left lateral position: the study showed no difference between these lateral positions. When cardiac output fell in either the supine or standing position, there were significant rises in systemic and pulmonary vascular resistance to maintain the respective arterial pressures. The rise in pulmonary vascular resistance was proportionately greater than that on the systemic side of the circulation [4]. Systemic vascular tone is reduced in the early stages of pregnancy leading to a widened pulse pressure and a fall in mean blood pressure but central venous pressure and pulmonary wedge pressure appear to remain within prepregnancy values.

Peripartum the cardiovascular changes are even more dramatic. There are yet further increases in cardiac output during the first, second and third stages of labour of some 25, 50 and 80% respectively. These additional rises are thought to be secondary to sympathetic stimulation and an autotransfusion of uteroplacental blood into the systemic circulation during contractions. After delivery the autotransfusion of approximately 500 ml of blood and the cessation of caval occlusion may lead to a 200–300% rise in cardiac output. Within an hour of delivery cardiac output falls to between 110–120% of prepregnancy values and then continues to fall at a much slower rate until it returns to normal by four to six weeks postpartum.

Symptoms and signs which occur during a normal pregnancy can mimic those of cardiac disease [5] and care must be taken to ensure that normal women are not labelled as having cardiac disease. Equally, in a patient with cardiac disease, these symptoms and signs must not be too readily diagnosed as the physiological effects of pregnancy lest a deterioration be missed. The normal increase in respiratory minute volume and symptoms such as fatigue, decreased exercise tolerance and peripheral oedema may be physiological or pathophysiological. Up to 80% of normal pregnant women may have peripheral oedema due to an increase in total body water and exchangeable sodium. The increased venous pressure in the lower limbs due to compression of the inferior vena cava by the gravid uterus may augment oedema in the legs [5]. After 20 weeks' gestation the jugular venous pulse is more conspicuous because rapid X and Y descents make the A and V waves more obvious. The right ventricular impulse may be felt on the chest wall and that of the left ventricle becomes hyperdynamic. The increase in left ventricular contractility produces a loud first heart sound and third heart sounds are often heard. Flow murmurs are common and a venous hum almost universal.

THE CONTRIBUTION OF CARDIAC DISEASE TO MATERNAL MORTALITY

The total number of cardiac deaths has remained fairly static since 1973 although, with the total number of maternal deaths and the maternal mortality rate both falling by approximately 50%, the relative proportion of maternal cardiac deaths has increased.

In the triennium 1988–1990 there were 21 maternal deaths from cardiac disease in the UK [6]. It was considered that almost all the women who died had received substandard care. Substandard care in this report included failures in the health-care system as well as situations where the mothers did not present for medical care or ignored the advice given to them. In the latter cases the authors of the report felt that the methods of advising could be improved [6]. Much of the substandard care was felt to be related to poor antenatal assessment; hence the need for good preconception counselling was stressed. For those who decide to go ahead with a pregnancy close supervision by both obstetrician and cardiologist is required. At some stage there must be anaesthetic involvement so that the

Table 7.1 General considerations for pregnant women with cardiac disease

- Should the pregnancy be allowed to continue?
- Symptoms and signs of worsening cardiac disease may mimic those of normal pregnancy and vice versa making assessment difficult but essential
- Need for a multidisciplinary team approach throughout. Team should include obstetrician, anaesthetist and cardiologist
- Plan for delivery, including anaesthesia and analgesia, should be clearly made. Should include action in event of foetal or maternal distress
- Management and delivery arranged in a unit capable of caring for high-risk patients: full intensive care unit backup required. Care closely supervised by senior medical and midwifery staff.
- There is no place for delivery in an isolated maternity unit
- Anticoagulation may be needed, e.g. for prosthetic valve or as prophylaxis against thromboembolic disease
- Antibiotic prophylaxis against subacute bacterial endocarditis is required if anatomy is abnormal. Local advice should be sought but usually ampicillin and gentamicin are used for labour, delivery and for at least eight hours postpartum

appropriate analgesic/anaesthetic methods can be clearly documented.

PRE-EXISTING HEART DISEASE

In 1878 Angus MacDonald, in the first book in English on cardiac disease and pregnancy, noted the large number of cases of rheumatic mitral valve disease in pregnant women [7]. Although there has been a dramatic decline in the incidence and severity of rheumatic fever and rheumatic heart disease, the latter is still the most common cause of heart disease in pregnancy. We now face management challenges that MacDonald could never have envisaged: advances in surgical and medical care lead to increasing numbers of women with congenital heart disease surviving to adulthood and becoming pregnant; there is an increase in coronary artery disease in young women, of multifactorial origin but largely due to an increase in smoking habits in this group; there is a tendency for working women to delay their pregnancies until they are older – not to mention the occasional phenomenon of women beyond the natural menopause becoming pregnant by *in vitro* fertilization and other assisted techniques.

Whatever the pathology there are common factors which must be considered when a woman with cardiac disease first presents (Table 7.1).

In an ideal world women with major cardiac disease will have been seen preconception and adequately advised. But pregnancies continue to occur when the risk of maternal mortality is so great that termination of pregnancy is recommended: examples include end-stage pulmonary hypertension, uncorrected severe mitral stenosis, Eisenmenger's syndrome and Marfan's syndrome. Case studies of successful outcomes in all these conditions have been reported so a careful discussion with each woman and her family is needed before final decisions are made.

Usually, to reduce the cardiac problems of pregnancy, any possible corrective surgery will be carried out before childbearing. Rarely is corrective surgery necessary during pregnancy but if the maternal condition is deteriorating, or is predicted to do so, in spite of aggressive medical management, then many would recommend surgery. This should be carried out in the late second trimester at a time when foetal organogenesis is complete, thus reducing the likelihood of teratogenicity and, from the maternal cardiovascular and uteroplacental function aspects, it is before marked caval occlusion comes into play. Although there is some foetal risk this is obviously less than if the pregnancy is terminated or if the maternal condition deteriorates and leads to maternal and foetal death.

Once the decision has been made to continue with the pregnancy, regular multidisciplinary follow up is required. Any existing drug therapy needs to be evaluated but is usually continued as the risks of foetal teratogenicity are small compared to the maternal (and therefore foetal) risks if therapy is stopped. The major exception to this is warfarin which is teratogenetic if taken in the first trimester. If it is avoided for the first six weeks of gestation this risk is almost abolished. Thus women taking anticoagulation therapy, usually for a prosthetic heart valve or previous thromboembolic disease, should be converted onto heparin before conception, or as early in pregnancy as possible. Since heparin needs to be given parenterally there may be problems with patient compliance. The importance of continuing co-operation should be stressed. Warfarin crosses the placenta and risks placental or foetal bleeding. Because of this heparin is preferable to warfarin in the third trimester. Although warfarin may be used in the second trimester some may elect to continue heparin throughout the pregnancy. Again, decisions should be made by the full multidisciplinary team, including senior haematological opinions.

Anaesthetic management will be geared to support the agreed mode of delivery: this may be either a planned vaginal delivery or an elective caesarean section. An epidural with slow, careful drug titration is a good method of analgesia or anaesthesia and will reduce cardiovascular demands arising from sympathetic reflexes. If an epidural is not possible then other methods will be required. Entonox, an example of patient-controlled analgesia which has been available for many years, may be used but is usually not enough. In anticoagulated patients the routine use of intramuscular analgesia is not recommended and intravenous analgesia should be arranged as required: this is best provided by patient-controlled intravenous analgesia (PCA). Anxieties

surrounding foetal depression have probably limited the use of conventional PCA on the labour ward but, in practice, such depression is not a significant problem with pethidine [8], nalbuphine [9] or fentanyl (local experience). The quality of analgesia is unlikely to approach that of epidural analgesia but is a considerable improvement over intramuscular injections.

Many teams will opt for delivery by elective caesarean section thus allowing the availability of the full senior team and intensive care support to be planned. The anaesthetic may be either a general or a regional technique. All techniques have their problems, and the advantages and disadvantages (Table 7.2) need to be considered in each case with reference to the individual pathophysiology as outlined later. In general, conditions in which the blood flow tends to be backwards (mitral or aortic regurgitation) benefit from a modest reduction in systemic vascular resistance to promote forward flow: a regional technique may be helpful here. Conditions in which forward flow is restricted (severe aortic stenosis) cannot compensate for a reduction in systemic vascular resistance and regional techniques should be used with great caution, if at all. Local infiltration for caesarean section is, in theory, an option if the mother is considered too unwell for a general or regional technique but few obstetricians have any experience of this: pain and fear experienced by the mother may elicit autonomic effects which could destabilize the cardiovascular system so careful additional supplementation with intravenous or inhalational analgesia or sedation may be required. Whichever technique is chosen, the woman should be induced in theatre with full monitoring in place, including central venous, direct arterial and pulmonary artery wedge pressures as indicated. The usual precautions including a lateral tilt or wedged position should be used and emergency drugs should be readily available. Paediatric support is needed, particularly if the mother is given a general anaesthetic with high-dose opioids.

Table 7.2 Factors to consider when deciding between regional and general anaesthesia

	Regional	*General*
Advantages	Continuous, gradually established Block reduces sympathetic stimulation and allows for cardiovascular stability Good postoperative pain control Mother able to be awake	Established technique in cardiac patients for cardiac or non-cardiac surgery
Disadvantages	If block develops too rapidly hypotension may cause rapid and perhaps untreatable decompensation	Intubation mandatory. Hypertensive response to intubation. Failed intubation with hypoxia and risk of gastric aspiration

The most likely contraindications to regional anaesthesia are anticoagulation or coagulopathy, abnormalities of the lumbar spine preventing successful access to the spinal canal, and situations where hypotension may be catastrophic (severe aortic stenosis). If a regional technique is employed its onset should be gradual with close cardiovascular monitoring, and vigorous prevention and treatment of hypotension. The use of a single-shot spinal or epidural should be avoided.

Because of the possibility of premature labour, or foetal or maternal problems prior to the planned day of delivery it is essential that the anaesthetic plan includes options for the emergency situation. This plan needs to be discussed with the obstetrician and the mother in advance. To prevent an inappropriate technique being used in an emergency the directives should be clearly laid out such that all staff in the unit are aware of them. It must be clear whether general anaesthesia or a single-shot spinal can be used in an emergency; if these techniques are considered too dangerous for the mother then this should apply whatever the state of the foetus, and the maternity team and mother should be made aware that rapid anaesthsia for foetal distress is not an option.

MITRAL VALVE DISEASE

In spite of its reduced prevalence, rheumatic heart disease still accounts for most cases of heart disease in pregnant patients. Mitral stenosis, followed by mitral regurgitation, is the most commonly encountered valve disease in pregnancy [10].

Mitral stenosis

As a result of the stenosed mitral valve, left ventricular filling (and therefore output) is reduced, and the increased left atrial pressure leads to pulmonary hypertension and eventually right ventricular failure. Patients with significant mitral stenosis have a fixed stroke volume and are unable to compensate for reduced left atrial filling (e.g. a fall in preload due to hypovolaemia). Tachycardia, by reducing the time for ventricular filling, is poorly tolerated. If the gradient across the stenosis is greater than 25 mm Hg or if atrial fibrillation coexists, decompensation is more likely.

Anaesthetic management is aimed at avoiding tachycardia and hypovolaemia. As well as avoiding obvious causes of tachycardia, sympathomimetic or antivagal drugs (e.g. pancuronium or atropine), it should be remembered that a reduced afterload may cause reflex tachycardia. Careful attention to fluid balance is required to avoid the dangers of both under and over-filling: the former will reduce left atrial and hence left ventricular filling whilst the latter predisposes to pulmonary oedema. Because the loss of an effective atrial contraction significantly reduces ventricular filling the onset of atrial fibrillation should be managed aggressively by digitalization or cardioversion: atrial fibrillation is associated with a higher mortality [11] than sinus rhythm.

Regional techniques should be used with caution so as to avoid a reduction in afterload. A continuous epidural for labour, particularly opioids and low-concentration local anaesthetic, is useful for avoiding increases in sympathetic activity (and therefore tachycardia) during labour and delivery. The epidural may also be used to provide anaesthesia for caesarian section with standard solutions such as 0.5% bupivacaine or 2% lignocaine, providing the block is established slowly. Since epidural adrenaline should be avoided to prevent tachycardia from systemic absorption it may be advantageous to add fentanyl to improve the efficacy of the block. Single-shot subarachnoid anaesthesia should be avoided because of the rapidity of cardiovascular changes and the inability of the mother, or anaesthetist, to compensate for this. Ephedrine, with its invariable tendency to cause tachycardia, is best substituted by phenylephrine.

Mitral incompetence

In mitral incompetence, blood regurgitates into the left atrium during systole. Although the atrium will tolerate this extra load initially, in chronic regurgitation left ventricular dilation and hypertrophy will result, eventually leading to left ventricular failure. Atrial fibrillation may result from the dilated atrium and, as with mitral stenosis, should be corrected because of the increased maternal mortality and morbidity associated with pulmonary oedema from the inefficient forward emptying

of the atrium. It is crucial to maintain the atrial filling pressure so if a regional technique is used an adequate fluid preload should be given and attention paid to correcting perioperative or peridelivery blood loss and fluid shifts. A modest reduction in afterload is well tolerated as it encourages forward flow from the ventricle into the systemic circulation rather than backward through the incompetent valve. Thus regional analgesia or anaesthesia, carefully performed and gradually built up, has much to recommend it.

AORTIC VALVE DISEASE

Aortic valve disease may result from rheumatic fever, congenital causes (stenosis), or be secondary to trauma (regurgitation).

Aortic stenosis

In aortic stenosis left ventricular hypertrophy develops to overcome the outflow obstruction but, in spite of this, the stroke volume is fixed in severe cases. The drop in pressure across the valve reduces the perfusion pressure at the origins of the coronary arteries. The hypertrophied ventricle requires a greater blood flow than normal and this, combined with the reduced perfusion pressure and increased intramural pressure, may lead to ischaemia and hence left ventricular failure. Pregnancy may precipitate a rapid deterioration. These patients are often asymptomatic until a critical pressure gradient is reached when symptoms of stenosis including angina, breathlessness or syncopal attacks may be experienced.

Management is directed toward the avoidance of both tachycardia and a reduced afterload. A slower heart rate allows more time for the ventricle to empty in systole and improves perfusion of the ventricular muscle in diastole. Regional techniques have been used for caesarean section [12] but many feel they should be avoided completely because of the rapid, and possibly irreversible, deterioration associated with hypotension and coronary ischaemia. An epidural is preferable to a spinal as the block can be built up slowly and haemodynamic stability maintained [12]. Even for labour, epidurals should be used with extreme caution. Hypotension should be treated aggressively with fluids and phenylephrine. Direct arterial pressure monitoring is useful as changes in blood pressure are seen immediately. Phenylephrine, an alpha stimulant, is preferred to ephedrine in outflow obstruction because it promotes a bradycardia rather than a tachycardia. Like other alpha agonists it may reduce uteroplacental blood flow in large doses, but studies have shown that when used in small doses in healthy women undergoing caesarean section there are no abnormalities in foetal acidbase status [13].

Aortic incompetence

In aortic regurgitation the abnormal valve allows backflow of blood into the left ventricle causing left ventricular dilation leading on to reduced left ventricular output, pulmonary hypertension and eventually biventricular failure.

Management is aimed at reducing systemic vascular resistance and avoiding bradycardia. This not only promotes forward flow into the systemic circulation but also limits the time available for backflow. Thus regional techniques are useful with ephedrine being an appropriate vasoconstrictor because it will maintain or increase the heart rate (in contrast to the use of phenylephrine to reduce the heart rate in aortic stenosis). Epidural anaesthesia is preferable to spinal anaesthesia: with the latter, changes in haemodynamic variables may occur too quickly for the mother to compensate. Even with an epidural caution is required as a large bolus of local anaesthetic may cause rapid hypotension: a bolus of 18 ml bupivacaine 0.5% epidurally followed by a further bolus of 6 ml for a caesarean section in a woman with aortic regurgitation resulted in maternal death [14]. Subsequent correspon-

dence was largely supportive of epidural anaesthesia in this situation but recommended smaller bolus doses of local anaesthetic, titrated to effect, and the use of invasive arterial and central venous pressure monitoring [15].

HYPERTROPHIC OBSTRUCTIVE CARDIOMYOPATHY

Hypertrophic obstructive cardiomyopathy (HOCM), also referred to as idiopathic hypertrophic subaortic stenosis (IHSS), results from an asymetric hypertrophy of the interventricular septum. There is left ventricular outflow obstruction and the degree of obstruction is increased by a low arterial pressure, a low ventricular volume and an increased ventricular ejection velocity. HOCM in pregnancy usually results in a favourable outcome although symptomatic worsening may occur [16]. Management of the condition, whether in the pregnant or non-pregnant state, is aimed at treating symptoms and preventing complications, especially sudden death. Beta blockers are widely used for arrhythmia control and are accepted as the drug of choice for heart failure associated with the condition [17], with or without atrial fibrillation. By their negative inotropic and chronotropic effects beta blockers reduce ventricular ejection velocity and so reduce the muscular obstruction, reduce heart rate thus increasing end diastolic ventricular volume, and reduce myocardial oxygen consumption. These effects protect against sudden death. During anaesthesia vasoconstrictors (e.g. phenylephrine) and cardiac depressant anaesthetics (e.g. halothane) have proved useful. As with aortic stenosis, hypotension, hypovolaemia and tachycardia should be avoided. Should mitral regurgitation coexist with HOCM care is required with drug therapy. Drugs have the opposite effect compared to other forms of mitral regurgitation: inotropes and vasodilators worsen and vasoconstrictors improve ventricular ejection.

RIGHT-SIDED HEART VALVULAR LESIONS

These are uncommon and present little problem to the pregnant woman other than at delivery when antibiotic prophylaxis is needed against bacterial endocarditis.

CONGENITAL HEART DISEASE

There are an enormous number of congenital heart lesions of various complexity; those of importance to the obstetric anaesthetist are the uncorrected ones likely to be found in women of childbearing years. These include both acyanotic heart conditions (e.g. ostium secundum atrial septal defect, patent ductus arteriosus, pulmonary valve stenosis, coarctation of the aorta and aortic valve disease), and cyanotic conditions involving right to left shunting (e.g. Fallot's tetralogy) [18].

In terms of the anaesthetic management the most important factors are the presence of a shunt and whether it is left-to-right or right-to-left.

Left-to-right shunt

These conditions include atrial or ventricular septal defects, and patent ductus arteriosus. In the early stages of the disease, blood flows from the left to right side of the heart down a pressure gradient through the defect and results in increased pulmonary blood flow. If uncorrected, right ventricular hypertrophy and pulmonary hypertension develop. Pregnancy, with its increased cardiovascular demands, may lead to right-sided heart failure or to a reversal of the shunt – Eisenmenger's syndrome. This latter occurs when the pregnancy-induced reduction in systemic vascular resistance (maximum reduction immediately post-partum) falls below the raised pulmonary artery pressure and causes blood to flow down a pressure gradient from the right side of the heart through the shunt into the systemic circulation. Increases in pulmonary vascular resistance accompanied by an increased right ventricular pressure occur secondary to pain in labour, further increasing the likelihood of shunt reversal.

Meticulous care is needed with vascular access and intravenous fluids to avoid air bubbles or thrombi being carried to the right heart and paradoxically embolizing through the defect to reach the cerebral circulation. Prophylaxis against bacterial endocarditis is mandatory and monitoring should include ECG and pulse oximetry; hypoxia measured by the latter may allow early detection of shunt reversal. Due to distortion of the cardiac anatomy and physiology, pulmonary artery flow catheters are often unhelpful: the position of the catheter tip cannot be known with certainty and the readings obtained will be unreliable; with correctly placed catheters optimal values for that patient are not known; the catheter may pass through the shunt causing anatomical damage and enlargement of the shunt.

Factors that increase pulmonary vascular pressure should be avoided or corrected: these include hypoxia, hypercarbia, acidosis and pain. As systemic hypotension may precipitate shunt reversal blood loss should be replaced and regional techniques used with great care. Although regional techniques are used widely in this group of conditions the loss of resistance to air technique for locating the epidural space is not recommended: up to 18% of epidurals may be associated with a 'bloody tap' [19] and there is a real possibility of intravenous air injection.

Right-to-left shunts

These include cyanotic heart diseases like Fallot's tetralogy, transposition of the great arteries in which a right-to-left shunt is present from birth and Eisenmenger's syndrome in which chronic disease progression or acute decompensation has reversed a left-to-right shunt. Women in whom surgery has been fully corrective require no special precautions other than prophylaxis against bacterial endocarditis. However, depending on the complexity of the lesion, surgery may not have been fully corrective and these women should be regarded as extremely high risk for pregnancy.

Almost all events in pregnancy conspire to worsen the shunting: a fall in systemic vascular resistance, hypotension with blood loss at delivery, stress and pain during labour causing an increase in pulmonary vascular resistance. Pain control, intravascular volume status, systemic blood pressure and oxygen saturation should all be monitored. With aggressive active control of these physiological variables general anaesthesia or carefully titrated regional techniques may be used for delivery.

Coarctation of the aorta

This is less common in women than men but is important because the changes in connective tissue which occur in pregnancy weaken the aortic wall and this, taken together with the increased cardiac output, increases the risk of aortic rupture. There is also a risk of rupture of associated aneurysms of the circle of Willis: at postmortem such aneurysms may be present in up to 25% of cases dying due to coarctation of the aorta [20]. While surgical correction of the coarctation solves one problem the risk from rupture of aneurysms of the circle of Willis will not have changed. In surgically uncorrected mothers mortality may be as high as 9% and foetal loss double this.

Systolic blood flow through the coarctation cannot increase and so cardiac output is rate limited. The progressive reduction in systemic vascular resistance of pregnancy is poorly tolerated as are tachycardia or bradycardia. Hypotension should be avoided because of the lack of compensation available but, conversely, a rise in blood pressure predisposes to aortic dissection or cerebral aneurysm rupture.

Anaesthesia of any sort is hazardous and cardiovascular stability should be monitored closely with direct arterial and pulmonary arterial catheters. The blood pressure at the heart and cerebral circulation should be measured invasively from a vessel arising proximal to the coarctation (e.g. the right radial artery rather than the left radial or lower limb arteries). Although the foetoplacental unit is distal to the coarctation and its perfusion pressure will be low (collateral flow may afford some compensation) we should not lose sight of the fact that increasing maternal blood pressure proximal to the coarctation may cause a maternal catastrophe and be even more detrimental to the foetus. Heart failure may develop and should be watched for. Antibacterial prophylaxis is indicated at delivery to prevent endocarditis in the coarctation.

Marfan's syndrome

If there is aortic root dilatation greater than 40 mm Marfan's syndrome in pregnancy is associated with an increased risk of aortic dissection and rupture [21]. As in coarctation of the aorta there is a risk of rupture of an associated aneurysm of the circle of Willis, particularly if blood pressure rises during pregnancy or delivery. Preconceptual counselling is of great importance as the mother's lifespan is reduced by some 50% and any child born has a 50% chance of inheriting the condition. Pregnancy should be avoided, or termination of pregnancy should be considered, if evidence of significant aortic root dilatation is present. It has been suggested that the root diameter should be assessed every six to eight weeks by echocardiography [22] since in the absence of aortic root dilatation pregnancy may continue without increased risk of aortic dissection. The greatest risk of rupture is in the third trimester and first postpartum month [22].

Management is directed towards strict control of blood pressure to prevent any rise. Functional aortic regurgitation or mitral valve prolapse with regurgitation may coexist and these should be managed appropriately. Regional anaesthesia may be technically more difficult because of the coexisting lumbar scoliosis and prior back surgery.

MYOCARDIAL INFARCTION

The first reported myocardial infarction during pregnancy was recorded by Katz in 1922 [23]. Since that time less than 100 cases have been recorded, although an incidence as high as 1 in 10 000 deliveries has been suggested [24]. Arteriosclerosis, delineated by angiography or autopsy, was found in 40% of women following infarction: the arteriosclerosis was not considered severe and the cause of infarction was thought to be thrombus and spasm [24]. With an increasing incidence of ischaemic heart disease in young women it may be assumed that more women will first present with coronary artery disease when they face the increased cardiovascular demands of a pregnancy.

Mortality following myocardial infarction during pregnancy averages 30% with a higher risk nearer to term [25]. Mortality is twice as high in the third trimester as at any other time and can be explained by the peak cardiovascular demand at this time. Because of the high mortality post infarction these women should be managed in an intensive care unit with invasive monitoring (arterial and pulmonary artery catheter) in order to stabilize the situation and prevent further infarction, arrhythmias etc. It is axiomatic that the supine position should be avoided at all times. As in the non-pregnant state treatment may include oxygen, narcotics, nitrates, calcium channel blockers and beta blockers: none of these drugs have been shown to result in adverse foetal effects in this setting although nitrates may relax uterine tone and slow the progress of spontaneous or induced labour [26]. These women are usually in a hypercoagulable state [27] and heparin therapy is recommended. Systemic streptokinase therapy tends not to be used in pregnancy because of the association with maternal haemorrhage, dysfunctional uterine contractions and premature labour. Full anticoagulation is required if there is severe hypokinesis of the ventricular wall, with or without mural thrombosis, otherwise prophylaxis against deep vein thrombosis is sufficient. When there is evidence of ongoing ischaemia, emergency angiography should be considered with angioplasty or coronary artery bypass grafting as required. If the mother continues to deteriorate or cannot be stabilized then delivery of the foetus should be considered to improve the chances of survival for both patients.

Should the woman survive the initial infarct in a good condition a decision needs to be made as to the timing and mode of delivery. The longer the interval between the infarct and delivery the less chance there is of complications from myocardial irritability and arrhythmias but this needs to be weighed against the increasing cardiovascular demands made later in pregnancy when the extra stress on the heart may lead to the possibility of further infarction. There are advocates for both caesarean section and vaginal delivery. Ginz [28], in a retrospective review of 39 cases of myocardial infarction in pregnancy, found higher maternal and foetal mortalities when delivery was by caesarean section compared to delivery by forceps: caesarean section 27% maternal and 9% foetal mortality; forceps 0% maternal or foetal mortality. Those women who laboured and delivered without forceps had a maternal mortality of 13% and infant mortality of 27%. Bembridge and Lyons [29] reported a favourable outcome for both mother and baby following a myocardial infarction complicated by cardiac arrest at 38 weeks' gestation: the mother was resuscitated from an 'in hospital' ventricular fibrillation arrest and transferred to intensive care for invasive monitoring and inotropic support. The spontaneous onset of labour was managed on the intensive care unit with a lumbar epidural topped up intermittently with 0.25% plain bupivacaine without cardiovascular instability and the mother was delivered electively by forceps. Both mother and baby did well. Although the numbers are small, these reports [28,29] support the argument for an assisted vaginal delivery. Whatever the mode of delivery or anaesthetic technique tachycardia and hypotension must be avoided so that myocardial blood flow and oxygen supply are maintained.

Increases in myocardial oxygen demand should be minimized by avoiding pain and shivering. The latter is often unexpected and may occur in 23% of healthy women without epidural blockade [30] and between 14 and 68% with an epidural block especially in the first 10 min after establishing the block [31]. Although the mechanism of postepidural shivering is unclear it can be reduced by warming intravenous [32] and epidural [33] solutions and by adding an opioid such as fentanyl to the epidural local anaesthetic solution [34]. Myocardial oxygen supply may be increased by a higher inspired oxygen tension, avoidance of hypovolaemia and treatment of ischaemia with nitrates.

During anaesthesia, maternal monitoring should include ECG, direct arterial and pulmonary artery pressures, pulse oximetry, temperature and, if a general anaesthetic is given, end-tidal carbon dioxide monitoring. The choice of volatile agent for general anaesthesia is not clear. Halothane will decrease cardiac work by reducing both myocardial contractility and systemic arterial blood pressure but, by sensitizing the heart to endogenous catecholamines, it is arrhythmogenic. Isoflurane may reduce systemic blood pressure by vasodilatation but is thought to induce a 'coronary steal' syndrome [35]: i.e. vasodilating healthy coronary arteries in preference to atherosclerotic vessels, diverting blood to healthy heart tissue at the expense of flow through the atherosclerotic vessels and thus making ischaemia worse. However others have shown that isoflurane anaesthesia in patients with coronary artery disease is no more likely to worsen ischaemia than other anaesthetic agents [36] and consequently it is still used widely.

ARRHYTHMIAS IN PREGNANCY

Benign arrhythmias, such as atrial premature contractions, are more common during pregnancy and are more likely to be noticed as palpitations. Serious arrhythmias are fortunately very rare; if they do occur they are treated in the same way as if they had occurred in the non-pregnant state. This includes checking for precipitating causes (e.g. thyrotoxicosis, or underlying heart disease). As with all prescribing issues in pregnancy, the potential foetal effects of any proposed drug therapy should be remembered and alternatives, including whether treatment is needed, considered. The safety of the mother is paramount. Deterioration in her health will jeopardize the foetus. Lignocaine, quinidine, procainamide, disopyramide, verapamil, digoxin and propranolol, to name some of the more commonly used agents, are all considered as probably safe. Phenytoin (with a high risk of foetal malformation) and amiodarone (with the possibility of foetal goitre) should only be used if other agents have failed [37]. The choice of treatment should always be made in conjunction with a cardiologist but possible agents for consideration appear in Table 7.3.

PERIPARTUM CARDIOMYOPATHY

Idiopathic cardiac failure associated with pregnancy and delivery was first described in the 19th century. Peripartum cardiomyopathy as a distinct entity was described in the 1950s and subsequently [38]. Cardiomyopathy presents as primary pump failure with high central venous and pulmonary wedge pressures and low cardiac output. The aetiology is unknown and diagnosis is by exclusion. It is more common in the over 30s and there is a weak association with multiparity, multiple pregnancies, obesity, and breast feeding. There is a high incidence in Nigeria thought to be related to a local ritual practice involving a high salt intake and remaining in a hot, humid room following delivery. Women who develop cardiomyopathy under these latter circumstances have higher levels of atrial natriuretic peptide and lower levels of aldosterone and renin than those exposed to the same conditions who did not develop the condition [39].

Table 7.3 Possible therapy for arrhythmias in pregnancy

Arrhythmia	Treatment
Sinus tachycardia	No specific treatment required in absence of hypotension, hypoxia, anaemia or fever
Sinus bradycardia	Very rare. Treat underlying cause (e.g. hypothyroidism, cardiomyopathy, drug effects). Atropine if hypotensive
Premature atrial contractions	Remove precipitating factor, e.g. caffeine consumption, alcohol consumption, fatigue, stress. May precede atrial fibrillation in women with rheumatic heart disease
Paroxysmal atrial tachycardia	Usually well tolerated unless underlying heart disease
Atrial flutter	Treat underlying condition, e.g. hyperthyroidism, pulmonary or cardiac disease. Consider synchronized DC shock – after anticoagulation if long-standing. Digoxin can control the ventricular rate
Atrial fibrillation	Rare except with mitral valve disease. Digoxin or verapamil may be used and anticoagulation should be considered
Supraventricular tachycardia	Usually self-limiting or resolved with (unilateral) carotid sinus massage. Adenosine may resolve it. If longer-acting agent required, digoxin or a beta blocker. Verapamil can be used in the absence of myocardial or valvular disease but **not** with a beta blocker because of the risk of hypotension and bradycardia.
Premature ventricular contractions	Remove precipitating causes (as for premature atrial contractions). Check for underlying cardiac disease
Ventricular tachycardia	DC cardioversion if haemodynamically unstable, otherwise lignocaine. Lignocaine prophylaxis against recurrent attacks may be needed
Ventricular fibrillation	DC shock

Cardiomyopathy occurs most commonly in the second postpartum month [38] but can occur in the antepartum period. There is an overall mortality of up to 60% with half the deaths occurring in the initial hospitalization period. There is no specific treatment and management is supportive but some cases have required heart transplantation. With antenatal cardiomyopathy the foetus should be delivered. If resolution has not taken place within six months the prognosis is very poor [40]: further pregnancies are associated with a recurrence or worsening of the disease, so women whose cardiomyopathy has not resolved should be categorically advised against further pregnancies. However there is a report of four women with fully resolved peripartum cardiomyopathy having subsequent uncomplicated pregnancies [41].

Both regional and general anaesthesia have been employed for delivery [42]. These women are usually anticoagulated and coagulation should be normalized before any attempt is made to use a regional technique. The anaesthetic options are either a carefully titrated regional technique or a 'cardiac' anaesthetic, both followed by postoperative intensive care.

HEART AND HEART–LUNG TRANSPLANTATION

Women of childbearing years (e.g. postpartum cardiomyopathy) are now receiving heart transplants and a few are embarking on pregnancy following this intervention. The potential problems are two-fold: firstly, graft function and secondly, the need for immunotherapy and the fine balance between graft rejection and infection. This latter problem is common to women with other allografts (e.g. renal transplants). Providing there is no rejection, graft function should be well maintained; the presence or absence of histological changes accompanying rejection will be monitored closely by intracardiac biopsies. Because the graft is denervated there is an absence of the usual dominant vagal tone and the resting heart beat is slightly faster than normal. There is no cardiac response to indirectly acting drugs like atropine or neostigmine and the latter, from the cardiac point of view, may be given without atropine or glycopyrrolate. On the other hand sympathetic denervation leads to up-regulation of beta adrenoceptors and extreme sensitivity to adrenaline or isoprenaline. A case report describes profound tachycardia requiring esmolol treatment after the use of epidural 2% lignocaine with 1 in 200 000 adrenaline for caesarean section [43]. General or regional anaesthesia may be used and both are well tolerated as long as the preload is not allowed to fall. Halothane will cause direct myocardial depression but the usual changes in heart rate due to volatile agents are not seen as they rely on an intact autonomic nervous system.

Wagoner *et al.* [44] reviewed 32 heart and heart–lung transplant recipients who had become pregnant: 29 had heart only and three had heart–lung transplants. Of these 32 pregnancies, five miscarried and 27 progressed to delivery (two sets of twins). There were no peripartum maternal or foetal deaths, although three late maternal deaths were reported. Thirty-three per cent were delivered by caesarean section. Premature labour leading on to delivery occured in almost half the total deliveries. Complications during pregnancy included hypertension in 50% and preeclampsia in 25%. Infection or graft rejection occurred in a few, requiring adjustment to the immunotherapy. The most frequent adjustment required was an increase in the dose of cyclosporin to compensate for the decreased plasma levels found in pregnancy. A few

needed alternations in steroid dosage. No foetal abnormalities or neonatal deaths were reported and all children were in good health three years later. Thus with the excellent posttransplantation care these women receive, pregnancy can be contemplated and, if achieved, is likely to have a successful outcome.

MATERNAL RESUSCITATION DURING PREGNANCY AND LABOUR

Cardiopulmonary resuscitation in pregnancy is fraught with problems, not least because it is usually unexpected by staff who have little exposure to such a situation. In addition, because of reduced functional residual capacity and increased oxygen consumption, the pregnant woman is disadvantaged by her tendency to become hypoxic more quickly. After approximately 20 weeks' gestation aortocaval compression becomes significant and reduces the maximum cardiac output achievable during cardiopulmonary resuscitation to a third or less of that achievable in the nonpregnant state [45]. Various manoeuvres have been suggested to reduce aortocaval compression in this setting but they can reduce the efficacy of external cardiac compression. The Cardiff resuscitation wedge has a 27 degrees left lateral inclination: during resuscitation about 80% of the compression force achieved in the supine position can be applied [46]. A human wedge is also described [47]: the patient is supported in a left semilateral position by assistants kneeling and sitting on their heels with the patient resting along their knees and thighs. Using a Laerdal Resusci Anne Skillmeter with this human wedge, both ventilation and external cardiac compressions were performed as well as in the supine position [47]. It should be noted that the photograph accompanying the article [47] has been reversed in printing and mistakenly shows the right lateral position!

As well as using a wedge of some sort the crucial factors in successfully resuscitating a

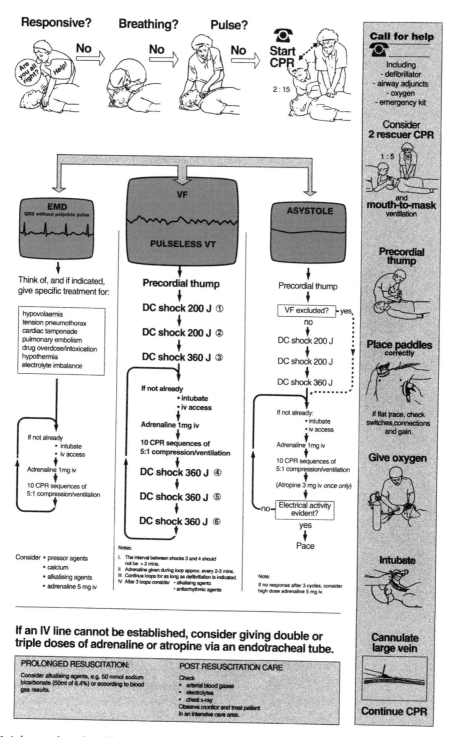

Figure 7.1 Advanced cardiac life support. Reproduced with permission from the European Resuscitation Council, reference [49].

Table 7.4 Successful maternal cardiopulmonary resuscitation needs

- A well-rehearsed team assessed regularly
- A patient wedged in the left lateral position
- Early intubation for oxygenation and protection against aspiration of gastric contents
- Early recourse to caesarean section if resuscitation attempts are not rapidly successful

pregnant woman include early intubation (because of the high risk of aspiration and low compliance of the lungs) and proceeding immediately to caesarean section if spontaneous cardiac output is not achieved within the first five minutes (Table 7.4, Figure 7.1). Delivery of the foetus is so essential to improve the chance of maternal and foetal survival that some units have a simple caesarean section pack on their maternity unit cardiac arrest trolley. Premature delivery of the foetus in this situation should not present an ethical dilemma in terms of foetal versus maternal survival since if the mother dies the foetus cannot survive *in utero*. Resuscitation of a pregnant woman should not be abandoned until after delivery of the infant. Even if this does not save the mother there is a chance that the foetus may survive. Marx reported a series of five women who arrested following the accidental intravenous injection of epidural bupivacaine for caesarean section [48]. Three mothers were delivered by caesarean section within minutes and all infants and mothers survived: the only after-effects were maternal amnesia. In the remaining two cases delivery was delayed for several minutes and although both mothers survived they suffered irreversible brain damage.

CONCLUSION

Pregnancy and delivery are considered by most women to be a normal part of their adult lives and few consider it unsafe. Many complications of pregnancy are unexpected and could not be anticipated preconception. However, women with pre-existing cardiac disease will benefit from preconceptual counselling as many of their cardiac complications can be predicted and managed appropriately by a knowledge of the underlying pathophysiology.

Although the probability of having to manage a complex obstetric cardiac case outwith a tertiary referral centre is small, obstetric anaesthetists should not be complacent. Pre-existing disease can be missed and cardiac problems may arise for the first time in pregnancy or labour. All anaesthetists should have the knowledge to care for these women, even if only during transfer to another unit, so that maternal and foetal survival may be optimized.

REFERENCES

1. Mabie, W.C., DiSessa, T.G., Crocker, L.G. *et al.* (1994) A longitudinal study of cardiac output in normal human pregnancy. *American Journal of Obstetrics and Gynecology*, **170**, 849–56.
2. Sadaniantz, A., Kocheril, A.G., Emaus, S.P. *et al.* (1992) Cardiovascular changes in pregnancy evaluated by two-dimensional and Doppler echocardiography. *American Journal of the Society for Echocardiography*, **5**, 253–8.
3. Mashini, I.S., Albazzaz, S.J. and Fadel, H.E. (1987) Serial non-invasive evaluation of cardiovascular hemodynamics during pregnancy. *American Journal of Obstetrics and Gynecology*, **156**, 1208–13.
4. Clark, S.L., Cotton, D.B., Pivarnik, J. *et al.* (1991) Position change and central hemodynamic profile during normal third-trimester pregnancy and post partum. *American Journal of Obstetrics and Gynecology*, **64**, 883–7.
5. Perloff, J.K. (1988) Pregnancy and cardiovascular disease, in *Heart Disease* (ed. E. Braunwald) W.B. Saunders, Philadelphia, pp. 246–51.
6. Department of Health Welsh Office, Scottish Office Home Health Department, Department of Health and Social Security Report on Health and Social Subjects (1994) *Report on Confidential Enquiries into Maternal Deaths in the United Kingdom 1988–1990*, HMSO, London.
7. MacDonald, A. (1878) *The Bearings of Chronic Disease of the Heart upon Pregnancy, Parturition and Childbed*, J. & A. Churchill, London.

8. Scott, J.S. (1970) Obstetric analgesia: A consideration of labor pain on a patient-controlled technique for its relief with meperidine. *American Journal of Obstetrics and Gynecology*, **106**, 959–78.

9. Podlas, J. and Breland, B.D. (1987) Patient-controlled analgesia with nalbuphine during labour. *Obstetrics and Gynecology*, **70**, 202–4.

10. Szekely, P., Turner, R. and Snaith, L. (1973) Pregnancy and the changing pattern of rheumatic heart disease. *British Heart Journal*, **35**, 1293–303.

11. Sullivan, J.M. and Ramanathan, K.B. (1985) Management of medical problems in pregnancy – severe cardiac disease. *New England Journal of Medicine* , **313**, 304–9.

12. Brian, Jr, J.E., Seifen, A.B., Clark, R.B. *et al.* (1993) Aortic stenosis, cesarean delivery, and epidural anesthesia. *Journal of Clinical Anesthesia*, **5**, 154–7.

13. Ramanathan, S. and Grant, G.J. (1988) Vasopressor therapy for hypotension due to epidural anaesthesia for caesarean section. *Acta Anaesthesiologica Scandinavica*, **32**, 559.

14. Alderson, J.D. (1987) Cardiovascular collapse following epidural anaesthesia for caesarean section in a patient with aortic incompetence. *Anaesthesia*, **42**, 643–5.

15. Mitchell, M.D. and Downing, J.W. (1987) Cardiovascular collapse following epidural anaesthesia for caesarean section. *Anaesthesia*, **42**, 1228–9.

16. Shah D.M. and Sundeji, S.G. (1985) Hypertrophic cardiomyopathy and pregnancy. Report of the maternal mortality and review of the literature. *Obstetrical and Gynecological Survey*, **40**, 444–8.

17. Waagstein, F. (1995) Adrenergic beta-blocking agents in congestive heart failure due to idiopathic dilated cardiomyopathy. *European Heart Journal*, **16**, Supplement O, 128–32.

18. Perloff, J.K. (1994) Congenital heart disease and pregnancy. *Clinical Cardiology*, **17**, 579–87.

19. McNeill, M.J. and Thorburn, J. (1988) Cannulation of the epidural space. *Anaesthesia*, **43**, 154–5.

20. Pitkin, R.M., Perloff, J.K., Koos, B.J. and Beall, M.H. (1990) Pregnancy and congenital heart disease. *Annals of Internal Medicine*, **112**, 445–54.

21. Murdock, J.L., Walker, B.A., Halpern, B.L. *et al.* (1972) Life expectancy and causes of death in the Marfan's syndrome. *New England Journal of Medicine*, **286**, 804–6.

22. Pyeritz, R.E. (1986) The Marfan syndrome. *American Family Physician*, **34**, 83–94.

23. Katz, H. (1922) About the sudden natural death in pregnancy: during delivery and the puerperium. *Archives of Gynaecology*, **115**, 283.

24. Hankins, G.D.V., Wendall, G.D., Leveno, K.H. and Stoneham, J. (1985) Myocardial infarction during pregnancy: a review. *Obstetrics and Gynecology*, **65** 139–46.

25. Sasse, L., Wagner, R., and Murray, F.E. (1975) Transmural myocardial infarction during pregnancy. *American Journal of Cardiology*, **35**, 448–52.

26. Briggs, G.G., Freeman, R.K. and Yaffe, S.J. (eds) (1986) *Drugs in Pregnancy and Lactation*, Williams and Williams, Baltimore.

27. Pfeifer, G.W. (1970) The use of thrombolytic therapy in obstetrics and gynaecology. *Australasian Annals of Medicine*, **19**, 1928–31.

28. Ginz, B. (1970) Myocardial infarction in pregnancy. *Journal of Obstetrics and Gynaecology of the British Commonwealth*, **77**, 610–5.

29. Bembridge, M. and Lyons, G. (1988) Myocardial infarction in the third trimester of pregnancy. *Anaesthesia*, **43**, 202–4.

30. Jaameri, K.E.U., Jahkola, A. and Perttu, J. (1966) On shivering in association with normal delivery. *Acta Obstetrica Gynaecologia Scandinavica*, **45**, 383–8.

31. Chan, V.W.S., Morley-Foster, P.K. and Vosu, H.A. (1987) Temperature changes and shivering after epidural anaesthesia for caesarean section. *Regional Anaesthesia*, **14**, 48–52.

32. Workhoven, M.N. (1986) Intravenous fluid temperature shivering and the parturient. *Anesthesia and Analgesia*, **65**, 496–8.

33. Ponte, J., Collett, B.J. and Walmsley, A. (1986) Anaesthetic temperature and shivering in epidural anaesthesia. *Acta Anaesthesiologica Scandinavica*, **30**, 584–7.

34. Shehabi, Y., Gatt, S., Buckman, T. *et al.* (1990) Effect of adrenaline, fentanyl and warming of injectate on shivering following extradural analgesia in labour. *Anaesthesia and Intensive Care*, **18**, 31–7.

35. Reiz, S., Balfors, E., Sorenson, M.B. *et al.* (1983) Insoflurane – a powerful coronary vasodilator in patients with coronary artery disease. *Anesthesiology*, **59**, 91–7.

36. Leung, J.M., Goehner, P., O'Kelly B.F. *et al.* (1991) Isoflurane anaesthesia and myocardial ischaemia: Comparative risk versus sufentanil anesthesia in patients undergoing coronary artery bypass graft surgery. *Anesthesiology*, **74**, 838–47.

37. *British National Formulary*, March 1996, appendix 4, p. 527.

38. Demakis, J.G. and Rahimtoola, S.H. (1971) Peripartum cardiomyopathy. *Circulation*, **44**, 964–8.

39. Adesonya, C.O., Anjorin, F.I., Sada, I.A. *et al.* (1991) Atrial natriuretic peptide, aldosterone and plasma renin activity in peripartum heart failure. *British Heart Journal*, **65**, 152–4.

40. Demakis, J.G., Rahimtoola, S.H., Sutton, G.C. *et al.* 1971. Natural course of peripartum cardiomyopathy. *Circulation*, **44**, 1053–9.

41. Sutton, M.S.J., Cole, P., Plappert, M. *et al.* (1991) Effects of subsequent pregnancy on left ventricular function in peripartum cardiomyopathy. *American Heart Journal*, **121**, 1776–8.

42. Malinow, A.M., Butterworth, J.F., Johnson, M.D. *et al.* (1985) Peripartum cardiomyopathy presenting at caesarean delivery. *Anesthesiology*, **63**, 545–7.

43. Camann, W.R., Goldman, G.A., Johnson, M.D. *et al.* (1989) Cesarean delivery in a patient with a transplanted heart. *Anesthesiology*, **71**, 618–20.

44. Wagoner, L.E., Taylor, D.O. and Olsen, S.L. (1993) Immunosuppressive therapy, management, and outcome of heart transplant recipients during pregnancy. *Journal of Heart and Lung Transplantation*, **12**, 993–1000.

45. Zakowski, M.I. and Ramanathan, S. (1990) CPR in pregnancy. *Current Review of Clinical Anesthesia*, **10**, 106–8.

46. Rees, G.A. and Willis, B.A. (1988) Resuscitation in late pregnancy. *Anaesthesia*, **43**, 347–9.

47. Goodwin, A.P. and Pearce, A.J. (1992) The human wedge. A manoeuvre to relieve aortocaval compression during resuscitation in late pregnancy. *Anaesthesia*, **47**, 433–4.

48. Marx, G.F. (1982) Cardiopulmonary resuscitation of late-pregnant women. *Anesthesiology*, **56**, 156.

49. Statement by the Advanced Life Support Working Party of the European Resuscitation Council (1992) *Resuscitation*, **24**, 111–21.

R.C. Wilson

INTRODUCTION

Pregnancy is usually associated with youth and good health but when medical problems do occur a significant proportion are due to immune disorders. A wide range of immune problems may occur (acute, subacute or chronic) and can lead to tissue damage which may be localized, organ specific or systemic.

This chapter outlines basic immunological principles and the effects of pregnancy and disease.

IMMUNOLOGY

PRINCIPLES OF IMMUNOLOGY

The immune system has the potential to recognize and respond to a large range of antigens and to distinguish between self and non-self [1]. End immune reactions are dependent either on antibody secreted by B lymphocytes and plasma cells (humoral response), or on T lymphocytes (cell-mediated response) [2].

B cells recognize antigen through their surface receptors known as immunoglobulins (Ig) and, while they can react with antigen in the native form, in general, require growth and differentiation factors (usually supplied by 'helper' T cells responding to the same antigen) in order to proliferate and secrete antibody. 'Helper' T cells (also known as CD4 cells or CD4+) respond to processed antigen associated with histocompatibility molecules (human leucocyte antigen, HLA) on specialized antigen-presenting cells. HLA molecules associate with foreign antigen to stimulate T cells. There are two types of HLA molecule: class I and class II molecules. Class I molecules, which are expressed by most nucleated cells, present peptide fragments derived from cytoplasmic proteins to cytotoxic T cells (most of these cytotoxic T cells are known as CD8+). On binding antigen at the cell surface these cytotoxic cells lyse the target cell. Class II molecules specifically interact with the CD4 antigen carried on 'helper' T cells. Class II molecules are carried on fewer types of cell (normally B lymphocytes and activated T cells), and are essential for the normal activation of B cells and cytotoxic cells. In response to antigen the activated helper T cells divide into two subpopulations, Th_1 and Th_2 cells, each releasing different lymphokines. Th_1 cells are required to initiate the cytotoxic T cell response as antigen presentation by class I or II HLA molecules alone is insufficient to initiate a T cell immune response. Th_1 cells are also responsible for producing delayed hypersensitivity reactions. Th_2

Clinical Problems in Obstetric Anaesthesia
Edited by Ian F. Russell and Gordon Lyons. Published in 1997 by Chapman & Hall, London. ISBN 0 412 71600 3.

cells stimulate antibody (B cell) responses. The final effector mechanism of the immune response is Th$_1$ cells or Th$_2$ cells or a mixture of both, determined by exogenous immunoregulatory factors such as steroids, prostaglandins and cytokines [3].

THE EFFECTS OF PREGNANCY

Fertilization, implantation and the development of the foetoplacental unit involve considerable modification of the immune system. During pregnancy there is a reduction in cell-mediated immunity. Both progesterone and oestrogen suppress T cell proliferation while oestrogen reduces the functional activity of CD8+ cells. There is a fall in the number of CD4+ cells, maximal at about seven months' gestation, rising again towards term to prepregnancy levels. As CD8 cell numbers are unchanged this alters the CD4:CD8 ratio. Pregnancy is a paradoxical state in which foreign tissue is not only tolerated but nurtured. The products of conception constitute an allogenic transplant and thus are potentially rejectable. However in the large majority of women the normally cytotoxic T cells are not generated, and a series of regulatory protective mechanisms is activated which allows the pregnancy to progress. This downregulation of the immune system is associated with the maintenance of, or increase in, maternofoetal defence mechanisms against infection, the latter being equally important in the survival of the pregnancy [4]. There is an increase not only in the number of maternal granulocytes and in the bactericidal and phagocytic properties of neutrophils but also in the concentrations of interferon and agents of inflammation.

Maternofoetal interactions which allow the survival of the foetal allograft include the vascular isolation of the foetus, the trophoblastic barrier, the transmission of passive immunity and the development of the foetal immune system [5].

The trophoblast, a tissue with exceptionally low immunogenicity, does not express cell surface antigens in a form that produces a reaction in the maternal immune system. The trophoblast is highly resistant to lysis by antibodies or immune effector cells and acts as a physical barrier between the mother and foetus preventing major exchanges of macromolecules. Along with the foetus, the trophoblast also produces suppressive factors which control the proliferation and activation of immune cells, thereby further increasing the resistance of trophoblast and foetal tissues to potential damage by the immune system.

The foetus is capable of producing IgM and IgA from about the 11th week of gestation and maternal IgG antibodies are actively transported across the placenta to reach maternal concentrations by 26 weeks. IgG autoantibodies in women with autoimmune disease may also pass into the foetus and produce disease, although the effects are usually transient. Amniotic fluid contributes to foetal protection with concentrations of IgG and IgA rising progressively throughout pregnancy until the 28–30th week. Full immune competence is not achieved until several months after birth.

AUTOIMMUNE DISEASE

Autoimmune disease (AID) occurs when the highly regulated immune response breaks down and becomes directed at self rather than at foreign antigens. AID is often associated with genetic or immunological abnormalities, or exogenous factors such as viruses. HLA class I genes are associated with the predominantly male spondyloarthropathies while class II diseases such as systemic lupus erythematosis (SLE) and myasthenia gravis (MG), are more common in female patients [6]. The pathogenesis of AID is related to autoantibody production and an alteration in the function and number of immunoregulatory T cells and/or the production of anti-idiotypic antibodies. The resulting pathology may affect a single organ (e.g. thyroid) or widespread targets (e.g. joint, muscle).

Expression of AID is influenced by endocrine, haematological and immunological alterations associated with the ovarian cycle, hormone treatment and pregnancy. For instance pregnancy often induces remission or stabilization of AID and relapse then occurs postpartum. Other interactions include the effect of the disease on the pregnancy.

IgE-mediated disease

One of the more common immune disorders occurring in pregnancy is anaphylaxis. True anaphylaxis is triggered by IgE and, on repeated exposure to antigen, produces an immediate and severe reaction involving bronchospasm, cardiovascular collapse and oedema secondary to the massive release of histamine, slow-reacting substance of anaphylaxis and other vasoactive amines. This reaction differs from the clinically similar anaphylactoid reaction, which is mediated by IgE but triggered by acute complement activation after exposure to various substances such as aspirin and non-steroidal anti-inflammatory drugs (NSAIDs). During pregnancy anaphylactic reactions may be triggered by parenteral drugs or solutions (parenteral iron, anaesthetic agents, dextran), and there is increasing awareness of latex exposure (examination gloves, catheters, endotracheal tubes) as a cause [7]. Even delivery itself and possibly amniotic fluid embolism have been implicated in such reactions [8, 9].

Antibody-mediated disease

Antibody-mediated disease is usually caused by the reaction of IgG antibodies with autoantigens, resulting either in complement activation and cell lysis or antibody-dependent cell-mediated cytotoxicity. Autoantigens may develop as a result of alteration by viruses or drugs, or cross-reactivity between extrinsic and intrinsic antigens. The autoantibodies produced may be directed against cell-surface receptors (e.g. Graves' disease, MG, idiopathic thrombocytopenic purpura and autoimmune haemolytic anaemia (AIHA)), adhesion molecules and extracellular matrix (e.g. pemphigus and Goodpasture's syndrome), circulating serum proteins (e.g. antiphospholipid syndrome), cytoplasmic antigens (e.g. diabetes and Wegeners granulomatosis) or nuclear antigens. Autoantibodies also result from exposure to intracellular antigens released by cell damage; these autoantibodies may act as markers for the disease.

Immune-complex-mediated disease

Immune-complex-mediated disease is the basis of the collagen vascular or connective tissue diseases. Circulating antigen–antibody complexes are formed when both antigen and antibody are unbound to tissue. As the immune complexes increase in size they become less soluble and eventually precipitate in various sites (capillary epithelium, renal basement membranes, the anterior chamber of the eye and serous cavities), where complement activation and ultimately cell destruction occur. Immune complex disease is associated with exogenous antigen (infective agents, drugs) as well as endogenous antigens such as nucleic and cytoplasmic components and tumours.

Cell-mediated disease

CD4+ T lymphocytes are involved in various immune effector mechanisms, but classical cell-mediated hypersensitivity is a delayed reaction involving CD4+ T cells, cytokine release and monocyte recruitment. It is the chief reaction against allografted tissue (e.g. renal transplant) and many infectious diseases.

The effects of anaesthesia on the immune system

Anaesthesia has been shown to impair cell-mediated immunity and interfere with natural killer cell activity [10, 11]. Halothane more than other volatile agents causes bone marrow suppression, inhibition of cell mitoses and has a negative effect on lymphocyte migration [12, 13]. Other substances such as sodium thiopentone and local anaesthetic agents also inhibit phagocytosis. The stress of surgery and anaesthesia suppresses lymphocyte function and adversely alters the CD4+/CD8+ ratio for days postoperatively [11].

THE RHEUMATIC DISEASES

The major rheumatic diseases are of particular importance to obstetric anaesthetists because they are common and most have a marked female preponderance, with a disease onset and/or duration that usually spans the reproductive years. The effects of pregnancy on the disease process, and the effects of the disease process on pregnancy, often results in greater morbidity and mortality for both mother and foetus.

There is considerable overlap between the various disorders especially of their systemic complications. The major disorders in this group, and the more common and serious disease manifestations of relevance to the anaesthetist, are described below.

SYSTEMIC LUPUS ERYTHEMATOSUS

Systemic lupus erythematosus (SLE) is the prototypical autoimmune disease. It affects about 1:2000 people but is even commoner in certain groups (e.g. 1:250 black women). The prevalence is far higher in women than men (9:1), especially during the reproductive years, when the ratio rises to about 15:1 affecting up to 1: 1500 pregnancies. The age of onset is usually between 15 and 25 years.

SLE is a systemic, chronic inflammatory disease characterized by exacerbations (flares) and remissions and, when fulminant, may rapidly lead to death, often from renal disease, intracerebral bleeding or status epilepticus. Virtually every organ system can be involved either by direct damage from autoantibodies,

or due to deposition of immune complexes. The commonest symptoms include arthralgia (in 90–100% of patients), rash (80%), fever (75%), neurological and psychiatric problems (60%), nephritis (50%) and pulmonary and pericardial effusions (40–60%). Mild anaemia is frequently found and occasionally a more severe Coombes positive haemolytic anaemia. Hypergammaglobulinaemia occurs associated with a low serum complement. The most common autoantibodies are antinuclear, with double-stranded DNA antibodies the most specific for SLE [14]. A number of other antibodies directed against nucleic and cytoplasmic components are frequently present, several of which are particularly important in obstetric patients (anticardiolipin, anti Ro(SS-A), antiphospholipid antibodies).

Effect of pregnancy on SLE

It is not fully established whether pregnancy exacerbates SLE. The reported incidence of flares during pregnancy varies considerably between studies (0 to 74%) and there appears to be a low risk of flare in the puerperium [15–18]. In common with most autoimmune disorders it is the disease state preconception that best predicts the course of the disease during pregnancy [19]. A first presentation of SLE during pregnancy or postpartum is often particularly severe and associated with a fulminant course but there is no evidence that termination of pregnancy improves maternal outcome [20]. Steroid dosage should not be modified, as a reduction is associated with exacerbation of disease [21]. In patients with lupus nephritis, pregnancy is more likely to be associated with flares and a permanent deterioration in renal function [22]. Hypertension, proteinuria and nephrotic syndrome may accompany lupus nephritis making it very difficult to distinguish from preeclampsia, a condition with an increased incidence (15–25%) in women with SLE. Complement and platelet levels may help differentiate the two conditions [23], allowing more appropriate medical management, for instance increasing doses of steroid in lupus flare [6].

Effect of SLE on pregnancy and the foetus

Women with SLE are at increased risk of early pregnancy loss (11–46%), intra-uterine growth retardation (IUGR) and premature labour. Neonatal lupus erythematosus (NLE) is associated with antibodies to the Ro(SS-A) ribonucleoprotein complex and/or the La(SS-B) protein. Affected infants (7–38%) may have cardiac, systemic or cutaneous manifestations. Congenital complete heart block is irreversible and fatal in approximately one third of those infants affected. There is no correlation with disease severity in the mother [24].

Antiphospholipid syndrome

Phospholipids are constituents of all cell membranes and antibodies to them (antiphospholipid antibodies, APAs) are produced as a result of endogenous and exogenous stimuli. It is those APAs resulting from endogenous stimuli that are associated with thrombosis and adverse pregnancy outcomes (late spontaneous abortion, IUGR, stillbirth) and maternal morbidity (preeclampsia (33%), arterial or venous thromboembolic disease (28–33%), thrombocytopenia and rarely vasculitis) [25]. Cerebral ischaemia, a common neurological manifestation of the syndrome, may be related to cerebral vessel thrombosis and/or cardiac valvular lesions [26]. Complications may also arise after delivery with the development of an autoimmune pleuropulmonary syndrome [27].

The two classes of APAs arising from endogenous stimuli include lupus anticoagulant (LAC) and anticardiolipin antibody (ACA). LAC prolongs phospholipid dependent *in vitro* clotting assays; ACA is recognized by immunoassays using cardiolipin [28]. These APAs occur singly or together in 10–34% of patients with SLE, although the antiphospholipid syndrome also occurs commonly in patients without SLE, or any other defined AID disorder, but in whom there are high levels of ACA or LAC activity. The inhibition of blood coagulation is detected in plasma primarily as an increase in activated partial thromboplastin time (APTT) . Coagulation factor deficiency can be excluded by retesting the sample mixed with normal plasma, when clotting times do not correct to normal. Clinically these results are not a problem as there is no associated *in vivo* bleeding tendency unless there are other antibodies to clotting factors present (e.g. factor VIII), an associated thrombocytopenia or patients are on anticoagulant therapy.

Anaesthetic considerations

Patients with SLE have reduced myocardial reserve often secondary to cardiomyopathy or pericarditis and may have valvular lesions (Libman–Sachs endocarditis). Renal reserve may be reduced and active nephritis should be distinguished from pregnancy-induced hypertension by the presence of renal casts and low complement levels. Other abnormalities include arthritis of the temporomandibular joint (TMJ), interstitial pneumonitis, pulmonary angiitis, thrombocytopenia and coagulation problems [29]. Drug therapy includes intravenous immunoglobulins, steroids, aspirin, anticoagulants and immunosuppressives [30]. Traditionally the presence of LAC, low platelets and aspirin therapy has strongly favoured general anaesthetic techniques [31], but the thromboelastogram (TEG) may permit more regional techniques to be used, with the associated benefits for an already compromised placenta. Neuropsychiatric disorders are common, causing diagnostic confusion with eclampsia if seizures occur, and make regional anaesthesia more challenging [32].

RHEUMATOID ARTHRITIS

Rheumatoid arthritis (RA) is a common condition affecting 1–2% of the population, three times commoner in women than men, and affecting approximately 1 in 1000–2000 pregnancies [6]. It can occur at any age (peak onset 35–50 years), although the juvenile form (JRA) is distinguished clinically from the adult form.

Rheumatoid arthritis is a chronic systemic disease characterized by a symmetrical peripheral polyarthritis, usually beginning with the small joints of the hand and wrist and ultimately affecting most of the joints of the upper and lower limb, the TMJ and the cervical spine. The initial inflammatory synovitis progresses to secondary destructive changes, with swollen painful joints becoming ankylosed or unstable and deformed. RA has a genetic predisposition and the disease is associated with characteristic IgM (classical rheumatoid factor) and IgG autoantibodies.

Effect of pregnancy on RA

Usually, most women with RA who become pregnant begin to improve symptomatically during the first trimester with maximum improvement occurring towards term. However over 90% of these women experience postpartum relapse, often with progression of joint disease. Factors reducing disease activity during pregnancy may include the decrease in cell-mediated immunity and inflammatory reactions, foetal suppression of maternal immunity, immune modification by the placenta, and humoral and circulating factors with anti-inflammatory and immunoregulatory activity, such as pregnancy specific proteins [15,33].

Effect of RA on pregnancy

There is no conclusive evidence that RA causes a significant increase in perinatal morbidity or mortality, although vaginal delivery may be particularly difficult and painful if there is hip involvement.

Anaesthetic considerations

The anaesthetic techniques used for labour and delivery will depend on the degree of the patient's disability as well as her wishes and any obstetric concerns. In addition to joint disease the major systemic manifestations include involvement of the cardiovascular, respiratory, neuromuscular and haematological systems [14].

Cardiovascular system

Pericarditis is common but frequently missed. Nodular disease is associated with an increased incidence of effusion and conduction defects.

Respiratory system

Pleural effusion is common, obstructive airways disease and interstitial fibrosis less frequent. Nodules are a potential cause of cavitation and haemoptysis. The pregnant patient with significant disease may have a marked restrictive defect; the upwardly displaced diaphragm which tends to reduce lung volume and vital capacity is normally accommodated by rib cage flare [34], but this flare can be limited by stiffness of the costochondral joints exacerbating the effects of other pulmonary abnormalities and kyphosis. Decreased diffusion capacity may also contribute to hypoxia.

Neuromuscular

Peripheral neuropathy may be a mild symmetrical glove and stocking type or a more severe sensorimotor mononeuritis multiplex probably secondary to vasculitis of the vasa nervorum. Other forms of neuropathy are secondary to nerve entrapment (particularly of the median, posterior tibial and ulnar nerves) and cervical spine disease. Muscle atrophy occurs due to a polymyositis-like syndrome, drug therapy (steroids, chloroquine) or secondary to joint destruction.

Haematological

A normochromic normocytic anaemia is common. The need for supplementary iron may be indicated by the absence of the often elevated serum ferritin occurring in RA. Thrombocytopenia and neutropenia may occur in Felty's syndrome (an association between RA, splenomegaly and leucopenia, particularly neutropenia). Hepatosplenomegaly occurs in about 11% of patients and mild renal impairment is common.

SYSTEMIC SCLEROSIS (SCLERODERMA)

Systemic sclerosis (SSc) is a multisystem disorder of connective tissue, characterized by abnormal collagen deposition and widespread vascular damage. There is a wide range of clinical expression of the disease including two major subsets: diffuse cutaneous SSc (dcSSc) and limited cutaneous SSc (lcSSc) [14]. The majority of patients are in the latter group with visceral involvement tending to occur after many years; dcSSc is more serious and may rapidly progress to death from cardiac, renal or pulmonary failure. SSc is an uncommon disease (incidence 2–14/million/year), however the problems facing the anaesthetist can be particularly severe. The peak age of onset is 40–50 years with a female:male ratio of 3:1 overall, rising to 10:1 during the reproductive years. The cause of SSc is obscure although genetic and immunological factors are involved, the most frequent abnormality being anticentromere antibodies in lcSSc. Cell-mediated cytotoxicity is implicated in the endothelial cell dysfunction which is central to the widespread microvascular injury.

The clinical course is a series of relapses and remissions and, as with SLE, assessing the effect of pregnancy on the course of the disease is difficult, but the best available evidence is that it has little or none [35]. The effect of SSc on pregnancy is likely to be an increase in foetal morbidity but reported rates vary greatly and have probably been overestimated in the past.

Anaesthetic considerations

The implications for the anaesthetist depend on the extent to which various organs are affected.

Skin

Sclerotic skin and chronic vasoconstriction make venous access difficult; all patients should be kept warm, the delivery room or operating theatre warmed and i.v. fluids warmed with i.v. access in as large and distal a vein as possible. Pulse oximetry and blood pressure recordings may be unreliable and standard monitoring equipment inadequate. An ultrasonic device (e.g. Dinamap®) has proved useful for recording blood pressure [36]. Peripheral vascular spasm makes direct arterial pressure monitoring especially hazardous. Skin contractures can severely limit mouth opening and neck movement making conventional intubation extremely difficult and facemasks fit poorly. Oral and nasal telangiectasias can cause substantial bleeding if traumatized. Sjögren's syndrome may add to difficulties with swallowing and intubation because of an excessively dry mouth and oesophagus.

Gastro-intestinal tract

Oesophageal dysmotility, reflux and gastro-oesophageal sphincter incompetence greatly increase the risk of pulmonary aspiration of gastric contents. Abdominal bloating and malabsorption (of vitamin K) may be significant.

Musculoskeletal

Arthralgia is common, especially of the small joints including the TMJ. Reduced joint mobility, contractures and skin changes may make positioning and performance of regional techniques difficult and these are patients in whom an inadvertent intravenous or intrathecal injection of a large bolus of local anaesthetic would be extremely hazardous. SSc patients may also have an abnormal sensitivity to local anaesthetics resulting in prolonged sensory blockade.

Renal

Renal involvement may occur at any time during pregnancy. It is manifested by hypertension, often of sudden onset. Renal crisis is the commonest cause of mortality in pregnant patients with SSc, presenting usually with accelerated hypertension, or less commonly with rapidly progressive renal failure, proteinuria and micro-angiopathic haemolytic anaemia. Angiotensin converting enzyme inhibitors are the first-line treatment to control hypertension and prevent deterioration in renal function although normally contraindicated in obstetric practice because of the possibilities of teratogenicity, neonatal renal failure and foetal death. As in SLE the distinction between SSc renal crisis and preeclampsia may not be clear clinically, however plasma renin activity will be markedly elevated in the former and low to normal in the latter.

Cardiac

The heart is involved in about 50% of patients, with manifestations including myocardial fibrosis, pericarditis, arrhythmias, conduction defects and pulmonary hypertension (most commonly in patients with lcSSc). Pulmonary hypertension associated with pregnancy has a maternal mortality over 40%.

Pulmonary

Fibrosis, concentrated mainly in the lower lungs, causes a restrictive defect with reduced lung compliance, reduced transfer factor and an increase in residual volume. Severely affected patients may be hypoxic at rest, particularly at term and when recumbent, and need high inflation pressures when ventilated. Aspiration pneumonia is not uncommon.

POLYARTERITIS NODOSA

Polyarteritis nodosa (PAN) is one of a number of systemic necrotizing vasculitides. Classical PAN is a rare multisystem connective tissue disease which is commoner in males (male:female ratio 2:1) with a peak age of onset at 40–50 years. Hence PAN is rare in pregnancy. The chief pathological characteristic is widespread inflammation of small and medium-sized arteries leading to aneurysm formation, thrombosis and infarction. Any part of the body may be affected, commonly kidney, skin, nerve, heart and gut, and the clinical picture is of systemic illness, organ infarction and haemorrhage, neuropathy and myalgia. Hypersensitivity reactions and circulating immune complexes may be causative factors; diagnosis is usually confirmed by biopsy and/or visceral angiography [14].

Very few cases of PAN associated with pregnancy have been reported, but maternal mortality was very high in those patients developing disease during pregnancy [35]. The outcome was better for those patients with established disease in remission at the time of conception. Death usually occurs secondary to renal and cardiac involvement. Treatment is with steroids, cytotoxic agents and immunosuppressives plus organ specific treatments such as antihypertensives.

Anaesthetic considerations

Anaesthetic considerations relate to managing a patient with severe systemic hypertension, renal failure and ischaemic heart disease. Peripheral neuropathy and mononeuritis multiplex occur commonly and should be clearly documented if regional anaesthesia is proposed.

POLYMYOSITIS

There are several clinical types of polymyositis (PM), an inflammatory disease of skeletal muscle characterized by a progressive symmetrical proximal muscle weakness. PM may be associated with cutaneous manifestations (**dermatomyositis**, DM), idiopathic, related to neoplasia or to another autoimmune disease. Apart from a childhood variant associated with vasculitis, the peak onset is between 30–60 years and occurs in females twice as often as males. It is uncommon and associated with genetic, immunological and viral factors. Diagnosis is made by muscle biopsy, electromyography and raised muscle enzymes. In addition there is the characteristic rash of DM [14].

Idiopathic PM or DM is rare in pregnant patients. When it does occur perinatal mortality is increased, and those developing the disease during pregnancy do considerably less well than those with established disease at the time of conception [37].

Anaesthetic considerations

Muscles are not usually tender, but become wasted and atrophic, eventually with contractures. Pharyngeal and respiratory muscle involvement, myocardial fibrosis and pulmonary infiltrates (acute or chronic fibrosing alveolitis) are of concern to anaesthetists, but are extremely uncommon in pregnant patients probably because of the short duration of disease in the relatively young. Difficult intubation is not a feature, but aspiration of pharyngeal secretions or gastric contents, vocal cord dysfunction and respiratory insufficiency may cause postoperative complications [38]. The smaller muscle mass and diminished sensitivity to relaxants mandate the use of neuromuscular monitoring when using these agents. Haematological abnormalities (leucopenia, thrombocytopenia and autoimmune haemolytic anaemia) often occur [39].

ANAESTHETIC MANAGEMENT OF THE COMPLICATIONS OF RHEUMATIC DISEASES

Clearly the overwhelming concerns for anaesthetists in most of these disorders are the potential difficulties with endotracheal intubation and/or adequate ventilation [30, 32, 36, 38, 40].

Musculoskeletal

Arthritis of the TMJ and the cervical spine may make mouth opening and neck extension extremely limited. Cricoarytenoid involvement can result in fixed adduction of the vocal cords or glottic stenosis. These common complications of RA make tracheal intubation, particularly in a patient requiring caesarian section, incomparably difficult and hazardous. If such a venture is proposed, a full assessment of the extent of damage to these structures is mandatory. If there is serious peripheral arthritis it should be assumed that the neck is potentially unstable. Signs and symptoms of possible problems include hoarseness, dysphagia, dyspnoea, stridor, neck pain, stiffness, visual or vestibular symptoms and sensory or motor disturbances. Mouth opening, neck movement and laryngeal function must be assessed and if there is concern about the neck the only safe options for general anaesthesia are an awake (preferably fibreoptic) intubation, or an elective tracheostomy. In an emergency, a percutaneous tracheostomy or cricothyroidotomy may be faster and safer (if appropriate expertise and equipment are available). As a last resort, a laryngeal mask or combined laryngeal mask and oesophageal tube (e.g. Combitube; Sheridan) may be placed and the patient kept as head up as possible [41].

Examination may need to include mouth opening (should be >4 cm), mandibular protrusion [42] and Mallampati scoring [43], indirect fibreoptic laryngoscopy and radiological studies [44, 45] of the cervical spine.

Anterior subluxation is present when the distance between the posterior arch of the axis and the anterior surface of the odontoid peg >3–4 mm. Subaxial subluxation is diagnosed by a loss of alignment >2 mm between the posterior surfaces of two adjacent vertebral bodies.

The use of a soft collar to act as a visual reminder to take particular care of the neck (even in the conscious patient) is recommended as the majority of patients with RA have involvement of the cervical spine even if asymptomatic [46]. Great care must be paid to protecting joints and other parts of the body from an unusual range of movement or weight bearing during anaesthesia. Involvement of the hips may limit flexion and abduction (stirrups!) and hinder positioning for regional anaesthesia. The sequelae of JRA commonly result in the need for operative delivery [47]. Muscles may be wasted and atrophic secondary to the disease process, drug therapy, neurological problems or painful and immobile joints. Pharyngeal and respiratory muscles are of particular concern as airway protection and adequate ventilation are problems exacerbated in the anaesthetized pregnant patient at term. Evidence of dysphagia and regurgitation should be sought and an assessment made of exercise tolerance and respiratory reserve, possibly with arterial blood gases and pulmonary function tests. Weakness of the muscles of respiration may cause respiratory insufficiency after general anaesthesia, following a high regional block or after opiate administration.

Cardiovascular

A degree of cardiac involvement is common even if subclinical, and should be looked for. Patients with SLE, SSc and JRA can have very serious cardiovascular pathology. Pericarditis and effusions, myocarditis and conduction defects will diminish myocardial reserve and valvulitis may result in mitral or aortic incompetence. An electrocardiogram and if necessary an echocardiogram should be obtained preoperatively. Patients should have their cardiac function optimized before surgery and monitored perioperatively, including a pulmonary artery catheter if necessary. The facility to pace the heart may be required. Regional blocks are often desirable and appropriate for

patients with significant cardiac disease but demand experienced personnel, invasive haemodynamic monitoring perioperatively, high-dependency care facilities and, above all, a flexible, cautious and titratable technique. Hypotension following a regional block can be catastrophic and irretrievable. A 'cardiac' general anaesthetic is sometimes preferable and the paediatricians should be warned to expect a narcotized baby. Antibiotic prophylaxis may be required for labour and delivery.

Vasculitis is common and, when severe, leads to visceral infarction, gangrene, organ failure and death. The skin and extremities need particular care when handling and positioning to avoid further damage especially from pressure effects. Patients should be kept warm and infused fluids should be warmed. Hypotension may be marked in patients who are chronically vasoconstricted.

Pulmonary

Given that a normal chest X-ray does not preclude significant lung disease pulmonary function tests and arterial blood gases may be indicated in addition to pulse oximetry prior to anaesthesia. Pulmonary function should be optimized preoperatively with treatment of infection, reversible airways disease and pleural effusions. An epidural is recommended for labour and delivery to avoid the use of opiates, and potentially deleterious episodes of desaturation associated with the hyper/hypoventilation cycle of painful contractions. Care must be taken with the upper level of a block in any patient whose ventilatory reserve gives cause for concern, and small or dilute doses and a titratable technique are advised. A single-shot spinal is not recommended and epidural blockade must be established only with great caution. Monitoring should include the upper level of the block, peak flow readings, respiratory rate and continuous pulse oximetry. A suitable technique for surgery in high-risk patients includes an intrathecal catheter and small incremental doses of bupivacaine (in concentration ≤0.5%) [48]. If a general anaesthetic is used as the primary technique the possibility of adjuvant epidural analgesia could be considered. The risks of respiratory depression and undue sedation with opiate analgesia may be reduced with a patient-controlled analgesia system (PCAS) and pulse oximetry monitoring. Post-operative supervision should continue for at least 24 hours and treatment with antibiotics, bronchodilators and physiotherapy should be maintained.

Renal

Control of hypertension can be a major problem particularly in patients with SLE, SSc and PAN. Epidural analgesia should be employed where possible to attenuate further rises in blood pressure associated with labour and delivery. Preeclampsia may co-exist in patients with renal disease and management requires careful attention to fluid balance, coagulation and drug therapy. In patients with mild renal impairment, NSAIDs often used for postoperative analgesia should be avoided, as should prolonged perioperative fluid restriction.

Haematological

Anaemia may require preoperative transfusion or necessitate having blood cross-matched and readily available on the delivery suite. Cross-matching can take longer than usual in some patients with significant antibodies (e.g. antiphospholipid syndrome). Thrombocytopenia and coagulation problems may preclude an epidural; a TEG is the investigation of choice if in doubt, rather than arbitrary limits on laboratory indices. A single-shot spinal with a fine (<25 G) pencil point needle may remain an option in experienced hands. Complex problems such as Felty's syndrome will require specialist advice and frequent monitoring of coagulation and platelets. A low white count exposes the patient to additional

risk of sepsis and scrupulous aseptic technique must be maintained for invasive procedures.

Drugs

As steroids, given in relatively large doses for prolonged periods, are the mainstay of therapy for most of these disorders, side effects should be expected: obesity, glucose intolerance, friable skin and blood vessels, osteoporosis, reduced resistance to infection and reduced wound healing. Steroid cover for operative procedures is usually necessary and great care must be taken to avoid infection. Immunosuppressant therapy is also common and increases the risk of infection. Caution may be required when using muscle relaxants because of reduced muscle mass or altered sensitivity, e.g. dermatomyositis, cyclosporin therapy.

Neurological

A variety of peripheral neuropathies occur commonly in immune disorders. Traditionally, pre-existing neurological pathology has often been seen as a contraindication to a neuraxial block, but the benefits of such techniques should not be denied to patients if the lesion(s) has been formally examined and documented and the risks fully explained. Appropriate follow-up is obviously necessary to record recovery or manage sequelae.

Gastro-intestinal

The dangers of gastric aspiration are exacerbated in patients with oropharyngeal pathology, cervical spine disease and dysmotility problems. The standard preoperative regimen of metoclopromide, H_2 antagonists and 0.3 M sodium citrate is mandatory, with preoperative stomach emptying as a bonus if it is possible. General anaesthesia requires meticulous attention to induction and emergence, with stomach emptying via a large-bore orogastric tube prior to extubation in the left lateral position, when adequate ventilation and protective airway reflexes have returned.

IMMUNODEFICIENCY SYNDROMES

HIV AND AIDS

Human immunodeficiency virus (HIV-1) was first described in 1981 and within a few years the acquired immunodeficiency syndrome (AIDS), the long term consequence of infection with HIV-1, has become a leading cause of death in women aged 15–44 years in some countries [49, 50]. The prevalence of HIV-1 in pregnant women in the UK has risen from 0.18% in 1990 to 0.26% in 1993 and is highest (0.3%) in women aged 20–30 years in London. The prevalence of HIV-1 in rural areas and of HIV-2 infection is much lower (0.007–0.002%) [51]. Globally, transmission of the virus in 70–80% of cases is sexual (mostly heterosexual), 8–15% parenterally from blood transfusion or intravenous drug use (IVDU) and 5–10% perinatally. In the UK more than half of the cases of AIDS in women since 1982 are due to heterosexual contact and less than a quarter due to IVDU [52].

HIV-1 and HIV-2 (identified in 1986 as serologically and molecularly different but producing the same disease) are cytopathic retroviruses which infect by binding to a receptor on a host target cell. The receptor for HIV is the CD4 molecule on T helper lymphocytes and other cells. HIV binds to CD4+ cells, kills them, and thus may interfere with all immune responses. Patients with HIV infection are asymptomatic for a variable time but eventually develop non-specific constitutional symptoms such as weight loss and malaise and progress to AIDS-defining conditions, which include central nervous system (CNS) disease, unusual tumours and opportunistic infections.

Zidovudine (azido thymidine, AZT) is the mainstay of treatment in pregnant women as it reduces the rate of perinatal virus transmission [53, 54], but it may be associated with anaemia,

neutropenia, thrombocytopenia and a myopathy. Other drug therapy is directed towards the prevention or treatment of active infection, the most common in pregnancy being *Pneumocystic carinii* pneumonia (PCP), herpes, toxoplasmosis, candidiasis and tuberculosis. Complications of infection or drug treatment may cause respiratory, cardiac, renal, hepatic or haematological dysfunction.

The effect of pregnancy on HIV/AIDS

During a normal pregnancy there is a fall in CD4 cell count compared to the postpartum period. The CD4+ lymphocyte count falls more rapidly in HIV positive pregnant women and tends not to rise in the postpartum period. If the count falls to a very low level (<200 cells/mm^3), the possibility of opportunistic infection, particularly PCP, is increased and prophylaxis with antiviral and anti-pneumocystis drugs should be considered [55, 56]. PCP is often fulminant in pregnancy with a high morbidity and mortality. Early studies suggested several factors may affect the progression of HIV infection to AIDS including pregnancy, age, drug use and smoking, but more recent work found that differences in disease progression were more likely due to differing medical care [57]. About 50% of patients with HIV infection will progress to AIDS in ten years; the one-year survival rate once AIDS has developed is only 50% and the three year survival rate is 20%. Pregnancy does not appear to influence the rate of disease progression. Short-term outcomes in pregnancy, such as birth weight and gestational age, are not substantially altered by HIV infection [58], although when clinical illness develops inevitably a pregnancy can be adversely affected.

The effect of HIV/AIDS on pregnancy

In women infected with HIV neither the early reports of a dysmorphic syndrome in their infants, nor the suspected increased rate of spontaneous abortion have been confirmed. When asymptomatic, and controlling for other factors such as drug abuse and poverty, there are only slight effects on the rates of preterm births, IUGR and foetal mortality [59]. Infection is a major concern given that the CD4 count is reduced in pregnancy anyway and the absolute number of CD4 lymphocytes is related to infection risk; a low CD4 count (<200–300 cells/mm^3) is associated with an increase in serious infections such as hepatitis B, cytomegalovirus (CMV), toxoplasmosis and PCP.

The chief problem of HIV infection in pregnancy is the risk of vertical viral transmission to the foetus. Reported rates range from 13% and increasing in Europe, to 40–50% in Africa [49, 60]. Viral transmission may occur *in utero*, intrapartum or postpartum (largely from breast feeding). The perinatal transmission rate increases the lower the maternal CD4 count, and the prognosis is worse for the infant the earlier in pregnancy the foetal infection occurs. The majority of transmissions occur at or near the time of birth. The mode of delivery does not appear to affect the intrapartum rate of infection, although there is a higher incidence of infection for first born twins during vaginal delivery [61]. The routine use of foetal scalp electrodes, scalp pH sampling and artificial rupturing of membranes should be avoided in infected mothers.

Anaesthetic considerations

Multiple organ systems may be affected. Respiratory infections of a severe and resistant nature are common and may be exacerbated by general anaesthesia. HIV infection is not transmitted by airborne particles but a filter capable of trapping small particles (down to 0.2 μm) placed between the patient and the anaesthetic machine should prevent contamination and is a sensible precaution [62]. (Recent recommendations are that an appropriate filter should be placed between the patient and the breathing system for every anaesthetized patient [63].)

Cardiac disease, especially valvular lesions associated with IVDU, may require perioperative medical management and invasive monitoring. Dysrhythmias and cardiomyopathy are also common in more advanced disease. Oropharyngeal lesions (candidiasis, Kaposi's sarcoma) may present difficulties with intubation, and debilitating diarrhoea and anorexia can produce fluid and electrolyte abnormalities which need preoperative correction [64]. Other concerns include the haematological manifestations of advanced HIV infection: anaemia, leucopenia and AIDS-related thrombocytopenia are common. Clinically similar to ITP, AIDS-related thrombocytopenia rapidly improves once treatment with AZT is started. A lupus-like anticoagulant has been described associated with malignancy and opportunistic infections causing a raised APTT and PT and abnormal platelet aggregation.

Previously spinal and epidural anaesthesia have been advised against because of the possible risk of introducing the virus into the CNS. It is now recognized that the CNS is involved very early in the natural course of HIV infection and by the time AIDS has developed the majority of patients will have neurological symptoms. The commonest problem is encephalopathy or dementia which can make communication and co-operation with patients difficult. Focal neurological signs occur secondary to vacuolar myelopathy or space-occupying lesions (e.g. tumours, toxoplasmosis), hence raised intracranial pressure is also a potential problem. Several different peripheral nervous system complications may occur, including a distal symmetrical polyneuropathy, mononeuritis multiplex and a demyelinating neuropathy. Neurological deficits should be sought and documented prior to regional anaesthesia and the risks and rewards of these techniques discussed. For example urinary retention related to peripheral nervous system damage by HIV has been reported presenting postpartum or after caesarian section [65], but could easily be confused with problems due to regional anaesthesia. Although the numbers are small to date, parturients managed with regional techniques have suffered no adverse disease progression, or infective or neurological sequelae as a consequence of anaesthetic interventions [66]. This includes the use of an autologous blood patch for post-dural puncture headache (PDPH) [67], albeit with the caveat that these studies have been performed on patients with relatively normal CD4 cell counts (>200 cells/mm^3); the consequences for patients with more advanced disease need further investigation. Whether there is a case for fresh donor blood for patching PDPH in more advanced cases is unknown. Every effort should be made to avoid factors known to increase the risk of PDPH during deliberate spinal puncture [68].

Obstetric patients with HIV infection requesting pain relief for labour or requiring anaesthesia should be offered the same choices as uninfected patients providing clinical circumstances permit. However it is possible that regional anaesthesia which attenuates the neuroendocrine stress response, would have the least deleterious effect on a compromised immune system. Avoidance of halothane anaesthesia or prolonged exposure to nitrous oxide is advisable because of their negative effects on lymphocyte function [69].

Prevention of HIV transmission to health care workers demands universal precautions.

1. Thorough and frequent handwashing after all patient or contaminated fluid contact.
2. Wear protective gowns, gloves, masks and eye protection.
3. Take particular care handling sharps (e.g. avoidance of resheathing needles, disposable containers). Consider double gloving.
4. Avoidance of mouth-to-mouth resuscitation and mouth-to-tube suction devices.
5. Health-care workers with breached or inflamed skin to avoid direct patient contact.

Additional precautions should be taken to reduce the risk of viral transmission to the infant at the time of delivery [70].

ORGAN TRANSPLANTATION

Advances in transplantation surgery have resulted in increasing numbers of women with successful allografts bearing children.

Renal

Improvements in reproductive function invariably follow renal transplantation and a successful pregnancy may result providing the graft is functioning well. There are definite risks for both mother and foetus but of the 65–75% of pregnancies which continue beyond the first trimester, over 90% end successfully despite preterm delivery occurring in 45–60% and IUGR in 20–30% [71]. Impairment in graft function before pregnancy doubles the perinatal mortality rate and the incidence of further deterioration in renal function is increased [72]. Overall, permanent impairment in graft function occurs in 15% of pregnancies, most commonly in those patients developing hypertension or preeclampsia during pregnancy and in those with episodes of rejection in the year prior to conception.

Liver

Pregnancy is also increasingly successful in women after orthotopic liver transplantation (OLT) [73] provided the OLT–conception period is at least 9–12 months, there is no active viral infection and graft function is good. Strict multidisciplinary surveillance is required in addition to the maintenance of immunosuppressive therapy: azothioprine, corticosteroids and cyclosporin A. Primary maternal complications include hypertension, preeclampsia, anaemia and hyperbilirubinaemia. The effects on the foetus can include preterm birth, IUGR and viral infection, particularly CMV. In general if the graft is functioning well, pregnancy appears to have little effect and rejection episodes are uncommon [74].

Anaesthetic considerations

Fluid retention and a hyperdynamic circulation are features of the third trimester of pregnancy, particularly in patients on steroids, and the risk of fluid overload must be balanced against the need for good uteroplacental flow and good blood flow through the graft. Management during anaesthesia requires additional invasive haemodynamic monitoring and careful management of cardiac output and blood pressure. Preeclampsia must be distinguished from hypertension as treatment differs substantially. High doses of corticosteroids and immunosuppressants may lead to electrolyte imbalance, hyperglycaemia and increased infection risk. Potentially nephrotoxic or hepatotoxic agents (e.g. NSAIDs, halothane) should be avoided. If coagulation is not a problem a careful regional technique is recommended but a high index of suspicion should be maintained for untoward events such as uterine rupture. Caesarian section is common because of hypertension, prematurity and premature rupture of membranes and may involve increased technical difficulty and blood loss; specialist advice should be obtained about transfusion requirements.

AUTOIMMUNE ENDOCRINE DISEASE

DIABETES MELLITUS

Diabetes may antedate pregnancy or first become manifest during pregnancy. Autoimmunity is predominantly associated with type 1b diabetes [75] which is clinically indistinguishable from the commoner type 1a (insulin-dependent, juvenile-onset diabetes); although females predominate, patients are usually older (30s) at presentation and have associated islet cell antibodies and sometimes other autoimmune endocrinopathies.

Effect of pregnancy on diabetes

Early in normal pregnancy plasma insulin decreases in line with a progressive decline in maternal plasma glucose but in the last half of pregnancy plasma insulin levels rise due to marked peripheral insulin resistance. Thus diabetic women may need to decrease their insulin dose in early pregnancy and continue to adjust it throughout pregnancy, often nearly doubling their prepregnancy insulin requirements in the third trimester. In general, good glycaemic control becomes more difficult during pregnancy, with adverse foetal consequences occurring in association with hypoglycaemia or with acute or chronic hyperglycaemia. Pregnancy may also accelerate retinopathy and nephropathy in the mother.

Effect of diabetes on pregnancy

Adverse effects on pregnancy are related to the severity, duration and management of the disease. Polyhydramnios, preeclampsia, infection, foetal macrosomia, intra-uterine death, congenital malformations and neonatal hypoglycaemia may occur [76, 77]. With careful planning of pregnancies and strict glycaemic control perinatal mortality has improved greatly but is still double the norm, and maternal mortality is increased compared with non-diabetic patients. The need for intensive insulin therapy to optimize pregnancy outcome must be balanced with the risks of potentially life-threatening hypoglycaemia. Other acute complications of diabetes include keto-acidosis, hyperosmolar non-ketotic syndrome and lactic acidosis [78]. Intensive insulin therapy may delay the onset and progression of chronic complications in the mother:

- coronary artery disease;
- cerebrovascular disease;
- peripheral arterial disease;
- cardiomyopathy;
- hypertension;

- nephropathy;
- peripheral neuropathy;
- autonomic neuropathy;
- proliferative retinopathy.

Anaesthetic considerations

During labour epidural analgesia is advisable to increase uteroplacental blood flow and reduce potential foetal acidosis. Regional anaesthesia is often preferable in diabetic patients scheduled for caesarean section since it may avoid prolonged perioperative fasting and does not mask hypoglycaemia like general anaesthesia. Prior to regional anaesthesia neurological problems should be sought and documented, with particular attention to sensorimotor deficits and autonomic dysfunction.

Common signs of autonomic neuropathy, including sinus tachycardia, gastroparesis and orthostatic hypotension, may also be present in normal pregnant women at term, especially if in labour. Autonomic neuropathy is commoner in hypertensive patients [79] and hypotension following a regional block or induction of general anaesthesia may be profound and prolonged. There is also a risk of refractory bradycardia which can lead to cardiac arrest. An epidural may be preferable to a one-shot spinal technique in diabetic patients with longstanding (>10 years) disease because of the risk of cardiomyopathy and autonomic neuropathy [80–82], although a further potential hazard to be aware of is anterior spinal artery thrombosis after epidural anaesthesia [83].

Monitoring of plasma glucose and electrolytes is important during any type of anaesthesia and a suitable insulin regimen should be established (e.g. Alberti's glucose–insulin–potassium [84] or separate insulin and glucose infusions). Insulin requirements decrease dramatically after delivery of the placenta.

In addition to the possible dangers of gastroparesis and cardiovascular instability at induction, stiff joint syndrome may make intubation hazardous. Stiff joint syndrome is a complication of diabetes and is associated with rapidly progressive microangiopathy, non-familial short stature, tight waxy skin and limited joint mobility [85]. Intubation difficulties are due to glycosylation of cervical and laryngeal tissues combined with microvascular disease of the atlanto-occipital joint. The prayer sign (palmar surfaces of the phalangeal joints cannot approximate) or defective palm prints are useful predictors of difficult intubation.

THYROID DISEASE

The incidence of autoimmune disease of the thyroid approaches 10% in women; Graves' disease (GD) and Hashimoto's thyroiditis are the two main disorders. Patients may be hyperthyroid, euthyroid or hypothyroid, depending on the balance of thyroid stimulating immunoglobulins (usually occurring in GD), which may stimulate or inhibit thyroid function, and antimicrosomal and antithyroglobulin antibodies (usually Hashimoto's) [15]. Autoimmune thyroid disease is also associated with an increased incidence of postpartum lymphocytic thyroiditis and hypothyroidism and a risk of accelerated thyroid neoplasia during pregnancy [86].

Levels of thyroid-stimulating hormone (TSH) are not altered in normal pregnancy, but total serum tri-iodothyronine (T_3) and thyroxine (T_4) are increased because oestrogen stimulates an increase in thyroid-binding globulin production; free T_3 and T_4 are in the normal range.

Hyperthyroidism occurs in 0.05–0.2% of pregnancies and may be due to GD, multinodular goitre or thyroiditis. As with most other autoimmune disorders amelioration during pregnancy is typically accompanied by exacerbation after delivery. Serious complications include congestive cardiac failure and thyroid crisis. Thyroid autoimmunity is associated with an increased risk of spontaneous abortion, prematurity and congenital malformations. Although maternal symptoms may be controlled, transplacental transfer of immuno-globulins may cause IUGR, IUD and neonatal thyrotoxicosis or hypothyroidism [24].

Maternal **hypothyroidism** is usually iatrogenic or due to Hashimoto's thyroiditis. It is rarely severe in pregnancy as hypothyroidism is associated with anovulation and infertility but when it does occur it is associated with preeclampsia, anaemia and haemorrhage. In women with autoimmune thyroid disease who are euthyroid at booking, subclinical hypothyroidism may develop progressively during pregnancy. An elevated TSH is a reliable sign of diminishing thyroid function.

Anaesthetic considerations

Patients may be on thioamides to inhibit thyroid hormone synthesis, β-blockers to control symptoms of thyrotoxicosis, as well as iodides, steroids or thyroxine replacement. If preeclampsia, anaemia and cardiac dysfunction develop they will need assessment and treatment before anaesthesia. Goitre or nodular disease of the thyroid may make intubation difficult and predispose to postoperative ventilatory problems. The possibility of concurrent steroid deficiency should be considered if the patient becomes unduly hypotensive perioperatively. Epidural analgesia is recommended for labour and delivery to blunt sympathomimetic responses.

CONCLUSION

This chapter outlines some principles of immunology. This is one of the fastest developing medical specialties and much of what readers may have learned at medical school will now be obsolete. The greater understanding of the immune system and its disorders has led to the identification and reclassification of some diseases and the potential for new therapies. As many of these medical conditions commonly occur in young women, it is particularly important for the obstetric anaesthetist to have a working knowledge of the range of possible problems and pathologies which may be encountered. Certain immune disorders such as MG, immune thrombocytopenic purpura and AIHA have been excluded here since they have been dealt with in other chapters relating to the organ system primarily affected. The most important point in managing the labour and delivery of women with these complications is good communication and co-operation between the anaesthetists, obstetricians and physicians who care for them.

REFERENCES

1. McMichael, A.J. (1995) Principles of immunology, in *Oxford Textbook of Medicine*, 3rd edn (eds D.J. Weatherall, J.G.G. Ledingham and D.A. Warrell), Oxford Medical Publications, Oxford, **1**(5.1), pp. 141–54.
2. Bell, J.I. and O'Hehir, R.E. (1995) Immune mechanisms of disease, in *Oxford Textbook of Medicine*, 3rd edn (eds D.J. Weatherall, J.G.G. Ledingham and D.A. Warrell), Oxford Medical Publications, Oxford, **1**(5.2), pp. 154–65.
3. Dudley, D.J. (1992) The immune system in health and disease. *Baillière's Clinical Obstetrics and Gynaecology*, **6**, 393–416.
4. Marsico, S., Pizzo, A., Grioli, M.F. and Scriva, D. (1994) Fisiologia e patologia immune della riproduzione. *Minerva Ginecologica*, **46**, 223–33.
5. Billington, W.D. (1992) The normal fetomaternal immune relationship. *Baillière's Clinical Obstetrics and Gynaecology*, **6**, 417–38.
6. Floyd, R.C. and Roberts, W.E. (1992) Autoimmune diseases in pregnancy. *Obstetrics and Gynecology Clinics of North America*, **19**, 719–32.
7. Stewart, P.D. and Bogod, D. (1995) Latex anaphylaxis during late pregnancy. *International Journal of Obstetric Anaesthesia*, **4**, 48–50.
8. Smith, H.S., Hare, M.J., Hoggarth, C.E. and Assem, E.S.K. (1985) Delivery as a cause of exercise-induced anaphylactoid reaction: a case report. *British Journal of Obstetic Gynaecology*, **92**, 1196–8.
9. Howes, L.J. (1995) Anaphylactoid reaction possibly caused by amniotic fluid embolism. *International Journal of Obstetric Anaesthesia*, **4**, 51–4.
10. Waymack, J.P., Warden, G.D., Alexander, J.W. *et al.* (1987) Effect of blood transfusion and anaesthesia on resistance to bacterial peritonitis. *Journal of Surgical Research*, **42**, 528–35.

11. Scannell, K. (1989) Surgery and human immunodeficiency virus disease. *Journal of Acquired Deficiency Syndromes,* **2,** 43–53.

12. Thomson, D.A. (1987) Anaesthesia and the immune system. *Journal of Burn Care and Rehabilitation,* **18,** 483–7.

13. Salo, M. (1992) Effects of anaesthesia and surgery on the immune response. *Acta Anaesthesiologica Scandinavia,* **36,** 201–20.

14. Maddison, P.J., Isenberg, D.A., Woo, P. and Glass, D.N. (eds) (1993) *Oxford Textbook of Rheumatology,* Oxford Medical Publications, Oxford.

15. Silver, R.M. and Ware Branch, D. (1992) Autoimmune disease in pregnancy. *Baillière's Clinical Obstetrics and Gynaecology,* **6,** 565–600.

16. Lockshin, M.D. (1989) Pregnancy does not cause systemic lupus erythematosus to worsen. *Arthritis and Rheumatism,* **32,** 665–70.

17. Lockshin, M.D., Reinits, E., Druzin, M.L. *et al.* (1984) Case-control prospective study demonstrating absence of lupus exacerbation during or after pregnancy. *American Journal of Medicine,* **77,** 893.

18. Nossent, H.C. and Swaak, T.J.G. (1990) SLE. VI. Analysis of the inter-relationship with pregnancy. *Journal of Rheumatology,* **17,** 771–6.

19. Ramsey-Goldman, R. (1988) Pregnancy in SLE. *Rheumatic Diseases Clinics of North America,* **14,** 169–85.

20. Zulman, J.I., Talal, N., Hoffman, G.S. *et al.* (1979) Problems associated with the management of pregnancies in patients with SLE. *Journal of Rheumatology,* **7,** 37–49.

21. Varner, M.W., Meehan, R.T., Syrop, C.H. *et al.* (1983) Pregnancy in patients with SLE. *American Journal of Obstetrics and Gynecology,* **145,** 1025–37.

22. Bobrie, G., Liote, F., Houillier, P., *et al.* (1987) Pregnancy in lupus nephritis and related disorders. *American Journal of Kidney Diseases,* **9,** 339–43.

23. Abramson, S.B. and Buyon, J.P. (1992) Activation of the complement pathway: comparison of normal pregnancy, preeclampsia, and systemic lupus erythematosus during pregnancy. *American Journal of Reproductive Immunology,* **28,** 183–7.

24. Giacoia, G.P. and Azubuike, K. (1991) Autoimmune diseases in pregnancy: their effect on the fetus and newborn. *Obstetrical and Gynecological Survey,* **46,** 723–31.

25. Pattison, N.S.P., Chamley, L.W., McKay, E.J. *et al.* (1993) Antiphospholipid antibodies in pregnancy: prevalence and clinical associations. *British Journal of Obstetrics and Gynaecology,* **100,** 909–13.

26. Hughes, G.R.V. (1993) The antiphospholipid syndrome: ten years on. *Lancet,* **342,** 341– 4.

27. Ayres, M.A. and Sulak, P.J. (1991) Pregnancy complicated by antiphospholipid antibodies. *Southern Medical Journal,* **84,** 266–9.

28. Lockwood, C.J. and Rand, J.H. (1994) The immunobiology and obstetrical consequences of antiphospholipid antibodies. *Obstetrical and Gynecological Survey,* **49,** 432–41.

29. Mills, J.A. (1994) Systemic lupus erythematosus. *New England Journal of Medicine,* **330,** 1871–9.

30. Milhet, E., Bouthors-Ducloy, A.S., Krivosic-Horber, R. *et al* (1991) Obstetric anaesthesia in patients with systemic lupus erythematosus. *Annales Franc D'Anesthes Reanimation,* **10,** 242–7.

31. Malinow, A.M., Rickford, W.J.K., Mokriski, B.L.K. *et al.* (1987) Lupus anticoagulant. Implications for obstetric anaesthetists. *Anaesthesia,* **42,** 1291–3.

32. Davies, S.R. (1991) Systemic lupus erythematosus and the obstetrical patient – implications for the anaesthetist. *Canadian Journal of Anaesthesia,* **38,** 790–6.

33. Gilbert, C. (1994) Neurotransmitter status and remission of rheumatoid arthritis in pregnancy. *Journal of Rheumatology,* **21,** 1056–60.

34. Gianopoulos, J.G. (1995) Establishing the criteria for anesthesia and other precautions for surgery during pregnancy. *Surgical Clinics of North America,* **75,** 33–45.

35. Friedman, S.A., Bernstein, M.S. and Kitzmiller, J.L. (1991) Pregnancy complicated by collagen vascular disease. *Obstetrics and Gynecology Clinics of North America,* **18,** 213–6.

36. Thompson, J. and Conklin, K.A. (1983) Anesthetic management of a pregnant patient with scleroderma. *Anesthesiology,* **59,** 69–71.

37. Gutierrez, G., Dagnino, R. and Mintz, G. (1984) Polymyositis/dermatomyositis and pregnancy. *Arthritis and Rheumatism,* **27,** 291–4.

38. Khan, F.A., Anjum, I. and Kamal, R.S. (1991) Anaesthetic hazards in dermatomyositis. *Journal of the Pakistan Medical Association,* **41,** 69–71.

39. Pinheiro, G. da RC., Goldenberg, J., Atra, E. *et al.* (1992) Juvenile dermatomyositis and pregnancy: report and literature review. *Journal of Rheumatology,* **19,** 1798–801.

40. Khanam, T. (1994) Anaesthetic risks in rheumatoid arthritis. *British Journal of Hospital Medicine,* **52,** 320–5.

41. Calder, I., Ordman, A.J., Jackowski, A. *et al.* (1990) The brain laryngeal mask airway. An alternative to emergency tracheal intubation. *Anaesthesia*, **45**, 137–9.

42. Calder, I. (1992) Predicting difficult intubation. *Anaesthesia*, **487**, 528–9.

43. Mallampati, S.R., Gatt, S.P., Gugino, L.D. *et al.* (1985) A clinical sign to predict difficult tracheal intubation: a prospective study. *Canadian Journal of Anaesthesia*, **32**, 429–34.

44. Sharp, J. and Purser D.W. (1961) Spontaneous atlanto-axial dislocation in ankylosing spondylitis and rheumatoid arthritis. *Annals of the Rheumatic Diseases*, **20**, 47–74.

45. Weissman, B.N., Aliabadi, P., Weinfield, M.S. *et al* (1982) Prognostic features of atlanto- axial subluxations in rheumatoid arthritis. *Radiology*, **144**, 745–51.

46. Conlan, P.N., Isdale, I.C. and Rose, B.S. (1971) Rheumatoid arthritis of the cervical spine. An analysis of 333 cases. *Annals of the Rheumatic Diseases*, **25**, 120–6.

47. Ostensen, M. (1991) Pregnancy in patients with a history of juvenile rheumatoid arthritis. *Arthritis and Rheumatism*, **34**, 881–7.

48. Dresner, M.R. and Maclean, A.R. (1995) Anaesthesia for Caesarian section in a patient with Klippel–Feil syndrome. The use of a microspinal catheter. *Anaesthesia*, **50**, 807–9.

49. Kesson, A.M. and Sorrell, T.C. (1993) Human immunodeficiency virus infection in pregnancy. *Baillière's Clinical Obstetrics and Gynaecology*, **7**, 45–74.

50. Priolo, L. and Minkoff, H.L. (1992) HIV infection in women. *Baillière's Clinical Obstetrics and Gynaecology*, **6**, 617–28.

51. Nicoll, A., Hutchinson, E., Soldan, K. *et al.* (1994) Survey of human immunodeficiency virus infection among pregnant women in England and Wales: 1990–1993. *Communicable Disease Report. CDR Review*, **4**, R115–120.

52. Johnson, A.M. (1992) Epidemiology of HIV infection in women. *Baillière's HIV Infection in Obstetrics and Gynaecology*, **6**, 13–33.

53. Connor, E.M., Sperling, R.S., Gelber, R. *et al.* (1994) Reduction of maternal–infant transmission of human immunodeficiency virus type 1 with zidovudine treatment. Paediatric AIDS Clinical Trials Group Protocol 076 Study Group. *New England of Medicine*, **331**, 1173–80.

54. Connor, E.M. and Mofenson, L.M. (1995) Zidovudine for the reduction of perinatal human immunodeficiency virus transmission: Paediatric AIDS Clinical Trials Group Protocol 076 – results and treatment recommendations. *Pediatric Infectious Disease Journal*, **14**, 536- -41.

55. Sperling, R.S. and Stratton, P. (1992) Treatment options for human immunodeficiency virus-infected pregnant women. Obstetric–Gynecologic Working Group of the AIDS Clinical Trials Group of the National Institute of Allergy and Infectious Diseases. *Obstetrics and Gynecology*, **79**, 443–8.

56. Vermund, S.H., Galbraith, M.A., Ebner, S.C. *et al.* (1992) Human immunodeficiency virus/acquired immunodeficiency syndrome in pregnant women. *Annals of Epidemiology*, **2**, 773–803.

57. Chaisson, R.E., Keruly, B.S.N. and Moore, R.D. (1995) Race, sex, drug use and progression of human immunodeficiency virus disease. *New England Journal of Medicine*, **333**, 751–6.

58. Minkoff, H.L., Henderson, C., Mendez, H. *et al.* (1990) Pregnancy outcomes among women infected with HIV and matched controls. *American Journal of Obstetrics and Gynecology*, **163**, 1598–603.

59. Walker, C.K. and Sweet, R.L. (1992) Pregnancy and paediatric HIV infection. *Current Opinion in Infectious Diseases*, **5**, 201–13.

60. Ades, A.E., Davison, C.F., Holland, F.J. *et al* (1993) Vertically transmitted HIV infection in the British Isles. *British Medical Journal*, **306**, 1296–9.

61. Goedert, J.J., Duliège, A.M., Amos, C.I. *et al.* and the International Registry of HIV- exposed twins (1991) High risk of HIV-1 infection for first born twins. *Lancet*, **38**, 1471–5.

62. Berry, A.J. and Nolte, F.S. (1991) An alternative strategy for infection control of anesthesia breathing circuits: A laboratory assessment of the PALL–HME filter. *Anesthesia and Analgesia*, **72**, 651–5.

63. A report received by the Council of the Association of Anaesthetists on blood borne viruses and anaesthesia. The Association of Anaesthetists of Great Britain and Ireland, January 1996.

64. Halpern, S. and Preston, R. (1994) HIV infection in the parturient. *International Anesthesiology Clinics*, **32**, 11–30.

65. Verkuyl, D.A. (1995) Practising obstetrics and gynaecology in areas with a high prevalence of HIV infection. *Lancet*, **346**, 293–6.

66. Hughes, S.C., Dailey, P.A., Landers, D. *et al.* (1995) Parturients infected with human

immunodeficiency virus and regional anesthesia. Clinical and immunological response. *Anesthesiology*, **82**, 32–7.

67. Tom, D.J., Gulevich, S.J., Shapiro, H.M. *et al.* (1992) Epidural blood patch in the HIV- positive patient: review of clinical experience. *Anesthesiology*, **76,** 943–7.

68. Cesarini, M., Torrielli, R., Lahaye, J.M. *et al.* (1990) Sprotte needle for intrathecal anaesthesia for caesarian section: incidence of postdural puncture headache. *Anaesthesia*, **45**, 656–8.

69. Stevenson, G.W., Hall, S.C., Rudnick, S. *et al.* (1990) The effect of anesthetic agents on the human immune response. *Anesthesiology*, **72**, 542–52.

70. Frost, E.A. (1994) Anaesthesia for the patient with acquired immune deficiency syndrome: a review. *Annals of the Academy of Medicine, Singapore*, **23** (6:Suppl), 14–19.

71. Davison, J.M. (1994) Pregnancy in renal allograft recipients: problems, prognosis and practicalities. *Clinical Obstetrics and Gynaecology*, **8**,501–25.

72. Cararach, V., Carmona, F., Monleon, F.J. and Andreu, J. (1993) Pregnancy after renal transplantation: 25 years experience in Spain. *British Journal of Obstetrics and Gynaecology*, **100**, 122–5.

73. Laifer, S.A., Darby, M.J., Scantlebury, V.P. *et al.* (1990) Pregnancy and liver transplantation. *Obstetrics and Gynaecology*, **76**, 1083–8.

74. Ville, Y., Fernandez, H., Samuel, D. *et al.* (1993) Pregnancy in liver transplant recipients: course and outcome in 19 cases. *American Journal of Obstetrics and Gynecology*, **168** (3 Pt 1), 896–902.

75. National Diabetes Group (1979) *Diabetes*, **28**, 1039–57.

76. Jarvis, G.J. (1994) Diabetes and pregnancy. *Obstetrics and Gynaecology. A Critical Approach to the Clinical Problems*, Oxford University Press, Oxford.

77. Greene, M.F. (1993) Prevention and diagnosis of congenital anomalies in diabetic pregnancy. *Clinics in Perinatology*, **20**, 533–47.

78. Ockert, D.B. and Hugo, J.M. (1992) Diabetic complications with special anaesthetic risk. *South African Journal of Surgery*, **30**, 90–4.

79. Maser, R.E., Pfeifer, M.A., Dorman, J.S. *et al.* (1990) Diabetic autonomic neuropathy and cardiovascular risk: Pittsburgh epidemiology of diabetes complications study III. *Archives of Internal Medicine*, **150**, 1218–22.

80. Airaksinen, K.E.J., Ikaheimo, M.J., Salmela, P.I. *et al.* (1986) Impaired cardiac adjustment to pregnancy in type 1 diabetes. *Diabetes Care*, **9**, 376–83.

81. Uusihipa, M.I., Mustonen, J.N. and Airaksinen, K.E.J. (1990) Diabetic heart muscle disease. *Annals of Medicine*, **22**, 377–86.

82. Airaksinen, K.E.J., Salmela, P.I. and Ikaheimo, M.J. (1987) Increase in heart rate in pregnancy blunted in diabetic women. *Diabetes Care*, **10**, 748–51.

83. Eastwood, D.W. (1991) Anterior spinal artery syndrome after epidural anaesthesia in a pregnant diabetic patient with sclerodema. *Anaesthesia and Analgesia*, **67**,1002–4.

84. Alberti, K.G.M.M. and Thomas, D.J.B. (1979) The management of diabetes during surgery. *British Journal of Anaesthesia*, **51,** 693–710.

85. Milaskiewicz, R.M. and Hall, G.M. (1992) Diabetes and anaesthesia: the past decade. *British Journal of Anaesthesia*, **68**,198–206.

86. Walker, R.P., Lawrence, M.D. and Paloyan, E. (1995) Nodular disease during pregnancy. *Surgical Clinics of North America*, **75**, 53–8.

THE FEBRILE OBSTETRIC PATIENT

L. Swanson and T.H. Madej

INTRODUCTION

While the use of regional analgesia in the presence of pyrexia is controversial, regional analgesia itself may cause pyrexia with consequent inappropriate therapy. In this chapter there is discussion of the complex relationship between body temperature, infection, regional analgesia and labour, together with a review of the management of patients with chorioamnionitis or significant viral infections including, herpes, measles, HIV and hepatitis.

THERMOREGULATION

Thermoregulation is achieved through the hypothalamus by autonomic and behavioural mechanisms. Basal metabolic heat production is lost mainly by convection, conduction and radiation but with exercise (or labour) evaporation of sweat and respiratory losses become more important. The normal diurnal rhythm (about 1°C) has other controlling factors superimposed on it (e.g. the response to ovulation). Various sites have been used as representative of core temperature [1]. Highest temperatures are found in the rectum and are influenced by the activity of gut flora and the temperature of venous blood from the legs. Oral temperatures are affected by the ingestion of fluids, mouth breathing, ambient temperature and hyper-

ventilation. Tympanic membrane temperature, now becoming widely used, correlates well with nasopharyngeal, oesophageal and bladder temperature. However, vaginal temperature may be a better reflection of foetal temperature as exemplified by two cases of foetal hyperthermia where maternal tympanic temperature was normal but vaginal temperature was >38.5°C [2].

MATERNAL TEMPERATURE IN LABOUR

The provision of analgesia affects temperature regulation. Women who hyperventilate and perspire in labour have lower core temperatures than those who receive adequate pain relief [2]. In a small study, using various analgesic methods, tympanic membrane temperature gradually increased as labour progressed, with superimposed peaks during contractions [3]. While both oral and vaginal temperatures were noted to rise within one hour of establishing epidural analgesia [4] no such increase was found in women receiving pethidine. Similarly, tympanic membrane temperatures have been reported to rise after epidural analgesia, although the rise was delayed for five hours [5]. The absolute rise in temperature was less than 1°C and it was poorly correlated with foetal heart rate [5].

Clinical Problems in Obstetric Anaesthesia
Edited by Ian F. Russell and Gordon Lyons. Published in 1997 by Chapman & Hall, London. ISBN 0 412 71600 3.

The relationship between oral and genital tract temperatures is not clear. Uterine temperatures were higher than oral temperatures in 95% of one study population, and only five of the 17 women with uterine temperatures greater than 37.4°C had raised oral temperatures [6]. These authors [6] also noted that temperature rose after instituting epidural analgesia and this was attributed to a lack of sweating, no hyperventilation, and vasodilatation in the presence of high ambient temperatures. Concern was also expressed for the foetuses, three (5%) of whom were calculated to have core temperatures of over 40°C [6]! The subject of temperature changes during labour with various forms of analgesia is an area in need of further detailed investigation.

PYREXIA, BACTERAEMIA AND THE WHITE CELL COUNT

During fever the thermoregulatory mechanisms behave as though the set point has been raised, resulting in heat conservation through vasoconstriction and decreased sweating together with heat generation through an increased metabolic rate. Interleukin 1 (a protein produced by phagocytes in response to a wide variety of infections, antibody–antigen reactions and tumour factors) acts upon the hypothalamus via intermediates to alter temperature regulation [7].

The commonest organisms cultured from the blood are said to be *E. coli*, group B *Streptococcus* and *Bacteroides* [8], but the incidence of bacteraemia is low (7.5 per 1000 obstetric admissions) [8–10]. Body temperature and bacteraemia are poorly correlated in that half the patients with positive cultures have temperatures below 38.8°C and only 10% of febrile patients grow organisms on blood culture [8]. Baker and Hubbell found positive blood cultures in 0.5–1.3% of labouring women, taking samples at and after delivery [9]. Another similar study yielded positive cultures in 3.6% of patients [10]. These authors [10] reviewed other published series and calculated an incidence of 2.15% bacteraemia in asymptomatic patients. Manual removal of the placenta was noted to cause bacteraemia and was associated with two cases of endocarditis [10].

The total white blood cell (wbc) count rises in pregnancy, mainly due to neutrophil polymorphonuclear leukocytes [11]. This occurs from the 45th day of pregnancy rising to a peak at 30 weeks; a plateau is reached during the third trimester with a mean wbc count of 9 × 10^9/l. During labour the total leukocyte count may reach 40 × 10^9/l but returns to non-pregnant levels by six weeks postpartum. Like body temperature, the wbc count seems of little predictive value since there is no correlation between the wbc count and the presence of bacteraemia [12]: a very wide range of wbc counts are observed in patients with sepsis [8].

Further evidence of the difficulties in defining significant infection can be found in studies of chorioamnionitis. Chorioamnionitis is diagnosed clinically by the presence of pyrexia, maternal or foetal tachycardia, uterine tenderness and raised white cell count. Its incidence is quoted as 1% of all pregnancies and of these some 8% will be bacteraemic [13]. Bader *et al.* [12] presented retrospective data of 319 women with chorioamnionitis of whom 253 received regional analgesia/anaesthesia. Three of these latter women were bacteraemic as proven by blood culture. No patient had any infective sequelae as a result of their regional block, and after reviewing the literature, these authors felt that 'the potential benefits of regional anaesthesia in this group of patients outweighs the theoretical risk of infectious complications' [12].

EPIDURAL ABSCESS

The main concern regarding regional anaesthesia in the presence of pyrexia, bacteraemia or a raised wbc count is that of causing an epidural abscess or meningitis, and evidence for this was sought in the literature. Epidural abscess is a rare condition with an incidence of 0.2–1.2 per 10 000 hospital admissions.

Spontaneous cases arise in patients with underlying medical conditions and organisms may originate from skin, soft tissues, the urinary tract; the respiratory tract and the genital tract: in up to one third of cases no source of infection is found. While the spectrum of causative organisms has become quite diverse, *Staphylococcus aureus* remains the most common.

Recent evidence for the occurrence of epidural abscess in the obstetric population is exceedingly rare, with only a handful of cases reported in the literature. Although Borum *et al.* [14] reported what they believed to be the fourth epidural abscess in association with epidural analgesia, there are undoubtedly other cases currently beyond the reach of computer searches (e.g. [15, 16]). A case was reported in the postal survey by Scott and Hibbard but no further details are available [17]. A second occurred five days following caesarean section under epidural analgesia: the catheter was removed after two days, 14 top-ups having been used for postoperative analgesia [18]. An initial diagnosis of endometritis was made but the organism cultured from the abscess was a *Staphylococcus aureus* of the same phage type as grown in blood cultures but different from the perineal swabs. A clinically similar case, described by Crawford [19], was found at surgery to have three small collections of sterile blood-stained watery fluid under pressure in the epidural space without evidence of abscess formation.

Epidural abscess related to regional block may occur directly due to introduction of organisms via the catheter or needle, via contaminated fluids or via local infection at the puncture site. Alternatively infection may be fortuitous and occur secondary to haematogenous spread from a distant focus of infection. Various aspects of the epidural technique have been investigated with regard to potential sources of infection. James *et al.* [20] found bupivacaine 0.25% at 37°C to be bactericidal to Gram positive bacilli including *S. epidermidis*. These authors [20], using in-line bacterial filters, noted that the epidural catheter tips from 101 labouring patients were sterile but five of the multi-use syringes were contaminated. Consequently, they recommended the use of a bacterial filter and a new sterile syringe for each injection [20]. In a study of 102 patients (63 obstetric cases) in which an in-line bacterial filter was not used, 9% of epidural catheter tips were contaminated [21]. In this study [21] paper tape was used to fix the catheters in place and it was noted that of the 53 vaginal deliveries a positive culture was obtained from 14 of the catheters at some point between the hub and the tip, but in the 10 women undergoing caesarean section there was no contamination of the catheter. Labouring women comprised 52% of the study population and accounted for 64% of the contaminated catheters. Although there were other confounding factors and the difference between labouring and non-labouring patients is not significant ($P = 0.22$) the authors used this data to recommend a waterproof dressing to protect the catheter [21]. In direct contrast Vasdev and Leicht advise against waterproof dressings because the environment under such dressings is warm and moist, ideal conditions for bacterial growth [22]. This information has led others to reconsider their practice [23].

When performing regional anaesthesia an aseptic technique with adequate skin preparation is mandatory. While there is general agreement that hands should be thoroughly cleaned and gloved there is less unanimity over other aspects of 'sterile' technique, e.g. the need for adhesive drapes, gown, mask or hat. However, the anaesthetist has been the source of infection on at least one occasion (nasal *Staphylococcus* of the same phage type) [24]. Abscess formation has been reported in non-obstetric cases following single-shot epidurals without catheterization but both of these involved steroid injection [25, 26]. It should also be borne in mind that epidural abscesses have been described in otherwise fit young women in the puerperium who had not received epidural analgesia [27, 28].

Table 9.1 Meningitis following obstetric regional anaesthesia

Type	Organism	Procedure	Reference
Septic	*Streptococcus sanguis*	Dural tap and 2 × blood patch	31
Septic	*Staphylococcus epidermis*	Epidural–spinal and blood patch	32
Septic	*Streptococcus faecalis*	Epidural	36
Septic	*Streptococcus uberis*	Epidural	36
Septic	*Streptococcus* beta-haemolytic	Epidural	37
Septic?	–	Spinal	33
Septic?	–	Spinal	34
Septic?	–	Dural tap	35
Aseptic	–	Spinal	32
Aseptic	Coxsackie virus	Epidural	38

MENINGITIS

Meningitis can be categorized as septic or aseptic. Both are associated with fever, headache, nausea, vomiting, neck stiffness and an increased wbc count of predominantly polymorphonucleocytes. Septic meningitis is caused by a bacterial infection, usually taking eight or more hours to develop and associated with a raised cerebral spinal fluid (CSF) pressure, a raised protein concentration and a reduced CSF glucose concentration. Aseptic meningitis is an inflammation of the meninges not due to bacterial infection: it may be due to chemicals, blood, pyrogens or viral infections [29]. Chemical aseptic meningitis is usually of more rapid onset with a benign course and the symptoms resolve rapidly without treatment. An initial CSF polymorpholeukocytosis is replaced by a predominance of mononucleocytes after 12–72 hours: like septic meningitis the CSF protein concentration is raised but the CSF glucose concentration is normal.

Infection may be borne into the CSF on needles or a core of skin may be carried in by a needle with a poorly fitting introducer [30]. Solutions used for cleaning the skin may be irritant, and these solutions, or indeed the drug for injection, may be infected or contain pyrogens. Blood, introduced by inadvertent puncture of a vessel or therapeutic epidural blood patch, may act as a focus for infection by organisms 'seeding' from distant sites by haematogenous spread.

Published reports of meningitis following obstetric regional block are listed in Table 9.1. Two cases of septic meningitis have been reported after epidural blood patch [31, 32]. The first patient had an accidental dural tap and two epidural blood patches for headache: she was apyrexial before the first blood patch, but following this she exhibited transient pyrexia and had an elevated wbc count after six hours; her temperature rose again three hours after the second blood patch; *Streptococcus sanguis* was grown from CSF cultures [31]. The second patient had a complex combined spinal–extradural procedure: this required resiting of the epidural followed by a repeat spinal and finally an epidural blood patch. She was apyrexial at the time of the blood patch but developed a temperature six hours later. *Staphylococcus epidermidis* was cultured subsequently from the CSF [32].

Two other examples of septic meningitis following repeated attempts at spinal anaesthesia were reported recently. Both developed symptoms within 24 hours of the regional block. No organisms were seen or cultured in either case but the CSF glucose concentrations were reduced [33, 34]. An even more confusing case of meningitis, thought to be bacterial in origin because of the delayed onset and sustained polymorpholeukocytosis in the CSF, followed accidental dural puncture, was later complicated by seizures and then administration of antibiotics before diagnostic lumbar puncture [35]. The incidence of aseptic meningitis has declined since the 1940s but a recent case was attributed to contamination of equipment by unstained chlorhexidine in alcohol [32].

Three cases of streptococcal meningitis following epidural analgesia have been reported. One involved use of an epidural catheter for elective caesarean section and 48 hours postoperative analgesia. As well as the usual symptoms and signs of meningitis, the patient developed an area of cellulitis at the insertion site of the epidural catheter which had been removed 84 hours previously. *Streptococcus faecalis* was cultured from the CSF [36]. The other two patients had normal vaginal deliveries and then developed meningitis 24–40 hours later. *Streptococcus uberis* and a beta-haemolytic *Streptococcus* were cultured from the CSF, blood and vagina [36, 37]. These latter two cases are though to be examples of haematological spread as there were no obvious risk factors or pre-existing pyrexia. Epidural block has also been followed by coincidental aseptic meningitis due to a Coxsackie B virus [38].

These examples emphasize the need for aseptic technique and a reliable source of sterile solutions and equipment uncontaminated by skin preparation fluids. Since epidural vein puncture creates a focus for infection, techniques which minimize its occurrence should be employed [39]. For similar reasons it may be best to avoid epidural blood patches in patients with local or systemic infection [40].

CONCLUSION

As discussed above the pathophysiological changes associated with infection are not clinically useful in diagnosing infection: temperature can rise in normal labour, there is little correlation between temperature and bacteraemia, bacteraemia can occur in asymptomatic

patients, and the wbc is too variable to be discriminating. It is difficult to assess the risk of pyrexia since the only means of finding complications is through published reports and there is no denominator. However, a pragmatic approach towards the use of regional techniques should be adopted, bearing in mind our inability to predict who will be bacteraemic and the probability that a proportion of patients who receive regional blocks will be asymptomatically bacteraemic. The risk of these major complications in an obstetric patient is very low and the benefit of any regional block should be weighed against this for each patient individually [41]. Since signs of epidural abscess or meningitis may not occur until after the patient has returned home it is axiomatic that anaesthetic involvement does not end with delivery of the infant. Guidelines should be in place so that late complications can be dealt with speedily and effectively.

VIRAL INFECTIONS

HERPES SIMPLEX

This virus exists in two forms, HVS II is responsible for 93% of primary genital infections and 98% of recurrences. Primary infection can cause systemic illness with fever, lymphadenopathy, hepatitis, aseptic meningitis and sacral nerve dysfunction. Presentation is often more severe in pregnancy and should a generalized, disseminated infection occur, a maternal mortality in excess of 50% may occur [42]. Recurrent lesions are present in 0.5–1% of the pregnant population and asymptomatic shedding of the virus occurs in another 0.6–1.4%. A prospective study of pregnant women with a history of infection demonstrated recurrence in 84% [42].

The foetus can be infected by transplacental spread in the primary infection. Vertical spread is possible in both primary and recurrent infection and, as a result, elective caesarean section is recommended in the presence of active lesions or recent positive culture.

Three retrospective studies, covering a total of 247 patients, have looked at the complications following regional techniques in association with HVS [43]. One patient who had an epidural had a recurrence which was attributed to antepartum steroids; no cases of meningitis or encephalitis were seen but epidural morphine was implicated in the recrudescence of oral herpes, perhaps secondary to facial itch. The situation is difficult to assess as recurrence may be delayed until the third day postpartum and there are other triggers including hormonal change, sunlight and stress. From the available data the use of regional anaesthesia for caesarean section in women with recurrent HVS infection appears to be safe as long as there are no lesions on the back. Unfortunately, there is a paucity of information on primary infection but of five patients thought to have primary infection one developed a transient neurological deficit of unknown aetiology [43].

VARICELLA-ZOSTER

Chicken-pox occurs in 1–5 per 10 000 pregnancies. Again there is an absence of data but regional anaesthesia seems unwise in the presence of systemic illness or lesions in the lumbar area. The incidence of herpes zoster in pregnancy is unknown. Herpes zoster recrudescence in association with spinal anaesthesia has been reported [41].

MEASLES

This is caused by a paramyxovirus; it is uncommon in adults and should become rarer with vaccination. In pregnancy there is increased risk of abortion, preterm labour pneumonitis and death [44]. There is no data on the use of regional anaesthesia.

HIV-1 AND AIDS

HIV is a retrovirus and the main target is the T lymphocyte with CD4 surface antigen. These lymphocytes are used as a marker of disease progression with counts falling as the immune system fails. Another marker is the p24 antigen which is a HIV-1 core protein and its presence in the blood has been associated with maternal foetal transmission. A wide range of risk is given for transmission to the foetus and there is evidence for vertical spread, and via breast milk.

The disease can affect many systems directly or indirectly and the patient needs careful assessment. The central nervous system is involved early with viral particles isolated from the CSF of otherwise well HIV positive patients [45]. Encephalitis, meningitis and demyelinating neuropathies can occur at the time of seroconversion. Poly or mononeuropathies have been reported in the latent phase. In advanced disease dementia, associated with cerebral hypoperfusion and increased sensitivity to benzodiazepines and opiates, is well recognized. Other dysfunctions of the central or peripheral nervous system may be due to HIV, associated infections or malignancies. Space-occupying lesions such as lymphoma and tuberculous abscess can be present and toxoplasmosis or cryptococcal infection can lead to raised intracranial pressure and impaired autoregulation. Cardiac involvement may include myocarditis, dilating myopathies, endo and pericarditis. The respiratory system may be impaired by previous or current infections. HIV thrombocytopenia with submucosal haemorrhages and epistaxis can occur but major haemorrhage is rare. The AIDS patient will often be on drug treatments which have adverse side effects and may have anaesthetic implications.

Hughes *et al.* [46] attempted to study the effects of regional analgesia and anaesthesia in 30 HIV positive parturients; 16 received epidurals, two spinals and the rest either opiates or no analgesia. There were no changes in immunological parameters, infections or neurological state up to six months postpartum. Other studies of small numbers have likewise observed no neurological sequaelae when regional anaesthesia was used in HIV positive women [47, 48]. Although blood patching is controversial in these patients, there have been no reports of adverse outcomes [48]. Theoretical concerns about the immunological effects of general anaesthesia have been expressed and, *in vitro*, opiates are known to reactivate and stimulate HIV reproduction in culture.

VIRAL HEPATITIS

This accounts for 40% of jaundice in pregnancy and can be due to the hepatitis virus group or as a complication of other viral illnesses [49]. There are at least five viruses in the hepatitis group. Hepatitis A and E are enteroviruses which cause acute illness only. Hepatitis B and C are haematologically spread and can cause chronic illness. The presence of hepatitis D with B is associated with more severe disease. Management is supportive, being aimed at confirming the diagnosis and preventing dehydration during the febrile stage. Anaesthesia and surgery should be avoided if possible during the acute phase as this can result in further deterioration of function. Particular care must be taken to avoid hypoperfusion, hypoxia and hepatic toxins. Coagulation, glucose homoeostasis and renal function can be disturbed and drug handling may be altered. Patients with chronic active hepatitis may have extrahepatic manifestations including cardiomyopathies and neuropathies.

CONCLUSION

While there is a paucity of reliable data, theoretical considerations would seem to warn against performing regional blocks in patients who are systemically unwell with bacterial or viral illness; however, examples are given of patients receiving regional blocks in the presence of chorioamnionitis or HIV with no untoward outcome. There may be situations where the theoretical risks of significant spinal canal infection are outweighed by real benefits but until more data is available from studies focusing on regional blocks performed in some of the circumstances outlined above it is not possible to give any accurate prediction of risk. Infected skin lesions are only a problem if they cannot be excluded from the cleaned area at, or immediately adjacent to, the puncture site. In some centripetal rashes (e.g. varicella) such an area may be impossible to produce.

REFERENCES

1. Imrie, M.M. and Hall, G.M. (1990) Body temperature and anaesthesia. *British Journal of Anaesthesia*, **64**, 346–54.
2. Goodlin, R.C. and Chapin, J.W. (1982) Determinants of maternal temperature during labor. *American Journal of Obstetrics and Gynecology*, **143**, 97–103.
3. Marx, G.F. and Loew, D.A.Y. (1975) Tympanic temperature during labour and parturition. *British Journal of Anaesthesia*, **47**, 600–2.
4. Fusi, L., Steer, P.J., Maresh, M.J.A. *et al.* (1989) Maternal pyrexia associated with the use of epidural analgesia in labour. *The Lancet*, **1**, 1250–2.
5. Camann, W.R., Hortvet, L.A., Hughes, N. *et al.* (1991) Maternal temperature regulation during extradural analgesia for labour. *British Journal of Anaesthesia*, **67**, 565–8.
6. Macaulay, J.H., Bond, K. and Steer, P.J. (1992) Epidural analgesia in labor and fetal hyperthermia. *Obstetrics and Gynecology*, **80**, 665–9.
7. Mitchell, D. and Laburn, H.P. (1985) Pathophysiology of temperature regulation. *The Physiologist*, **28**, 507–17.
8. Blanco, J.D., Gibbs, R.S. and Castaneda, Y.S. (1981) Bacteremia in obstetrics: clinical course. *Obstetrics and Gynecology*, **58**, 621–5.
9. Baker, T.H. and Hubbell, R. (1967) Reappraisal of asymptomatic bacteremia. *American Journal of Obstetrics and Gynecology*, **97**, 575–6.
10. Sugrue, D., Blake, S., Troy, P. *et al.* (1980) Antibiotic prophylaxis against infective endocarditis after normal delivery – is it necessary? *British Heart Journal*, **44**, 499–502.

11. Hytten, F. and Chamberlain, G. (eds) (1990) *Clinical Physiology in Obstetrics*. Blackwell Scientific, London.

12. Bader, A.M., Gilbertson, L., Kirz, L. *et al.* (1992) Regional anesthesia in women with chorioamnionitis. *Regional Anesthesia*, **17**, 84–6.

13. Gibbs, R.S., Castillo, M.S. and Rodgers, P.J. (1980) Management of acute chorioamnionitis. *American Journal of Obstetrics and Gynecology*, **136**, 709–13.

14. Borum, S.E., McLeskey, C.H., Williamson, J.B. *et al.* (1995) Epidural abscess after obstetric epidural analgesia. *Anesthesiology*, **82**, 1523–6.

15. Usubiaga, J.E. (1975) Neurological complications following epidural anesthesia. *International Anesthesiology Clinics*, **13**, 33–84.

16. Dhillon, A.R. and Russell, I.F. (1995) Epidural abscess in association with obstetric epidural analgesia. Personal communication.

17. Scott, D.B. and Hibbard, B.M. (1990) Serious non-fatal complications associated with extradural block in obstetric practice. *British Journal of Anaesthesia*, **64**, 537–41.

18. Ngan Kee, W.D., Jones, M.R., Thomas, P. *et al.* (1992) Extradural abscess complicating extradural anaesthesia for Caesarean section. *British Journal of Anaesthesia*, **69**, 647–52.

19. Crawford, J.S. (1975) Pathology in the extradural space. *British Journal of Anaesthesia*, **47**, 412–4.

20. James, F.M., George, R.H., Naiem, H. *et al.* (1976) Bacteriological aspects of epidural anaesthesia. *Anesthesia and Analgesia*, **55**, 187–90.

21. Hunt, J.R., Rigor, B.M. and Collins J.R. (1977) The potential for contamination of continuous epidural catheters. *Anesthesia and Analgesia*, **56**, 222–5.

22. Vasdev, G.M.S. and Leicht, C.H. (1993) Extradural abscess in the postpartum period. *British Journal of Anaesthesia*, **70**, 703.

23. Ngan Kee, W.D. (1993) Extradural abscess in the postpartum period. *British Journal of Anaesthesia*, **70**, 704.

24. North, J.B. and Brophy, B.P. (1979) A hazard of spinal epidural analgesia. *Australia and New Zealand Journal of Surgery*, **44**, 484–5.

25. Gouke, C.R. and Graziotti, P. (1990) Extradural abscess following local anaesthetic and steroid injection for chronic low back pain. *British Journal of Anaesthesia*, **65**, 427–9.

26. Chan, S.T. and Leung, S. (1989) Spinal epidural abscess following steroid injection for sciatica. *Spine*, **14**, 106–8.

27. Kitching, A.J. and Rice, A.S.C. (1993) Extradural abscess in the postpartum period. *British Journal of Anaesthesia*, **70**, 703.

28. Male, C.G. and Martin, R. (1973) Puerperal spinal epidural abscess. *The Lancet*, **1**, 608–9.

29. Phillips, O.C. (1970) Aseptic meningitis following spinal anesthesia. *Anesthesia and Analgesia*, **49**, 866–71.

30. Brandus, V. (1968) The spinal needle as a carrier of foreign material. *Canadian Anaesthetists Society Journal*, **15**, 197–201.

31. Berga, S. and Trierweiller, M.W. (1989) Bacterial meningitis following epidural anesthesia for vaginal delivery. *Obstetrics and Gynecology*, **74**, 437–9.

32. Harding, S.A., Collis, R.E. and Morgan, B.M. (1994) Meningitis after combined spinal–epidural anaesthesia in obstetrics. *British Journal of Anaesthesia*, **73**, 545–7.

33. Lee, J.J. and Parry, H. (1991) Bacterial meningitis following spinal anaesthesia for Caesarean section. *British Journal of Anaesthesia*, **66**, 383–6.

34. Roberts, S.P. and Petts, H.V. (1990) Meningitis after obstetric spinal anaesthesia. *Anaesthesia*, **45**, 376–7.

35. Sansome, A.J.T., Barnes, G.R. and Barrett, R.F. (1991) An unusual presentation of meningitis as a consequence of inadvertent dural puncture. *International Journal of Obstetric Anaesthesia*, **1**, 35–7.

36. Ready, L.B. and Helfer, D. (1989) Bacterial meningitis in parturients after epidural anesthesia. *Anesthesiology*, **71**, 988–90.

37. Davis, L., Hargraves, C. and Robinson, P.N. (1993) Postpartum meningitis. *Anaesthesia*, **48**, 788–9.

38. Neumark, J., Feichtinger, W. and Gassner, A. (1980) Epidural block in obstetrics followed by aseptic meningoencephalitis. *Anesthesiology*, **52**, 518–9.

39. Mannion, D. Walker, R. and Clayton, K. (1991) Extradural vein puncture – avoidable complication. *Anaesthesia*, **46**, 585–7.

40. Abouleish, E., de la Vega, S., Blendinger, I. *et al.* (1975) Long term follow-up of epidural blood patch. *Anesthesia and Analgesia*, **54**, 459–63.

41. Davies, J.M. and Thistlewood, J.M. (1988) Infections and the parturient. *Canadian Journal of Anaesthesia*, **35**, 270–2.

42. Stagno, S. and Whitley, R.J. (1985) Herpes virus infections of pregnancy. *New England Journal of Medicine*, **313**, 1327–30.

43. Bader, A.M., Camann, W.R. and Datta, S. (1990)

Anesthesia for cesarean delivery in patients with herpes simplex virus type II infections. *Regional Anesthesia*, **15**, 261–3.

44. Almar, R.L., Englund, J.A. and Hammill, H.(1992) Complications of measles during pregnancy. *Clinical Infectious Diseases*, **14**, 217–26.

45. Shapiro, H.M., Grant, I. and Weinger, M.B. (1994) AIDS and the central nervous system. *Anesthesiology*, **80**, 187–200.

46. Hughes, S.C., Dailey, P.A., Landers, D. *et al.* (1995) Parturients infected with human immunodeficiency virus and regional anesthesia. *Anesthesiology*, **82**, 32–7.

47. Gershon, R.Y., Manning-Williams, D.M., Berry, A.J. *et al.* (1991) The effect of anesthesia on the HIV infected parturient. *Anesthesiology*, **77**, A1037.

48. Birnbach, D.J., Bourlier, R.A., Choi, R. and Thys, D.M. (1995) Anaesthetic management of caesarean section in a patient with active recurrent genital herpes and AIDS-related dementia. *British Journal of Anaesthesia*, **75**, 639–41.

49. Pastorek, J.G. (1993) The ABCs of hepatitis in pregnancy. *Clinical Obstetrics and Gynecology*, **36**, 843–54.

E. McGrady

INTRODUCTION

Although anaesthesia-related maternal mortality has fallen in recent years, problems with intubation are still responsible for the majority of deaths [1–3]. Unexpected difficult intubation can lead to disaster, and many ways of predicting and managing difficult or failed intubation have been described [4, 5]. Compared to the general surgical population, the incidence of failed intubation is some eight times higher in the parturient: 1 in 300 versus 1 in 2230 [6, 7].

MATERNAL MORTALITY

In the 1982–1984 report on confidential enquiries into maternal deaths (CEMD) in England and Wales 19 mothers died as a result of anaesthesia, the third commonest cause of maternal death. Sixteen of these deaths were directly related to general anaesthesia: five women succumbed to the acid aspiration syndrome with a further 10 dying due to problems with endotracheal intubation (two of these women also aspirated) [1].

The two most recent confidential enquiries into maternal deaths in the UK (CEMDUK) have shown a reassuring reduction in anaesthetic-related maternal mortality, although seven out of eight [2] and four out of five [3] deaths were still due to problems occurring during induction or maintenance of general anaesthesia.

DIFFICULT INTUBATION IN THE OBSTETRIC POPULATION

A number of factors contribute to intubation difficulties in obstetrics (Table 10.1).

ANATOMICAL

A full set of teeth, breast engorgement and the presence of the hand applying cricoid pressure can make insertion of the laryngoscope blade difficult. Pregnant women have increased total body water, fat deposition and mucosal capillary engorgement, and many have frank oedema which may cause some subtle changes in anatomy and in soft tissue mobility. Laryngeal oedema is a known complication of pregnancy-induced hypertension [8] but can occur after strenuous pushing in the second stage [9]. During induction of anaesthesia women will be placed in a lateral tilt position or a wedge will be inserted, to avoid aortocaval occlusion: either of these manoeuvres may make laryngoscopy awkward.

Clinical Problems in Obstetric Anaesthesia
Edited by Ian F. Russell and Gordon Lyons. Published in 1997 by Chapman & Hall, London. ISBN 0 412 71600 3.

Table 10.1 Causes of difficult intubation in obstetrics

Anatomical
Full dentition
Breast engorgement
Left lateral tilt, or presence of wedge
Increased total body water
Laryngeal oedema
Engorgement of capillary mucosa
Cricoid pressure

Physiological
Factors leading to increased risk of regurgitation
  Reduced barrier pressure
  Delayed gastric emptying – opioid
    administration, labour
Factors leading to increased risk of hypoxia
  Reduced functional residual capacity
  Increased maternal O_2 consumption

Miscellaneous
Anaesthetist inexperience
Anaesthetist anxiety
Inadequate resources – monitoring, equipment,
  anaesthetic assistance

The application of cricoid pressure can distort anatomy: when single-handed cricoid pressure is applied with the mother in the left lateral position it is possible to push the larynx to one side rather than straight back against cervical vertebrae.

PHYSIOLOGICAL

Increased risk of regurgitation

Although serum gastrin concentration is increased in pregnancy [10], gastric secretion is probably unchanged. Intragastric pressure is raised [11] and this predisposes to regurgitation of gastric contents into the oesophagus. Pregnant women with heartburn – 80% at term [12] – have decreased lower oesophageal sphincter (LOS) pressures, with a corresponding fall in barrier pressure (LOS pressure minus intragastric pressure), and therefore the

symptom of heartburn is a warning of a woman being at increased risk of gastro-oesophageal reflux [11].

Gastric emptying is unaffected by pregnancy *per se* [13], but the administration of opioid drugs in labour, either intramuscular [14] or epidural [15], does cause delay. Delayed gastric emptying has been reported in mothers within two hours of normal vaginal delivery, some of whom (four out of 17) had received pethidine, though it had returned to normal by 18 hours postpartum [16]

Increased risk of hypoxia

With a reduced functional residual capacity and an increased oxygen consumption [17] maternal hypoxia develops rapidly if the lungs cannot be ventilated, particularly if a period of pre-oxygenation has been omitted.

Miscellaneous

Anaesthetist inexperience

Many emergency caesarean sections are performed during the night, when the only anaesthetist on site is a trainee. In this situation there may be little time for preoperative assessment and senior anaesthetic assistance may not be immediately available. Furthermore, in those units with very high regional anaesthesia (RA) rates for caesarean section, trainees may have had limited practical experience of general anaesthesia (GA) under consultant supervision.

Anaesthetist anxiety

In the presence of foetal distress there is pressure on the anaesthetist to induce anaesthesia rapidly. Not only is this stressful, but it limits the time available for detailed preoperative assessment and equipment checks. Trainees often attempt intubation too early, before suxamethonium has had time to act, thus self-inflicted difficulty engenders further anxiety.

Inadequate resources

Staff shortages, poorly trained staff and inadequate monitoring or anaesthetic equipment can all contribute to a disaster.

REDUCING THE RISK

While anaesthesia-related maternal mortality is falling, the reason is not clear: the two most common suggestions are (1) fewer women now receive general anaesthesia and (2) standards of care have improved. Two studies shed some light on this debate [18, 19]. Scottish data for 1993 showed that only 33.9% of women requiring emergency caesarean section and 13.7% of those having elective caesarean section received GA [18], although there was a large variation between units. A recent survey of UK obstetric units showed that in 31 units with accurate data over an 11-year period, 85% of 5832 (4983) women having an emergency caesarean section in 1982 received general anaesthesia compared with 54% of 9069 (4900) women in 1992 [19]; a further survey confirms this high rate of general anaesthesia for emergency caesarean section [20]. If these data [18–20] reflect nationwide practice then, although the GA **rate** has fallen significantly, the rise in the number of caesarean sections, emergencies in particular, means the actual **number** of GAs given over this time scale may have reduced very little if at all. Therefore there appears to be a real reduction in the death rate per number of GAs given, and possible factors contributing to this are shown in Table 10.2.

PREDICTION OF DIFFICULT INTUBATION

Methods for predicting difficult intubation are reviewed elsewhere [4, 21], but important factors in detecting potential intubation problems include the following.

Improved communication between midwives, obstetricians and anaesthetists

Anaesthetists do not, as a routine, see women in early pregnancy. Since many emergency sections are performed at the end of the second or beginning of the third trimester it is essential that those providing the antenatal care (i.e. obstetricians and midwives) not only elicit any history of a previous difficult or failed intubation but also detect any anatomical defect that may lead to difficult intubation and refer these women for anaesthetic assessment **early** in pregnancy. Current changes in midwifery training and practice have considerable implications for anaesthetists: midwives now receive little general nursing training and their knowledge of anaesthesia and its risks will be even more limited; very soon midwives will become the only health professional caring for a significant proportion of women throughout their pregnancy. When a woman is referred for anaesthetic assessment, a history should be taken, examination performed and previous anaesthetic records accessed before a management plan is prepared and written clearly in the case notes in readiness for some unforeseen anaesthetic requirement. Potential intubation problems, their implication, and the advantages of regional analgesia in labour should be discussed with the woman and obstetricians. Elective induction of labour or elective caesarean section should be considered in women with definite airway problems and the case notes of high-risk women should be 'flagged'. Since a woman confirmed as being at 'anaesthetic risk' will probably require obstetrician-led care it is to be hoped that conflict between professional groups (principally midwives and obstetricians) will not prevent appropriate anaesthetic referrals being made.

Airway assessment

Many methods have been devised, but all have similar failings. Both the **sensitivity** of the tests and the **positive predictive value** (PPV) are low. (Sensitivity is the proportion of difficult intubations actually predicted by the test to be difficult, i.e. if out of 100 difficult intubations, only 50 had been predicted by the test, the sensitivity would be 0.5. The PPV is

Table 10.2 Reducing the risk of problems at intubation

Prediction of a problem	
Obstetricians, midwives, anaesthetists	Improved communications, timely referrals
Antenatal assessment	Mallampati, Wilson rank sum
Airway assessment	Examination of back/RA contraindicated?
Labour ward assessment	Contingency plan prepared
	Avoidance of GA in high-risk cases
Prevention of aspiration	
Reduce gastric contents	Fasting? – low volume, but low pH
	Metoclopramide, domperidone
	Avoid opioid analgesia
	Stomach tube, apomorphine
	H_2 antagonists, omeprazole
Raise pH gastric contents	H_2 antagonists
	Omeprazole
	Non-particulate antacids – sodium citrate
Maximize barrier pressure	Avoid opioids, benzodiazepines, atropine
	Give metoclopramide
	Avoid lithotomy position
Prevent regurgitation	Cricoid pressure: correct position and force
Improved training	
Increased consultant presence	Preparation of failed intubation protocol
	Practice of failed intubation protocol
	Adequate equipment, monitoring facilities
Adequate trainee experience	At least one year's general experience
Anaesthetic technique	
	Adequate denitrogenation
	Adequate induction of anaesthesia
	Correct application of cricoid pressure
	Oxygenation between intubation attempts
	Recognize failed intubation (three attempts)
	Assessment of neuromuscular block
Trained anaesthetic assistance	To a nationally or regionally agreed standard

the proportion of subjects predicted by the test to be difficult who actually **were** difficult to intubate, i.e. if the test predicted that 100 subjects would be difficult to intubate but only 10 were then the PPV would be 0.1.) Increasing the sensitivity of a test in order to detect more difficult intubations leads to more false positives.

Samsoon and Young's modification of Mallampati's airway assessment is based on the theory that if the base of the tongue is disproportionately large it will obscure the view of the larynx at laryngoscopy [7, 22]. The patient sits upright, opens the mouth as wide as possible and maximally protrudes the tongue; the examiner, sitting opposite, assesses the visible pharyngeal structures as follows (Figure 10.1).

Class 1: soft palate, fauces, uvula and tonsillar pillars visible
Class 2: soft palate, fauces, and uvula only seen
Class 3: soft palate, base of uvula seen
Class 4: soft palate not visible at all

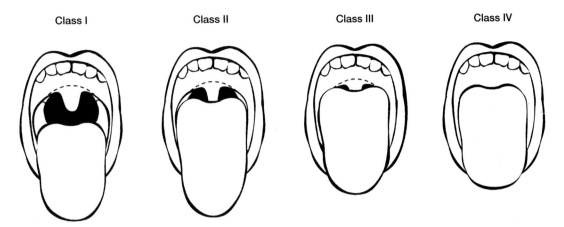

Figure 10.1 Pictorial classification of pharyngeal structures. Reproduced with permission from Samsoon, G.L.T. and Young, J.R.B. (1987) Difficult tracheal intubation: a retrospective study. *Anaesthesia*, **42**, 487—90.

Mallampati showed a good correlation between this classification and the view of the larynx at laryngoscopy, graded on a scale of one to four as follows [23] (Figure 10.2).

Grade 1: full view of the glottis
Grade 2: only the posterior commissure of the glottis seen
Grade 3: no view of the glottis – corniculate cartilages only seen
Grade 4: neither glottis or corniculate cartilages seen.

However a comparison of the Mallampati assessment with the Wilson risk sum assessment [24], which scores five risk factors including weight, head, neck and jaw mobility, mandibular recession, and presence of buck teeth, showed that both tests predicted less than 50% of difficult intubations and the false positive rates were high [25]. The Mallampati score is subject to inter observer variation, may be affected by phonation during the test [26] or by strenuous pushing in labour [27] and does not take into account risk factors such as limited neck mobility or obesity.

Rocke and coworkers assessed 1500 women before they received general anaesthesia for caesarean section, and graded the view at laryngoscopy and the difficulty of intubation [28]. Airway assessment included a modified Mallampati test, and examination for eight potential risk factors as follows: short neck, obesity, missing maxillary incisors, protruding maxillary teeth, single maxillary tooth, receding mandible (thyromental distance – distance between the thyroid cartilage and mentum),

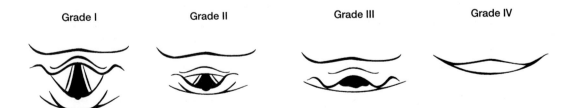

Figure 10.2 Classification of laryngoscopic views. Reproduced with permission from Samsoon, G.L.T. and Young, J.R.B. (1987) Difficult tracheal intubation: a retrospective study. *Anaesthesia*, **42**, 487—90.

facial oedema and a swollen tongue. Some 26.5% of women were graded as class 3 or 4 airways, but only 10% of these women had grade 3 or 4 views on laryngoscopy. The relative risk of a difficult intubation occurring was calculated for different risk factors: class 3 and class 4 airways had risks 7.58 and 11.2 greater than class 1 airways. The combination of a class 4 airway and a short neck (1.2% of women) was associated with a 15% probability of a difficult intubation.

Given the high false positive rate of the Mallampati classification it would seem unwise to label a woman as a 'difficult intubation' on the basis of this alone; however a class 3 or 4 airway, in combination with another strong risk factor, e.g. short neck or receding mandible, should not be ignored. Regional analgesia should be recommended for labour particularly if there are obstetric risk factors. All women requiring anaesthesia should have a Mallampati airway assessment together with an assessment of other anatomical features.

PREVENTION OF ASPIRATION

In Mendelson's description of aspiration of gastric contents into the lungs during obstetric GA only two of the 66 women he reported actually died, both having asphyxiated following airway obstruction by solid material [29]. Between 1982 and 1990 ten anaesthetic maternal deaths were due to aspiration of stomach contents – three of these were in the postoperative period [1–3].

Reduce gastric contents

Fasting during labour

Aspiration of gastric contents (AGC) was so common in earlier CEMDs that it became established practice to fast women during labour. While some now question this routine, on the grounds that several women who died from AGC had fasted throughout labour, the mortality from aspiration has fallen substantially and fasting of women in labour may have contributed to this. Gastric emptying appears to be delayed in labour; in one study, 50% of women in active labour had solid food in the stomach despite fasting for 8-24 hours [30]. However, when the risk of a woman requiring GA for caesarean section is low (as in many units with high RA rates) and the risk of actually aspirating is low, most women are being fasted to prevent a rare complication.

Studies of more liberal eating and drinking policies in labour are under way and future practice will be guided by these results. Unless these studies show an increased morbidity or mortality in women eating and drinking more freely in labour, units may have to introduce a feeding policy where there is at least the opportunity to advise certain women to fast. If hospitals maintain a rigid fasting policy there is a danger that some women will ignore it, and 'high risk' women who have been eating in labour may present for caesarean section. A 1991 survey showed that 96% of obstetric units in England and Wales allowed some form of oral intake, 68% using a selection policy based on the perceived risk of obstetric complications [31]. In hospitals with low GA rates, many women who receive GA for caesarean section are emergencies who have not been fasted in any case.

Metoclopramide

Metoclopramide promotes gastric emptying though this effect is obtunded by the administration of opioid analgesics in labour [14]. Its use as part of an antacid protocol has been recommended [32].

Avoidance of opioid analgesics

Intramuscular opioids delay gastric emptying [14] as do bolus doses of epidural opioids [15] although the initial 100 µg of fentanyl in a low-dose opioid epidural infusion (2 µg/ml) appears to have minimal effect on gastric emptying [33]. All three women dying from aspiration of gastric contents in the last two triennial reports had received systemic opioids during labour [2, 3]; thus a very strong argument can be made for fasting women who have received systemic opioids during labour.

Histamine₂ antagonists and omeprazole

Histamine₂ antagonists and omeprazole both reduce the volume of gastric contents

Active emptying

Insertion of a wide-bore stomach tube [3] or the administration of the emetic apomorphine to empty the stomach have been recommended in the past [34]. Both techniques are unpleasant, could cause morbidity, will not reliably empty the stomach and are not recommended.

Raising the pH of gastric contents

Histamine₂ receptor antagonists

Almost all obstetric units in the UK use H_2 receptor antagonists as part of their antacid policy for women undergoing caesarean section; ranitidine is the preferred drug [20]. H_2 receptor antagonists raise the pH and reduce the volume of intragastric contents, though at least 30 minutes is required for this effect. When intravenous ranitidine was given with oral sodium citrate to 292 women presenting for emergency section only 0.7% of women had a gastric pH < 2.5, the so-called critical pH (the safety of a pH of 2.5 has been questioned) – none of the women given ranitidine more than 30 minutes before induction of anaesthesia had a gastric pH < 3.5, or a volume >25 ml [35]. In the UK the use of routine antacid prophylaxis throughout labour is declining: only 57% of UK obstetric units adopt a routine antacid policy for labour and some 18% provide selective prophylaxis for high-risk women only [20]. Policies dictating that all labouring women receive

drugs with potential side effects [36] to prevent a complication they are unlikely to be exposed to, are being questioned.

Antacid therapy

H_2 antagonists may not have time to work in mothers presenting for emergency section and an oral antacid therapy should be used; recommended therapy is 30 ml 0.3M sodium citrate given within 30 minutes of GA induction. Nevertheless, the H_2 antagonist should still be given to optimize the intragastric conditions for extubation. Over 90% of UK obstetric units now use sodium citrate in contrast to a survey in 1984 when magnesium trisilicate was the preferred antacid [20]. The risks of particulate antacids have been well documented.

Omeprazole

Omeprazole, a parietal cell proton pump inhibitor, raises the pH of gastric content and may also reduce gastric volume. Studies in the parturient have shown conflicting results [37, 38]. Omeprazole is not routinely used in UK obstetric practice.

Maximizing barrier pressure

It is important to minimize intragastric pressure (e.g. by avoiding inducing anaesthesia in the lithotomy position) and to maximize the barrier pressure. Drugs lowering the LOS pressure should be avoided, and the use of those which increase tone should be considered (Table 10.3). Barrier pressure falls at induction of anaesthesia with thiopentone, so cricoid pressure should be applied as thiopentone is given. Suxamethonium causes a greater rise in LOS pressure than in intragastric pressure, so barrier pressure is increased [39].

IMPROVED TRAINING OF ANAESTHETISTS

As recommendations both to reduce the number of small and isolated units and to

Table 10.3 Drug effects on lower oesophageal sphincter pressure

Drugs increasing LOS pressure	Drugs decreasing LOS pressure
Metoclopramide	Atropine
Domperidone	Glycopyrrolate
Prochlorperazine	Ethanol
Neostigmine	Opiates
Suxamethonium	Thiopentone
	Diazepam
	Nitroglycerin

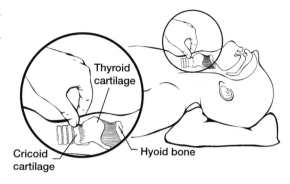

Figure 10.3 Single-handed application of cricoid pressure — note that the neck is flexed on the shoulders and the head extended on the neck, with the head on a pillow.

improve consultant anaesthetist input to obstetric units are implemented, the training and supervision of anaesthetic, midwifery and other staff should improve [40]. Current recommendations suggest that anaesthetic trainees should not work unsupervised in an obstetric unit till they have undergone a minimum of one year general training supplemented by appropriate obstetric anaesthesia training.

Consultant anaesthetists are responsible for preparing failed intubation protocols, and ensuring that trainees and other personnel are familiar with their use. While failed intubation protocols are now available in most obstetric units, unfortunately, they are rarely rehearsed [41]. Anaesthetic equipment and monitoring facilities must conform to published standards [42, 43], e.g. monitoring of carbon dioxide in respiratory gases from intubated patients is now mandatory. Although unrecognized oesophageal intubation caused five of the eight anaesthetic-related maternal deaths in the 1985–1987 triennium there were no deaths attributed to this cause in the 1988–1990 report. It is unlikely that CO_2 monitoring contributed significantly to this reduction since the recommendations could not have been implemented by this time [2, 3].

ANAESTHETIC TECHNIQUE

Important aspects of technique must be emphasized to trainees.

1. Premature attempts to pass an endotracheal tube (ETT) in an inadequately anaesthetized or paralysed woman may predispose to regurgitation and aspiration of gastric contents [44]. Although prompted by anxieties about awareness rather than regurgitation, trainees are now taught to give adequate doses of induction and maintenance agents [45].

2. Incorrectly applied cricoid pressure may contribute to difficulties at intubation [46]. The upper oesophageal sphincter relaxes when muscle relaxants are used, and aspiration can occur unless cricoid pressure is applied properly. Although in Sellick's original description of cricoid pressure the head and neck were fully extended in the tonsillectomy position [47], it is recognized that flexing the neck on the shoulders and extending the head on the neck, with a pillow beneath the occiput, is the optimum position for intubation (Figure 10.3). The 1988–1990 CEMDUK recommends that a trained midwife applies bimanual cricoid pressure while an anaesthetic assistant assists the anaesthetist, but in a small survey (44 obstetric units) only six units reported always using bimanual cricoid pressure [48]. It is unlikely that many units have the manpower to provide two trained assistants for the anaesthetist. The use of a cuboid of

rubber behind the neck [49] or a cricoid yoke has been described as an alternative [50].

3. An appropriate period of denitrogenation prior to induction of anaesthesia is an essential feature of any general anaesthesia technique. The combination of reduced FRC and increased alveolar ventilation facilitates denitrogenation and 95% of pregnant women should be adequately denitrogenated after two minutes of normal breathing from a Magill breathing system **with a prefilled reservoir bag**, provided care is taken to avoid leaks round the facemask [51].

4. A number of women have died because of undetected inadequate reversal of muscle relaxants at the end of anaesthesia. Profound muscle relaxation is not required for caesarean section, and peripheral nerve stimulators should be available, and used, to confirm adequate reversal.

Assistance for the anaesthetist

Recent recommendations are that anaesthetic assistants should be trained to a regionally or nationally agreed standard [43]. A recent survey of all UK obstetric units revealed that, while most units have adopted that standard, 9.3% of units still have midwives assisting the anaesthetist [41].

FAILED INTUBATION PROTOCOLS

Unexpected failed intubations will always occur and the anaesthetist must know and understand a protocol to assist in the management of these difficult cases [52, 53]. It is important to accept the diagnosis of failed intubation early: repeated attempts to intubate by a variety of anaesthetists are not acceptable. Not more than three attempts at tracheal intubation should be allowed, with oxygenation and maintained cricoid pressure between attempts. It is advisable that a stylet be used as a routine rather than make the observation during the first attempt that a stylet would have been

useful. Flow diagrams of various complexity have been published; the current Glasgow Royal Maternity Hospital failed intubation protocol is shown (Figure 10.4).

FAILED INTUBATION – NON-URGENT SECTION

Senior anaesthetic help should be summoned immediately by someone not immediately involved. Equipment must be available to facilitate ventilation of the mother's lungs until she reverts to spontaneous ventilation and recovers consciousness, when a regional anaesthetic technique can be used (Table 10.4). Cricoid pressure should be maintained until recovery of consciousness.

FAILED INTUBATION – URGENT SECTION OR CONTRAINDICATION TO REGIONAL TECHNIQUE

A failed intubation may occur when a regional technique is considered inappropriate, e.g. massive antepartum haemorrhage or a preoperative coagulopathy. The airway may be maintained and the lungs oxygenated with a facemask and oral or nasal airway (NB engorgement of mucosal capillaries in pregnancy may make epistaxis more likely if a nasopharyngeal airway is used). Alternatively a laryngeal mask airway (LMA) may be used. It has been suggested that a long size 6 mm ETT may be passed blindly through the laryngeal mask into the trachea but there is a risk of laryngospasm if the woman is recovering from induction at this point. When the mother reverts to spontaneous ventilation, anaesthesia can be maintained with inhalational agents. It is essential that no further muscle relaxants are given, and the surgeon must accept the muscle relaxation provided by inhalational agents.

It has been recommended that the woman should be turned into the left lateral, head down position and a wide-bore stomach tube inserted to empty the stomach [52]. While this may reduce the risk of aspiration of gastric

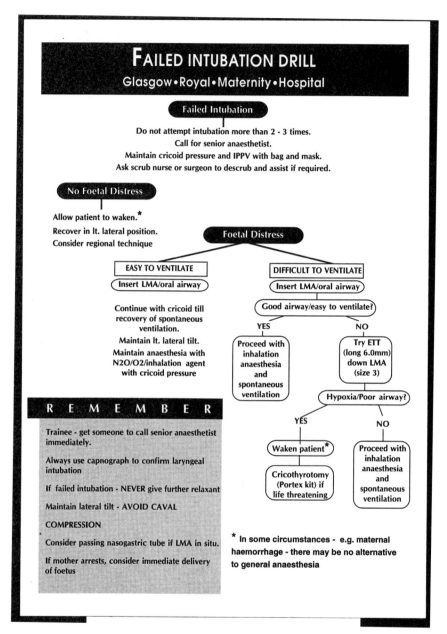

Figure 10.4 Glasgow Royal Maternity Hospital failed intubation protocol, 1995.

contents [53], cricoid pressure will be difficult to maintain while turning a woman into or maintaining this position. Insertion of an orogastric tube creates its own problems: it may provoke either regurgitation by compromising the lower oesophageal sphincter or vomiting if the woman is lightly anaesthetized. Furthermore, an orogastric tube does not guarantee an empty stomach, and ventilation of the lungs will be difficult during insertion and aspiration

Table 10.4 Equipment for difficult intubation cart

Essential	Optional
Range of ETTs – minimum 6 mm	McCoy laryngoscope
Two standard Macintosh laryngoscopes	Short-handled laryngoscope, Belscope laryngoscope
Size 3 and 4 blades, polio blade	Fibreoptic laryngoscope
Introducer stylets (use routinely)	Oesophageal gastric tube airway
Gum elastic bougie	
Oro- and nasopharyngeal airways	
Laryngeal mask airway size 3 or 4	
Cricothyrotomy equipment	
Large-bore orogastric tubes	

of such a tube leading to the risk of hypoxia. This author would recommend keeping the woman in the left lateral tilt and maintaining cricoid pressure, unless this was thought to be compromising the airway.

The LMA will not prevent regurgitated gastric contents entering the lungs. In a cadaver study cricoid pressure prevented gastric contents entering the airway when an LMA was in place [54]. Cricoid pressure may prevent adequate placement and/or ventilation through the LMA; consequently it is suggested that cricoid pressure should be released before LMA placement, and reapplied once the LMA is *in situ* [55], although attempted tracheal intubation through the LMA may be more difficult in the presence of cricoid pressure [56].

The insertion of an oesophageal tube to occlude the oesophagus and prevent aspiration has been described [53]; this may have a place in the management of women who have recently eaten a meal.

FAILED INTUBATION – VENTILATION OF LUNGS DIFFICULT

If oxygen saturation cannot be maintained, maternal safety should take precedence over foetal safety. Even in the presence of foetal distress the mother should be allowed to recover and a regional anaesthetic technique used. Rarely, hypoxia may occur before spontaneous ventilation returns; in these circumstances

transtracheal ventilation should be instituted (see below), the mother woken and a regional anaesthetic technique used. Emergency cricothyrotomy is probably safer than emergency tracheostomy particularly if the surgeon has little or no tracheostomy experience.

MANAGEMENT OF THE RECOGNIZED DIFFICULT INTUBATION

ELECTIVE CAESAREAN SECTION

Regional anaesthesia is the preferred option. Anxieties about excessively high blocks compromising respiratory function or protective airway reflexes should be abolished by a consultant anaesthetist supervising every aspect of patient management throughout induction of regional block and surgery. It is inappropriate for a trainee to manage these high-risk cases unsupervised. The last two CEMDUKs report women dying after unsupervised junior anaesthetists attempted regional blocks on women known to be high risk [2, 3].

There is little reliable evidence that 'single shot' spinals are unpredictable, but if an epidural is felt to be safer then it should be topped up with 3 ml increments every two minutes, with each increment being assessed to ensure that inadvertent subarachnoid injection has not taken place. A combined spinal epidural technique or spinal catheter may offer extra flexibility in experienced hands.

EMERGENCY CAESAREAN SECTION – EPIDURAL ANALGESIA IN LABOUR

Women who are known to have, or are predicted to have, intubation problems should have the risks of general anaesthesia explained to them. They should be encouraged to accept an epidural in labour. It is essential that a good bilateral block is confirmed; the analgesic block can be rapidly extended to an anaesthetic block for surgery if this is required [57].

EMERGENCY CAESAREAN SECTION – NO EPIDURAL IN LABOUR

Consultant assistance should be requested immediately. A regional technique is preferred. While a combined spinal–epidural technique or a spinal catheter will both give a rapid onset of sensory block and provide the opportunity to supplement the block should anaesthesia be inadequate, they are not as quick as a single shot spinal. If the woman is known to have experienced a previous failed intubation it is imperative that the risks of GA are explained to her and the obstetricians – in these unusual circumstances a delay for induction of a regional block and for senior assistance to arrive would seem justified even in the presence of foetal distress.

REGIONAL BLOCK CONTRAINDICATED

If there is a contraindication to RA (in these circumstances it may only be a relative contraindication) or immediate surgery is required to save the mother and the baby, e.g. massive haemorrhage, the decision on anaesthetic technique depends on the magnitude of risk. In a woman with gross anatomical abnormalities or a previous history of failed intubation, either awake fibreoptic intubation, tracheostomy insertion under local anaesthesia, or local anaesthetic infiltration of the abdominal wall will have to be considered [58]. If the risk is of a lower magnitude, such as Mallampati class 4 airway and a short neck, with no previous

history of problems, it would be reasonable to proceed with induction of GA after appropriate preparation. Anaesthetists working in the obstetric unit must be familiar with the failed intubation protocol, and the equipment provided for managing these problem cases.

ADJUNCTS TO INTUBATION

Techniques for facilitating endotracheal intubation in recognized difficult airways have been described in more detail elsewhere [5]. In obstetric practice they should rarely be used as RA is the preferred option.

AWAKE INTUBATION

Endotracheal intubation under local infiltration and sedation

Sedation may compromise both maternal protective airway reflexes and the foetus. Surface analgesia is achieved with local anaesthetic sprays, lozenges, or topical cocaine. Benumof has described techniques for relevant nerve blocks [5]. Intubation can proceed as a blind nasal intubation, or the laryngoscope can be introduced gradually through the mouth, spraying local anaesthetic as it is advanced. A gum elastic bougie can be used.

Fibreoptic intubation – local infiltration and sedation

Techniques for providing surface analgesia are as above, and oxygen supplementation should be used. Nasal intubation is probably easier, though epistaxis subsequent to nasal mucosal engorgement may make visualization of the larynx impossible. A fibreoptic scope can be passed through a LMA.

Retrograde intubation

A catheter or guide wire is introduced percutaneously from below the vocal cords, brought out through the mouth or nose, and used as a stylet for subsequent endotracheal intubation. This technique is useful when blood in the airway obscures the view but it can be difficult to railroad the endotracheal tube over the stylet [5]. Cricotracheal puncture may offer some advantages over cricothyroid puncture [59].

All these techniques require time and expertise, neither of which may be available in an obstetric unit when urgent delivery of the foetus is required.

EQUIPMENT

Gum elastic bougie

This should be available in all theatres. It can be passed blindly into the larynx and the ETT railroaded over it.

Laryngoscopes

A variety of laryngoscopes are now available. Difficulties encountered inserting the laryngoscope blade into the mouth can be overcome by inserting clip-on or screw-on blades before fixing to the handle. Newer short handled [60] or polio laryngoscopes may overcome such insertion problems without the need for blade detachment. The tip of the McCoy laryngoscope blade can lever the epiglottis out of the way to facilitate visualization of the larynx if the epiglottis is obscuring the view [61]. Straight-bladed laryngoscopes and Macintosh size 4 blades should be available. The Belscope laryngoscope has had favourable reports [62].

Transtracheal ventilation

Equipment must be available to perform transtracheal ventilation in the rare case when oxygenation of the lungs cannot be maintained by other means. The Portex minitracheostomy kit provides a guarded scalpel blade to penetrate the cricothyroid membrane: a size 4 mm

uncuffed ETT is passed over an introducer (Portex Ltd, Hythe, Kent, UK). The ETT has a standard connector which can be connected to a conventional anaesthetic circuit; this should maintain oxygenation of the mother. Other commercial kits which allow for the passage of larger tubes are described elsewhere [21].

Transtracheal jet ventilation involves the insertion of a large bore cannula (12 or 14 gauge) through the cricothyroid membrane and attaching this to a high pressure oxygen source, e.g. the emergency oxygen supply on the standard anaesthetic machine. A length of rigid tubing should connect the oxygen outlet and the cannula via a Luer lock [21]. It is essential to confirm correct catheter placement and ensure the lungs deflate after inflation since transtracheal ventilation may not be straightforward; life-threatening or fatal complications including haemorrhage, subcutaneous emphysema and barotrauma may occur.

Oesophageal gastric tube airway

Deliberate oesophageal intubation with a cuffed tube prevents pulmonary aspiration of gastric contents and can improve the airway [63].

All of this equipment is useless if the anaesthetist is unfamiliar with it. Anaesthetists should practice using the left lateral position, different laryngoscopes and gum elastic bougies on straightforward general surgical intubations. Experience with fibreoptic intubation and cricothyroid ventilation is inevitably limited, but anaesthetists should familiarize themselves with the equipment available; the anaesthetist most experienced with these techniques should be called.

CONCLUSION

The administration of general anaesthesia for emergency caesarean section can be difficult and challenging: these will be some of the most stressful cases an anaesthetist encounters. A sense of false security may develop among obstetricians, midwives, managers, and even anaesthetists themselves, as the number of anaesthetic disasters declines. New challenges lie ahead with changes in the ethos of childbirth, midwife training, midwife led care, a trend toward home deliveries and pressures on our own staffing levels. Constant vigilance is required by obstetric anaesthetists to maintain or, indeed, improve standards of care in order to sustain the current low rates of anaesthesia-related maternal mortality.

REFERENCES

1. Department of Health and Social Security Report on Health and Social Subjects, Number 34 (1989) *Report on Confidential Enquiries into Maternal Deaths in England and Wales 1982–1984*, HMSO, London.
2. Department of Health Welsh Office, Scottish Office Home Health Department, Department of Health and Social Security Report on Health and Social Subjects (1991) *Report on Confidential Enquiries into Maternal Deaths in England and Wales 1985–1987*, HMSO, London.
3. Department of Health Welsh Office, Scottish Home Health Department, Department of Health and Social Security Report on Health and Social Subjects, Number 34 (1994) *Report on Confidential Enquiries into Maternal Deaths in England and Wales 1988–1990*, HMSO, London.
4. Cobley, M. and Vaughan, R.S. (1992) Recognition and management of difficult airway problems. *British Journal of Anaesthesia*, **68**, 90–7.
5. Benumof, J.L. (1991) Management of the difficult adult airway. *Anesthesiology*, **75**, 1087–1110.
6. Lyons, G. (1985) Failed intubation. Six years' experience in a teaching maternity unit. *Anaesthesia*, **40**, 759–62.
7. Samsoon, G.L.T. and Young, J.R.B. (1987) Difficult tracheal intubation: a retrospective study. *Anaesthesia*, **42**, 487–90.
8. Rocke, D.A. and Scoones, G.P. (1992) Rapidly progressive laryngeal oedema associated with pregnancy aggravated hypertension. *Anaesthesia*, **47**, 141–3.
9. Joupilla, R., Joupilla, P. and Hollmen, A. (1980) Laryngeal oedema as an obstetric anaesthesia complication. *Acta Anaesthesiologica Scandinavica*, **24**, 97–8.
10. Attia, R.R., Ebeid, A.M., Fischer, J.E. and Goudsouzian, N.G. (1982) Maternal, fetal and placental gastrin concentrations. *Anaesthesia*, **37**, 18–21.
11. Dow, T.G.B., Brock-Utne, J.G., Rubin, J. *et al.* (1978) The effect of atropine on the lower esophageal sphincter in late pregnancy. *Obstetrics and Gynecology*, **51**, 426–30.
12. Vanner, R.G. and Goodman, N.W. (1989) Gastro-oesophageal reflux in pregnancy at term and after delivery. *Anaesthesia*, **44**, 808–11.
13. Macfie, A.G., Magides, A.D., Richmond, M.N. and Reilly, C.S. (1991) Gastric emptying in pregnancy. *British Journal of Anaesthesia*, **67**, 54–7.
14. Nimmo, W.S., Wilson, J. and Prescott, L.F. (1975) Narcotic analgesics and delayed gastric emptying during labour. *Lancet*, **1**, 890–3.
15. Wright, P.M.C., Allen, R.W., Moore, J. and Donnelly, J.P. (1992) Gastric emptying during lumbar extradural analgesia in labour: effect of fentanyl supplementation. *British Journal of Anaesthesia*, **68**, 248–51.
16. Whitehead, E.M., Smith, M., Dean, Y. and O'Sullivan, G. (1993) An evaluation of gastric emptying times in pregnancy and the puerperium. *Anaesthesia*, **48**, 53–7.
17. Knuttgen, H.G. and Emerson, K (1975) Physiologic response to pregnancy at rest and during exercise. *Journal of Applied Physiology*, **36**, 549.
18. CRAG Framework for Action Working Group for Maternity Services (1996) Report on pain relief in Labour.
19. Brown, G. and Russell, I.F. (1995) A survey of obstetric anaesthesia. *International Journal of Obstetric Anaesthesia*, **4**, 214–8.
20. Greiff, G.M.C., Tordoff, S.G., Griffiths, R. and May, A.E. (1994) Acid aspiration prophylaxis in 202 obstetric units in the UK. *International Journal of Obstetric Anaesthesia*, **3**, 137–42.
21. King, T.A. and Adams, A.P. (1990) Failed tracheal intubation. *British Journal of Anaesthesia*, **65**, 400–14.
22. Mallampati, S.R., Gatt, S.P., Gugino, L.D. *et al.* (1985) A clinical sign to predict difficult intubation: a prospective study. *Canadian Anaesthetists Society Journal*, **32(4)**, 429–34.
23. Cormack, R.S. and Lehane, J. (1984) Difficult intubation in obstetrics. *Anaesthesia*, **39**, 1105–11.
24. Wilson, M.E., Speiglhalter, D., Robertson, J.A. and Lesser, P. (1988) Predicting difficult intubation. *British Journal of Anaesthesia*, **61**, 211–6.
25. Oates, J.D.L., Macleod, A.D., Oates, P.D. *et al.* (1991) Comparison of two methods for

predicting difficult intubation. *British Journal of Anaesthesia*, **66**, 305–9.

26. Tham, E.J., Gildersleve, C.D., Saunders, L.D. *et al.* (1992) Effects of posture, phonation, and observer on Mallampati classification. *British Journal of Anaesthesia*, **68**, 32–8.

27. Farcon, E.L., Kim, M.H. and Marx, G.F. (1994) Changing Mallampati score during labour. *Canadian Journal of Anaesthesia*, **41**, 50–1.

28. Rocke, D.A., Murray, W.B., Rout, C.C. and Gouws, E. (1992) Relative risk analysis of factors associated with difficult intubation in obstetric anaesthesia. *Anesthesiology*, **77**, 67–73.

29. Mendelson, C.L. (1945) The aspiration of stomach contents into the lungs during obstetric anesthesia. *American Journal of Obstetrics and Gynecology*, **52**, 191–205.

30. Carp, H., Jayram, A. and Stoll, M. (1992) Ultrasound examination of the stomach contents of parturients. *Anesthesia and Analgesia*, **74**, 683–7.

31. Michael, S., Reilly, C.S. and Caunt, J.A. (1991) Policies for oral intake during labour. A survey of maternity units in England and Wales. *Anaesthesia*, **46**, 1071–3.

32. Thomas, T.A. (1994) Maternal mortality. *International Journal of Obstetric Anaesthesia*, **3**, 125–6.

33. O'Sullivan, G. (1995) Mendelson's Syndrome 1946 – feeding in labour 1996. Obstetric Anaesthesia Conference, Rotunda Hospital, Dublin, September 1995.

34. Holdsworth, J.D., Furness, R.M.B. and Roulston, R.G. (1974) A comparison of apomorphine and stomach tube for emptying the stomach before general anaesthesia in obstetrics. *British Journal of Anaesthesia*, **46**, 526 – 9.

35. Rout, C.C., Rocke, D.A. and Gouws, E. (1993) Intravenous ranitidine reduces the risk of acid aspiration of gastric contents at emergency caesarean section. *Anesthesia and Analgesia*, **76**, 156–61.

36. Powell, J.A. and Maycock, E.J. (1993) Anaphylactoid reaction to ranitidine in an obstetric patient. *Anaesthesia and Intensive Care*, **21**, 702–3.

37. Ewart, M.C., Yau, G., Gin, T. *et al.* (1990) A comparison of the effects of omeprazole and ranitidine on gastric secretion in women undergoing elective caesarean section. *Anaesthesia*, **45**, 527–30.

38. Rocke, A., Rout, C.C. and Gouws, E. (1994) Intravenous administration of the proton pump inhibitor omeprazole reduces the risk of acid aspiration at emergency caesarean section. *Anesthesia and Analgesia*, **78**, 1093–8.

39. Cotton, B.R. and Smith, G. (1984) The lower oesophageal sphincter and anaesthesia. *British Journal of Anaesthesia*, **56**, 37–46.

40. Association of Anaesthetists of Great Britain and Ireland (1987) *Anaesthetic Services for Obstetrics – a Plan for the Future*, Association of Anaesthetists of Great Britain and Ireland, London.

41. Cook, T.M. and McCirrick, A. (1994) A survey of airway management during induction of general anaesthesia in obstetrics. *International Journal of Obstetric Anaesthesia*, **3**, 143–5.

42. Association of Anaesthetists of Great Britain and Ireland (1994) *Recommendations for Standards of Monitoring during Anaesthesia and Recovery*, Association of Anaesthetists of Great Britain and Ireland, London.

43. Obstetric Anaesthetists Association (1995) *Recommended Minimum Standards for Obstetric Anaesthesia Services*, Obstetric Anaesthetists Association, OAA Secretariat, P.O. Box 3219, London.

44. Reynolds, F. (1990) It is essential that antacid prophylaxis is given to all women in labour – Arguments against, in *Controversies in Obstetric Anaesthesia Number 1* (ed. B Morgan), Edward Arnold, Kent, pp. 43–7.

45. Lyons, G. and Macdonald, R. (1991) Awareness during Caesarean section. *Anaesthesia*, **46**, 62–4.

46. Howells, T.H., Chamney, A.R., Wraight, W.J. and Simons, R.S. (1983) The application of cricoid pressure. *Anaesthesia*, **38**, 457–60.

47. Sellick, B.A. (1961) Cricoid pressure to control regurgitation of stomach contents during induction of anaesthesia: preliminary communication. *Lancet*, **2**, 404–6.

48. Sajjad, T. (1994) Survey of the provision of anaesthetic cover and aspects of the anaesthetic management of obstetric emergencies. *International Journal of Obstetric Anaesthesia*, **3**, 179–80.

49. Crawford, J.S. (1982) The contracricoid cuboid aid to tracheal intubation. *Anaesthesia*, **37**, 345.

50. Vanner, R.G., O'Dwyer, J.P., Pryle, B.J. and Reynolds, F. (1992) Upper oesophageal sphincter pressure and the effect of cricoid pressure. *Anaesthesia*, **47**, 95–100.

51. Russell, G.N., Smith, C.L., Snowdon, S.L. and Bryson, T.H.L. (1987) Pre-oxygenation and the parturient patient. *Anaesthesia*, **42**, 346–51.

52. Tunstall, M.E. (1976) Failed intubation drill. *Anaesthesia*, **31**, 850.

53. Tunstall, M.E. (1989) Failed intubation in the parturient. *Canadian Journal of Anaesthesia*, **36**, 611–3.

54. Strang, T.I. (1992) Does the laryngeal mask airway compromise cricoid pressure? *Anaesthesia*, **47**, 829–31.

55. Asai, T. and Morris, S. (1994) The laryngeal mask airway: its features, effects and role. *Canadian Journal of Anaesthesia*, **41**, 930–60.

56. Asai, T., Barclay, K., Power, I. and Vaughan, R.S. (1994) Cricoid pressure impedes placement of the laryngeal mask airway and subsequent tracheal intubation through the mask. *British Journal of Anaesthesia*, **72**, 47–51.

57. Price, M.L., Reynolds, F. and Morgan, B.M. (1991) Extending epidural blockade for emergency caesarean section. Evaluation of 2% lignocaine with adrenaline. *International Journal of Obstetric Anaesthesia*, **1**, 13–8.

58. Barth, W.H. (1992) Local infiltration for cesarean delivery, in *Manual of Obstetric Anesthesia*, 2nd edn (ed. G.W. Ostheimer), Churchill Livingstone, New York, pp. 202–8.

59. Shanther, T.R. (1992) Retrograde intubation using the subcricoid region. *British Journal of Anaesthesia*, **68**, 109–12.

60. Camann, W.R. and Ostheimer, G.W. (1992) Physiologic adaptations during pregnancy, *in Manual of Obstetric Anesthesia*, 2nd edn (ed. GW Ostheimer), Churchill Livingstone, New York, p. 7.

61. McCoy, E.P. and Mirakhur, R.K. (1993) The levering laryngoscope. *Anaesthesia*, **48**, 516–9.

62. Hodges, U.M., O'Flaherty, D. and Adams, A.P. (1993) Tracheal intubation in a mannikin: comparison of the Belscope with the Macintosh laryngoscope. *British Journal of Anaesthesia*, **71**, 905–7.

63. Tunstall, M.E. and Geddes, C. (1988) Emergency caesarean section – tracheal intubation or oesophageal gastric tube airway. *British Journal of Anaesthesia*, **60**, 476.

I.F. Russell

INTRODUCTION

The pregnant or postpartum woman may suffer from all the neurological diseases of her non-pregnant sister and the interested reader is referred to recent books for a more detailed discussion of general neurology specifically related to pregnancy [1, 2]. Similarly, in terms of the myriad anaesthetic causes of nerve injury not specifically related to obstetrics but which could occur in the course of obstetric anaesthesia the reader is referred to other reviews [3, 4]. This chapter is intended to draw to the attention of the reader both those postpartum neurological problems often blamed on regional anaesthesia, but which are invariably due to the pathophysiological process of pregnancy or labour, and the more unusual problems which may be secondary to regional anaesthesia.

Although postpartum obstetric palsies were first described in 1838 and were well recognized in the early part of this century [5], obstetric or neurological texts usually devote little if any space to the topic. Adornato and Carlini believe that as a consequence, today there is often a general lack of knowledge that 'compressive neuropathies can occur as a result of natural childbirth – free of instrumentation or anaesthesia' [6]. My own experience over the past 15 years is entirely in agreement with these authors. This is illustrated by a solicitor's letter alleging his client must have had an epidural performed negligently during her labour, some six months previously, as she was now unable to walk properly. Review of the obstetric notes revealed that the patient never had any actual or proposed regional, local or general anaesthesia whatsoever! The propensity to blame regional anaesthesia for any unusual neurological symptom in the puerperium is an important reason for ensuring that all women who have had any anaesthetic involvement are seen at least once within 24–48 hours after delivery and that accurate contemporaneous notes are always kept. It behoves the obstetric anaesthetist to be aware of the range of neurological problems which can arise postpartum and to become intimately involved in their diagnosis to ensure that regional anaesthesia is not blamed unfairly. Once the 'seed' is sown in the patient's mind, there is considerable potential for prolonged and costly medico-legal debate. Showing the patient a description of her complaint in a book can prove invaluable.

Any postpartum neurological problem requires immediate attention with detailed ongoing evaluation while the complaint persists. A thorough history and neurological

Clinical Problems in Obstetric Anaesthesia
Edited by Ian F. Russell and Gordon Lyons. Published in 1997 by Chapman & Hall, London. ISBN 0 412 71600 3.

examination are required to delineate the extent, site and aetiology of the symptoms so as to guide specific and supportive treatment. Careful mapping of any sensory or motor deficits will help to establish whether the lesion is segmental or peripheral in character. Nerve conduction studies and electromyography are an extension of the physical examination and are the prime methods used to confirm abnormalities of the peripheral nervous system [7]. These investigations not only accurately define the site of the lesion, but also indicate the age of the lesion, the prognosis for recovery, the rate of recovery and ultimately the extent of the recovery. Further evidence of the importance of such investigations can be seen in an analysis of 482 patients (all non-obstetric) whose neurological complaint had been attributed to spinal anaesthesia: all but four had an entirely unrelated neurological condition [8].

Neurological problems divide into two broad categories, central and peripheral. The former requires urgent diagnosis and treatment since delay significantly reduces the chance of recovery. In general, the sensory and motor abnormality found with peripheral nerve lesions follows the distribution of the affected part of the peripheral nervous system rather than involving an entire extremity.

PERIPHERAL NERVE INJURIES

These are the most common of the obstetric-related neurological problems and exist as one of three types.

- Neurapraxia: The nerve and its axonal sheath are intact and recover their function in a very short time, e.g. compression for a short time causes ischaemic paralysis with numbness and tingling. True ischaemic block even up to four hours usually recovers in minutes but compressive injuries also cause mechanical deformation of the nerve localized to the site of compression. This resultant damage, which includes localized oedema, white cell infiltration and loss of myelin, may take several weeks to repair but then full recovery occurs rapidly.
- Axonotmesis: Injury causing axonal degeneration, but the sheath remains intact, e.g. prolonged ischaemia or compression. Recovery will usually be complete, but slow as the axon only regenerates at the rate of about 1 mm/day. Patients with neuritis or vitamin B deficiencies tend to be more susceptible to both neurapraxia and axonotmesis [9].
- Neurotmesis: Both axon and axon sheath are disrupted, e.g. as a result of cutting, stretching or shearing forces There is little chance of full recovery since not only do the axons have to regenerate but they must also grow down their correct axon sheath.

NERVE ROOTS

Epidural or spinal needles may cause direct damage to nerve roots or the spinal cord. Should fluid be injected into the substance of the nerve or spinal cord then nerve fibres or tracts will be disrupted. Such direct trauma is invariably accompanied by severe lancinating pain, at which point further instrumentation or injection should cease, the needle or catheter should be withdrawn immediately and resited elsewhere. Residual paraesthesia, hypoalgesia and motor weakness may occur depending on the extent of the damage. The resolution of these symptoms is variable, some making a full recovery in a few weeks, but others are permanent. The importance of gentle controlled advance of needles and catheters cannot be overemphasized.

LUMBOSACRAL TRUNK

Lumbosacral trunk lesions occur secondary to direct pressure on these nerves within the pelvis, either by the baby's head or by obstetric forceps. The most susceptible portion is the lower lumbosacral plexus, composed of the 4th and 5th lumbar roots, and the higher sacral roots [7], supplying the sciatic and the gluteal nerves. The fibres which ultimately create the peroneal nerve are affected more often than the tibial components [7, 10]; hence foot drop is one of the most common findings. It may be important to differentiate between foot drop caused by foetal head pressure on the lumbosacral trunk from foot drop caused by pressure on the peroneal nerve as it courses round the head of the fibula (see below). In the latter situation pain is unusual whereas pain is common with lumbosacral plexus injury [11]. Other unusual causes may mimic lumbosacral plexus injury: one patient, unable to walk post-delivery, was diagnosed as having bilateral iliopsoas muscle strain but unfortunately no nerve conduction or electromyogram studies were obtained and the patient made a rapid recovery within a week [12]; multiple intramuscular injections in the buttocks of a labouring woman have resulted in bilateral sciatic nerve compression and several days of weakness [13]; prolonged nursing of a thin labouring woman (with an epidural *in situ*) in a reclining position has resulted in sciatic nerve damage [14].

PERONEAL NERVES

The common peroneal nerve, the smaller of the terminal branches of the sciatic nerve, forms at or above the apex of the popliteal fossa. Bilateral common peroneal palsies have been described following 'natural childbirth' in both supine [6] and squatting [15] positions. The aetiology suggested in these cases is either direct compression of the nerve as it courses round the head of the fibula (e.g. by the patient's hands [6]), or a stretching injury [15], or a compartment-like syndrome as the nerve passes through a fibrous tunnel under the origin of peroneus longus [16]. Deep peroneal nerve injuries secondary to prolonged squatting are a recognized occupational hazard in the Far East [16]. A patient from the author's unit who had been in receipt of an epidural for labour was referred following a complaint of

foot drop. This had first developed some months after delivery. Nerve conduction studies revealed deep peroneal nerve damage compatible with the mother spending prolonged periods in the squatting position with her newborn baby and older toddler.

FEMORAL NERVE

Within the body of the psoas muscle the femoral nerve is formed from fibres of the 2nd, 3rd and 4th lumbar nerves. It then courses between the psoas and the iliacus muscles across the wings of the ilia (the false pelvis) to pass under the inguinal ligament into the thigh. There have been many reports of femoral nerve damage during childbirth but a review suggests the incidence has declined considerably since the beginning of this century, possibly due to shorter labours and the greater use of caesarean section [17]. There is debate about the exact aetiology of damage to the nerve. Although in certain circumstances direct pressure from self-retaining abdominal retractors or compression under the inguinal ligament due to the lithotomy position is possible (flexing, abducting and externally rotating the thighs forces the femoral nerve into an 80–90% angulation on the inguinal ligament) [18], it seems likely that the most common cause during childbirth is a proximal lesion arising within the pelvis due to direct pressure by the foetal head [19]. Occasionally the neurological deficit displays a high degree of bilateral symmetry suggesting the possibility of a central lesion [20, 21]; in these circumstances it is only too easy to assume a central lesion and blame regional anaesthesia unless adequate investigations are performed. The symptoms of femoral nerve palsy will depend on the exact site of the lesion, but may include limited thigh flexion, loss of quadriceps power, absent or reduced knee jerk reflex (the most reliable objective sign of femoral neuropathy) and loss of sensation over the femoral nerve distribution. The patient may be able to walk on the level provided she locks her knee in hyperextension, but if the knee is at all bent the leg will give way, making it impossible to climb stairs or rise from a squatting position.

OBTURATOR NERVE

Like the femoral nerve, the obturator nerve is formed from fibres of the 2nd, 3rd and 4th lumbar nerves within the psoas muscle. The nerve may be injured by direct pressure within the pelvis or by acute angulation, induced by the lithotomy position, as it passes through the obturator foramen. Symptoms of obturator nerve injury may be minimal and difficult to detect: sensory loss is limited to the medial side of the thigh and, since adductor magnus also receives a nerve supply from the sciatic nerve, adduction is still present but weakened. The effect of the weakened adductor muscle may be seen during walking when the leg tends to swing outward.

LATERAL FEMORAL CUTANEOUS NERVE OF THE THIGH

Damage to this nerve gives rise to the syndrome of meralgia paraesthetica. The nerve is entirely sensory and arises from the L2 and L3 nerve roots. It emerges from the lateral border of psoas at the iliac crest and runs across the iliacus muscle to enter the thigh under the inguinal ligament just medial to the anterior superior iliac spine. The lesion may be proximal (i.e. within the pelvis, either as the nerve angulates over the sacro-iliac joint [1, 2] or by direct pressure from the foetal head) or peripheral (occasionally the nerve passes through a canal formed by an anterior and posterior fasciculus of the inguinal ligament: these latter patients are particularly susceptible to nerve damage [22]). Meralgia paraesthetica is an unpleasant sensation, variously described as numbness, burning, dysaesthesia or pain over the anterolateral aspect of the thigh. The symptoms are exacerbated by walking, standing or extending the hips [23]. The onset of the symptomatology is often associated with rapid

weight gain, possibly due to traction of panniculi on the nerve or to an associated lumbar lordosis [22]. While the enlarging uterus cannot exert direct pressure on the nerve it seems likely that increased tension in the abdominal fascia and muscles can create a shutter-like action where the nerve passes under the inguinal ligament [22]. Meralgia paraesthetica, when it occurs, is usually described during the antenatal period and should not contraindicate the use of regional anaesthesia [24]. While the above references all relate to the antenatal period the author is aware of several cases where symptoms were first complained of in the postnatal period. All had received epidural analgesia for labour and when the epidural wore off they became aware of altered sensation over the anterolateral aspect of the thigh. Their symptoms resolved over days to months. Not all of these women had their legs in lithotomy stirrups, but all had their feet placed on midwives' hips during delivery with the thighs hyper-flexed during pushing

RADIAL NERVE

Bilateral radial nerve palsies have been described following use of a 'birth frame' during 'natural childbirth': women were encouraged to hang their arms over the back of the frame to support their weight in a semi-squatting position. Initially, the numbness of the hands was attributed to hyperventilation, but after delivery the correct diagnosis of bilateral radial nerve palsy was made. EMG studies suggested that recovery would be expected, but the patient never returned for follow-up [25].

ULNAR NERVE

The ulnar nerve is susceptible to compression at both the elbow and the wrist, and symptoms have been reported in up to 2% of pregnant women [26] but in a recent survey of some 48 000 women only one postpartum ulnar nerve lesion was reported [27].

CARPAL TUNNEL SYNDROME

This is probably the most common compression syndrome in pregnancy [1, 2] with some 25% of postpartum women reporting symptoms [28]. Symptoms may include numbness, weakness or painful burning/tingling in the hands with a deep ache along the inner aspect of the forearm. Oedema may be a precipitating factor. The rate of ring removal for swelling of the fingers during pregnancy is twice as great for women with carpal tunnel syndrome as for non-symptomatic women. The tarsal tunnel syndrome is the equivalent lesion in the lower limb and is due to compression of the posterior tibial nerve at the ankle [2].

SPECIFIC CRANIAL NERVE LESIONS

Although the cranial nerves are within the skull, apart from the optic nerve, they are in fact classified as peripheral nerves. Cranial nerve paralysis is an infrequent but well-recognized complication of spinal anaesthesia or dural puncture and involvement of every cranial nerve except the olfactory, glossopharyngeal and vagus has been reported [29]. Several mechanisms have been suggested: the symptoms are often preceded by post-dural puncture headache (PDPH) and one theory is that a low cerebral spinal fluid (CSF) pressure allows downward displacement of the brain with resultant traction on the cranial nerves leading to stretching of individual nerves over bony prominences at the base of the skull; alternatively there may be restriction of the blood supply to the nerve, secondary to stretching or compression, as the nerve passes through some restricted area. With regard to auditory disturbances, it should be remembered that there is a direct communication between the CSF and the endolymph within the cochlea and changes in CSF pressure may have a direct effect on middle ear function. Sometimes, like PDPH, the symptoms referable to the cranial nerves are postural. Apart from treating the PDPH with a

blood patch there is no other specific treatment for any of these nerve palsies.

Optic nerve (2nd cranial)

Since the optic nerve is a tract of the brain rather than a peripheral nerve (the dura fuses with the sclera), changes in CSF pressure may affect the nerve or the central retinal vessels directly. De Lange *et al.* [30] describe two patients who complained of headache and black spots in their fields of vision after spinal anaesthesia for caesarean section (22 gauge needles). No specific treatment for the headaches was mentioned in the report, and both patients developed permanent pericentral ring scotoma. Traction on the optic nerves was postulated, but profound hypotension with ventricular fibrillation in one case probably made a significant contribution.

Trigeminal nerve (5th cranial nerve)

The trigeminal nerve is the largest cranial nerve, connected to the side of the pons by two roots: a large sensory root and a much smaller motor root. The sensory root arises from the trigeminal ganglion which in turn is made up from the afferent fibres of the three divisions of the trigeminal nerve: the mandibular, the maxillary and the ophthalmic. The mandibular nerve passes down through the foramen ovale and is joined immediately outside the skull by the small motor root of the trigeminal nerve. Of the three branches, the mandibular is said to be the most frequently involved in stretching injuries, possibly because of its angulation over the petrous bone and a sharp curve after it passes through the foramen ovale [29]. Symptoms will obviously depend on which particular branch is involved. Lee and Roberts [29] describe a patient with headache, left-sided facial numbness (also affecting the posterior two thirds of the tongue) and pain referred to the left neck and shoulder. These symptoms resolved soon after specific treatment for her headache (intravenous fluid and a tight abdominal binder). Numbness in the trigeminal distribution may also be found with high spinal or epidural blocks [31, personal observation].

Abducens nerve (6th cranial)

The nucleus of the 6th nerve lies in the floor of the fourth ventricle in direct contact with CSF. The nerve has a long and tortuous course over the temporal bone before passing through the cavernous sinus to innervate the lateral rectus muscle of the eye. Paralysis of the abducens nerve is reported more often than any other cranial nerve: in complete paralysis there will be a medial squint of the affected eye and double vision. With partial paralysis there will be weakness of the muscle: looking toward the ipsilateral side with the affected eye will cause double vision. The diplopia may last for several weeks to months. Other than epidural blood patch to treat the PDPH there is no specific treatment. Symptomatic therapy includes alternate eye patches or a prism to preserve/provide binocular vision. Other causes of bilateral 6th nerve palsy include diabetes, myasthenia gravis, herpes zoster, pseudotumour cerebri, cavernous sinus thrombosis and thyroid disease [32].

Facial nerve (7th cranial)

The facial nerve arises at the lower border of the pons and is mostly composed of motor fibres, although it has a small sensory component to the soft palate as well as carrying taste sensations from the anterior third of the tongue. The nerve passes through the internal acoustic meatus to enter the long and tortuous facial canal within the temporal bone. The incidence of idiopathic facial nerve paralysis (Bell's palsy) is more than three times greater during pregnancy than in the non-pregnant state. Coventry [33] described facial nerve paralysis in association with epidural analgesia for labour in a patient with preeclampsia, but whether this was purely coincidental is

unknown. Two recent cases of facial nerve paralysis after an epidural blood patch have been described [34, 35]. It is thought that the long course through the narrow facial canal may facilitate both nerve traction injuries and compression/ischaemia following a rapid rise in CSF pressure after a blood patch. Recurrent lower motor neurone facial paralysis has also been reported in consecutive pregnancies [36]. Despite the association of facial nerve paralysis and pregnancy it is felt that Bell's palsy in a pregnant woman should not be a contraindication to regional anaesthesia [37].

Vestibulocochlear nerve (8th cranial)

The 8th cranial nerve has a very short course from its origin at the lower edge of the pons in the cerebellar pontine angle to the internal auditory meatus. While traction on the intracranial nerve may be the cause of symptoms, it should be remembered that changes in CSF pressure (e.g. following a dural tap or blood patch) may cause endolymphatic pressure changes within the inner ear. Pressure changes in the endolymph may cause diminished hearing, tinnitus, popping and buzzing noises, as well as problems with balance akin to Menière's disease. These symptoms are usually transient, but may take several months to subside.

Finally, it should be remembered that mixed cranial nerve lesions are possible. Some 24 hours after a dural tap a patient in the author's unit complained of headache with hearing loss and tinnitus. A blood patch was performed, but due to technical problems only 10 ml could be injected. This did not completely relieve the headache or the auditory symptoms. When seen by the author some 24 hours later she still had a headache, hearing loss and tinnitus, although all were improved. A repeat blood patch was discussed, but it then emerged that for several hours after her original blood patch she had noted left-sided facial numbness. At this point we were both somewhat reluctant to attempt a further blood patch. The headache subsided over a further 24 hours, normal hearing returned within three to six months but tinnitus has persisted.

CENTRAL INJURIES

HEADACHE

There is a wide differential diagnosis of headache during pregnancy, childbirth and the puerperium. Khurana [38] gives an excellent and short review of the commoner headaches affected by pregnancy. These include vascular headaches (e.g. migraine, hypertensive), muscle contraction headaches (e.g. tension, cervical osteoarthritis), traction and inflammatory type headaches (e.g. tumour, arteritis, occlusive vascular disease), metabolic (e.g. postpartum exhaustion, hypoglycaemia), toxic effects from infective processes (e.g. wound abscess, intrauterine infection), preeclampsia, pseudotumour cerebri and intracranial haemorrhage. Myofascial pain is common after vaginal deliveries, resembles PDPH but is not postural. Headache due to air injection during epidural insertion may occur: a trainee under direct supervision unexpectedly injected the air remaining in the syringe (5–7 ml) after obtaining loss of resistance. The labouring patient was in a sitting position and unfortunately a dural tap had occurred. Before the catheter could be threaded into the CSF the patient complained of a severe headache. Neck pain with or without crepitus has been described after difficult epidurals in labouring patients when loss of resistance to air was used [39–41]. Air trapped within the skull or tissues may increase in volume and/or pressure when nitrous oxide is breathed: neck pain following Entonox has been described in this situation [39]. Some advise against using nitrous oxide at all after a loss of resistance to air technique [42].

CORTICAL VEIN THROMBOSIS

Spontaneous thrombosis of a cerebral vein or sinus may occur, usually within two weeks of delivery but occasionally before delivery. The pathogenesis is believed due to the triad of endothelial damage, venous stasis and hypercoagulability. The first two may be secondary to surges in intracranial venous pressure associated with expulsive efforts. Headache due to cortical vein thrombosis may be very difficult to differentiate from PDPH, but there may be subtle differences. With thrombosis the headaches are intensely throbbing, increasing in intensity and frequently associated with sweating, nausea and vomiting [43, 44]. There is usually progress to focal or generalized seizures within one to three days. This combination of symptoms warrants exclusion of venous thrombosis by radiography before an epidural blood patch is placed. In two case reports [43, 44] plain computed tomography (CT) scans were normal, but repeat scans with contrast revealed the cortical vein thrombosis (magnetic resonance imaging (MRI) would confirm the diagnosis today). Treatment is symptomatic with bed rest and anticonvulsants but patients usually suffer little or no permanent disability. Heparin prophylaxis is controversial as it may cause bleeding in infarcted areas, but heparin is indicated if a cerebral thrombosis has happened in a previous pregnancy [43, 44]. Although the patients in some case reports had received regional anaesthesia (RA) there are many cases where RA was not involved [44]. In the immediate postpartum period arterial obstruction is much more common than venous thrombosis and an accurate diagnosis is felt to be of more than academic interest since some of the arterial problems may be treatable by surgery [45].

EPIDURAL ABSCESS

The reported incidence of epidural abscess varies widely in obstetric patients: from 1 in 26 490 [46] to 1 in 505 000 [47]. Three more recent surveys reported no cases of epidural abscess in 13 636 [27], or 122 989 [48] or 288 351 [49] obstetric regional anaesthetic procedures.

In 1992 it was suggested that only five cases of epidural abscess in association with obstetric RA had occurred [50]. In non-obstetric patients *Staphylococcus aureus* is the most common organism in the UK, but tubercle bacillus is said to be more prevalent in developing countries. Epidural abscesses are an uncommon complication of RA and the anaesthetic technique may be implicated if other, more obvious, sources cannot be found. It is important to remember that an epidural abscess may arise following childbirth in the absence of RA [51, 52]. Arguments for and against the implication of the RA technique are exemplified in case reports and subsequent discussion [53–56]. Similar discussions occurred recently when one of our patients developed a pneumococcal epidural abscess some seven to 10 days post vaginal delivery. Bacteriological opinion favoured haematogenous spread, but neurosurgical opinion implicated the RA technique and suggested direct introduction of infection by the epidural instrumentation. Early symptoms of epidural abscess are fever, malaise, back pain and headache; bladder and bowel dysfunction, lower extremity pain and weakness/paralysis occur as late signs. The outstanding clinical feature is spinal pain and marked local tenderness of the spine at the level of the abscess formation: lightly tapping the spinous process with a tendon hammer may elicit this and indicate the pathological diagnosis [57]. A complaint of spinal pain, particularly in a younger patient (or of thoracic pain in all patients), should be regarded seriously rather than assuming the symptom is 'mechanical dysfunction'. High-grade MRI is the definitive diagnosis and treatment is by decompressive laminectomy [57].

EPIDURAL HAEMATOMA

When this subject is discussed, even in relation to obstetric anaesthesia, the multiple references provided almost invariably turn out to be non-obstetric cases with specific predisposing factors, e.g. bleeding diathesis and/or anticoagulant drugs. Although spontaneous epidural haematomas during pregnancy have been described in the absence of regional anaesthesia [58, 59], a 1989 review of the literature claimed that there were no cases of epidural haematoma in parturients who had received regional block [60]. One case of bilateral leg weakness said to be due to a haematoma was disputed because of lack of evidence [61] and no cases were found in a large French survey [49] or a Canadian survey [62]. Since 1989 only one case has been reported in association with RA [47] but since no details were provided it is not possible to say if there were any predisposing factors. One is led to the conclusion that the risk of epidural haematoma in the obstetric population is extremely small.

SUBDURAL HAEMATOMA

These fall into two categories: cranial subdural and spinal subdural. The former are particularly liable to occur in association with dural tap and headache. Cranial subdural haematoma may present as acute [63] or chronic with variable symptoms [64–66] including headache or psychiatric pathology. The accepted aetiology is low CSF pressure following dural puncture leading to traction and tearing of thin-walled dural blood vessels. Although rare, spinal subdural haematomata following epidural anaesthesia have been reported but the presentations were complex. One was thought to have occurred spontaneously before admission to hospital [67] and two others were found at surgery to be associated with ependymoma [68, 69].

ANTERIOR SPINAL ARTERY SYNDROME

The conus medullaris receives a dual blood supply: from above via the artery of Adamkiewicz; from below via a spinal branch of the internal iliac artery. In some 85% of the population the artery of Adamkiewicz arises from the aorta between T9 and L3 and supplies the bulk of the conus medullaris; the ascending contribution from the spinal branches of the iliac arteries is minimal. In the remaining 15% of the population the artery of Adamkiewicz arises much higher (T5) and the respective contributions of descending and ascending arteries are reversed. In these latter patients the principal blood supply now arises from branches of the internal iliac artery lying on the posterior wall of the pelvis and crossing in front of the ala of the sacrum. These vessels are exposed and in danger of compression by the foetal head, particularly if there is disproportion and prolonged labour. In a Nigerian survey Bademosi and colleagues [70] described 34 cases of maternal obstetric neurapraxia, five (15%) of which were permanent paraplegia. None of these women had received any RA [71]. One case of anterior spinal artery syndrome has been described in association with epidural anaesthesia [72]. In the UK three cases of permanent cord damage occurring in association with epidural anaesthesia in obstetrics are known to the author. In all three cases the anaesthetists were unable to prove their innocence because conclusive evidence as to the cause of the lesions was absent, but an anterior spinal artery syndrome did not find favour with legal opinion. A further possible vascular cause of spinal cord damage is a direct toxic effect secondary to retrograde flow from an accidental intra-arterial injection of a toxic substance into one of the branches of the gluteal arteries [73].

SPINAL CORD DAMAGE

As for spinal nerve roots, direct damage to the cord may occur from needles and catheters and on occasion this can give rise to a cauda equina syndrome secondary to direct disruption of the spinal cord from injected fluid. Alternatively, there may be a direct effect from a neurotoxic agent. There has been a sudden increase in cauda equina syndrome since the advent of spinal microcatheters with 10 of 11 reported cases being associated with 5% lignocaine in dextrose. Lignocaine 5% has since been shown to be neurotoxic. These patients were all supine while multiple injections were made in attempts to obtain adequate analgesia. Current opinion suggests that the aetiology of the cauda equina syndrome in these cases was secondary to pooling of heavy lignocaine within the sacral curvature leading to high local concentrations of drug. Symptoms are confined to areas innervated by the lumbosacral nerves and may include autonomic dysfunction with abnormal sweating and temperature control, loss of bowel or bladder control, motor weakness and sensory loss.

ARACHNOIDITIS

This is caused by irritant substances within the subarachnoid space and the injection of these substances is often painful at the time. The onset may be slow and painful, taking days to develop fully. Intact dura serves a protective function, and contaminants which are innocuous within the epidural space may become highly toxic within the subarachnoid space.

CONCLUSION

As the above discussion indicates, neurological complications during labour are not uncommon and are frequently associated with prolonged or difficult labour. These are just the kind of women most likely to be in receipt of regional analgesia and anaesthesia, particularly in maternity units providing a limited obstetric analgesia services. Thus, today, significant obstetric neurological complications may rarely be observed except in association with regional anaesthesia. In the absence of widespread knowledge in the community regarding the aetiology of obstetric neurological problems it is all too easy for the anaesthetic to be blamed. When compared to the neurological sequelae of pregnancy regional anaesthesia in the pregnant patient is a safe procedure.

However, when a neurological problem does arise, whatever its suspected aetiology, not only is it essential to perform a detailed and early examination of the patient but appropriate investigations must also be made to enable an accurate diagnosis and referral to the relevant specialty for further assessment and treatment. As described above, in today's medico-legal climate, the absence of an accurate diagnosis makes an effective defence virtually impossible.

REFERENCES

1. Donaldson, J.O. (1989) *Neurology of Pregnancy*, 2nd edn, W.B. Saunders, London.
2. Goldstein, P.J. and Stern, B.J. (eds) (1992) *Neurological Disorders of Pregnancy*, Futura Publishing Company, Mount Kisco.
3. Dornette, W.H.L. (1986) Compression neuropathies: medical aspects and legal implications, in *Neurological and Psychological Complications of Surgery and Anesthesia* (ed. B.J. Hindman), Little Brown and Company, Boston. *International Anesthesiology Clinics*, **24**, 201–9.
4. Vandam, L. (1986) Neurological sequelae of spinal and epidural anesthesia, in *Neurological and Psychological Complications of Surgery and Anesthesia* (ed. B.J. Hindman), Little Brown and Company, Boston. *International Anesthesiology Clinics*, **24**, 231–55.
5. Cole, J.T. (1946) Maternal obstetric paralysis. *American Journal of Obstetrics and Gynecology*, **52**, 372–85.
6. Adornato, B.T. and Carlini, W.G. (1992) 'Pushing palsy': A case of self induced bilateral peroneal palsy during natural childbirth. *Neurology*, **42**, 936–7.
7. Felsenthal, G. (1992) Peripheral nervous system disorders and pregnancy, in *Neurological Disorders of Pregnancy* (eds P.J. Goldstein, P.J. and B.J. Stern), Futura Publishing Company, Mount Kisco, pp. 223–67.
8. Maranacci, A.A. and Courville, C.B. (1958) Electromyogram in evaluation of neurological complications of spinal anesthesia. *Journal of the American Medical Association*, **168**, 1337–45.
9. Dornette, W.H.L. (1986) Compression neuropathies: Medical aspects and legal implications, in *Neurological and Psychological Complications of Surgery and Anaesthesia* (ed. B.J. Hindman), Little Brown and Company, Boston. *International Anaesthesiology Clinics*, **24**, 201–29.
10. Hill, E.C. (1962) Maternal obstetric palsies. *American Journal of Obstetrics and Gynecology*, **83**, 1452–60.
11. Murray, R.R. (1964) Maternal obstetric paralysis. *American Journal of Obstetrics and Gynecology*, **88**, 399–403.
12. Shin, Y.K., Lee, V.C. and Kim, Y.D. (1985) Unusual cause of weakness of the lower extremity following vaginal delivery under epidural analgesia: illiopsoas muscle strain. *Anesthesiology*, **63**, 531–3.
13. Ravindran, R.S. and Viegas, O.J. (1981) Transient lower extremity weakness in an obstetric patient unrelated to epidural anesthesia. *Anesthesia and Analgesia*, **60**, 527–8.
14. Reynolds, F. (1995) personal communication.
15. Reif, M.E. (1988) Bilateral common peroneal palsy secondary to prolonged squatting in natural childbirth. *Birth*, **15**, 100–2.
16. Sandu, H.S. and Sandey, B.S. (1976) Occupational compression of the common peroneal nerve at the neck of the fibula. *Australian and New Zealand Journal of Surgery*, **46**, 160–3.
17. Vargo, M.M., Robinson, L.R., Nicholas, J.J. and Rulin, M.C. (1990) Postpartum femoral neuropathy: relic of an earlier era. *Archives of Physical Medicine and Rehabilitation*, **71**, 591–5.
18. Hopper, C.L. and Baker, J.B. (1968) Bilateral femoral neuropathy complicating vaginal hysterectomy. *Obstetrics and Gynecology*, **32**, 543–7.
19. Donaldson, J.O., Wirz, D. and Mashman, J. (1985) Bilateral postpartum femoral neuropathy. *Connecticut Medicine*, **49**, 496–8.
20. Adelman, J.U., Goldberg, G.S. and Puckett, J.D. (1973) Postpartum bilateral femoral neuropathy. *Obstetrics and Gynecology*, **42**, 845–50.
21. Pham, L.H.T., Bulich, L.A. and Datta, S. (1995) Bilateral postpartum femoral neuropathy. *Anesthesia and Analgesia*, **80**, 1036–7.
22. Pearson, M.G. (1957) Meralgia paraesthetica. With reference to its occurrence in pregnancy. *Journal of Obstetrics and Gynaecology*, **64**, 427–30.
23. Dureja, G.P., Gulaya, V., Jayalakshmi, T.S. and Mandal, P. (1995) Management of meralgia paresthetica: A multimodality regimen. *Anesthesia and Analgesia*, **80**, 1060–1.
24. Van Diver, T. and Camann, W. (1995) Meralgia paresthetica in the parturient: Review article. *International Journal of Obstetric Anaesthesia*, **4**, 109–12.

25. Nichols, C.R. (1992) Bilateral radial nerve palsies from use of a birth frame. *Australian and New Zealand Journal of Obstetrics and Gynaecology*, **32**, 380.

26. McLennon, H.G., Oates, J.N. and Walstab, J.E. (1987) Survey of hand symptoms in pregnancy. *Medical Journal of Australia*, **147**, 542–4.

27. Holdcroft, A., Gibberd, F.B., Hargrove, R.L. *et al.* (1995) Neurological complications associated with pregnancy. *British Journal of Anaesthesia*, **75**, 522–6.

28. Voitk, A.J., Mueller, J.C., Farlinger, D.E. and Johnston, R.U. (1983) Carpal tunnel syndrome in pregnancy. *Canadian Medical Association Journal*, **128**, 277–81.

29. Lee, J.J. and Roberts, R.B. (1978) Paresis of the fifth cranial nerve following spinal anesthesia. *Anesthesiology*, **49**, 217–8.

30. De Lange, J.J., Stilma, J.S. and Crezee, F. (1988) Visual disturbance after spinal anaesthesia. *Anaesthesia*, **43**, 570–2.

31. Sprung, J., Haddox, J.D. and Maitra-D'Cruze, A.M. (1991) Horner's syndrome and trigeminal nerve palsy following epidural anaesthesia for obstetrics. *Canadian Journal of Anaesthesia*, **38**, 767–71.

32. Heyman, H.J., Salem, M.R and Klimov, I. (1982) Persistent sixth cranial nerve paresis following blood patch for postdural puncture headache. *Anesthesia and Analgesia*, **61**, 948–9.

33. Coventry D.M. (1986) Bell's palsy during epidural anaesthesia. *Anaesthesia*, **41**, 764.

34. Lowe, D.M. and McCullough, A.M. (1990) 7th nerve palsy after extradural blood patch. *British Journal of Anaesthesia*, **65**, 721–2.

35. Perez, M., Olmos, M. and Garrido F.J. (1993) Facial nerve paralysis after epidural blood patch. *Regional Anaesthesia*, **18**, 196–8.

36. Gbolade, B.A. (1994) Recurrent lower motor neurone facial paralysis in four successive pregnancies. *Journal of Laryngology and Otology*, **108**, 587–8.

37. Dorsey, D.L. and Camann, W.R. (1993) Obstetric anesthesia in patients with idiopathic facial paralysis (Bell's Palsy): A 10-year survey. *Anesthesia and Analgesia*, **77**, 81–3.

38. Khurana, R. (1992) Headache, in *Neurological Disorders of Pregnancy* (eds P.J. Goldstein and B.J. Stern), Futura Publishing Company, Mount Kisco, pp. 223–67.

39. Munro, H.M. (1990) Pain in the neck. *Anaesthesia*, **45**, 173.

40. Kilpatrick, S.M. (1984) Emphysema of the neck after epidural anaesthesia. *Anaesthesia*, **39**, 499–500.

41. Carter, M.I. (1984) Cervical surgical emphysema following extradural analgesia. *Anaesthesia*, **39**, 1115–6.

42. Gonzáles-Carrasco, F.J., Aguilar J.L., Llubiá, C. *et al.* (1993) Pneumocephalus after accidental dural puncture during epidural anaesthesia. *Regional Anaesthesia*, **18**, 193–5.

43. Gewirtz, E.C., Costin, M. and Marx, G.F. (1987) Cortical vein thrombosis may mimic postdural puncture headache. *Regional Anesthesia*, **12**, 188–90.

44. Ravindran, R.S., Zandstra, G.C. and Viegas, O.J. (1989) Postpartum headache following regional analgesia; a symptom of cerebral venous thrombosis. *Canadian Journal of Anaesthesia*, **36**, 705–7.

45. Cross, J.N., Castro, P.O. and Jennett, W.B. (1968) Cerebral strokes associated with pregnancy and the puerperium. *British Medical Journal*, **3**, 214–8.

46. Crawford, J.S. (1985) Some maternal complications of epidural analgesia for labour. *Anaesthesia*, **40**, 1219–25.

47. Scott, D.B. and Hibbard, B.M. (1990) Serious non-fatal complications associated with extradural block in obstetric practice. *British Journal of Anaesthesia*, **64**, 537–41.

48. Scott, D.B. and Tunstall, M.E. (1995) Serious complications associated with epidural/spinal blockade in obstetrics: a two year prospective study. *International Journal of Obstetric Anaesthesia*, **4**, 133–9.

49. Palot, M., Visseaux, H., Botmans, C. and Pire, J.C. (1994) Epidémiologie des complications de l'analgésie péridurale obstétricale. *Cahiers d'Anesthésiologie*, **42**, 229–33.

50. Borum, S.E., McLeskey, C.H., Williamson, J.B. *et al.* (1995) Epidural abscess after obstetric analgesia. *Anesthesiology*, **82**, 1523–6.

51. Male, C.G. and Martin, R. (1973) Puerperal spinal epidural abscess. *Lancet*, **1**, 608–9.

52. Van Winter, J.T., Nielsen, S.N.J. and Ogburn, P.L. (1991) Epidural abscess associated with intravenous drug abuse in a pregnant patient. *Mayo Clinical Proceedings*, **66**, 1036–9.

53. Ngan Kee, W.D., Jones, M.R., Thomas, P. and Worth, R.J. (1992) Extradural abscess complicating extradural anaesthesia for caesarean section. *British Journal of Anaesthesia*, **69**, 647–52.

54. Kitching, A.J. and Rice, A.S.C. (1993) Extradural abscess in the postpartum period. *British Journal of Anaesthesia*, **70**, 703.

55. Vasdev, G.M.S. and Leicht, C.H. (1993) Extradural abscess in the postpartum period. *British Journal of Anaesthesia,* **70,** 703–4.
56. Ngan Kee, W.D. (1993) Extradural abscess in the postpartum period. *British Journal of Anaesthesia,* **70,** 704.
57. Johnson, R.A. (1994) Acute spinal cord compression, in *Neurological Emergencies* (ed. R.A.C. Hughes), British Medical Journal Publishing Group, London, pp. 268–90.
58. Crawford, J.S. (1975) Pathology in the extradural space. *British Journal of Anaesthesia,* **47,** 412–5.
59. Bidzinski, J. (1966) Spontaneous spinal epidural hematoma during pregnancy. *Journal of Neurosurgery,* **24,** 1017.
60. Rasmus, K.T. (1989) Unrecognised thrombocytopenia and regional anesthesia: A retrospective review. *Obstetrics and Gynecology,* **74,** 972.
61. Ballin, V.C. (1981) Paraplegia following epidural analgesia. *Anaesthesia,* **36,** 952–3.
62. Ong, B.Y., Cohen, M.M., Esmail, A. *et al.* (1987) Paresthesias and motor dysfunction after labor and delivery. *Anesthesia and Analgesia,* **66,** 18-22.
63. Pavlin, D.J., McDonald, J.S., Child, B. and Rusch, V. (1979) Acute subdural hematoma – an unusual sequela to lumbar puncture. *Anesthesiology,* **51,** 338–40.
64. Jack, T.M. (1979) Post-partum intracranial subdural haematoma. A possible complication of epidural analgesia. *Anaesthesia,* **34,** 176–80.
65. Miyazaki, S., Fukushima, H., Kamata, K. and Ishii, S. (1983) Chronic subdural hematoma after lumbar-subarachnoid analgesia for cesarean section. *Surgical Neurology,* **19,** 459–60.
66. Campbell, D.A. and Varma, T.R.K. (1993) Chronic subdural haematoma following epidural anaesthesia, presenting as puerperal psychosis. *British Journal of Obstetrics and Gynaecology,* **100,** 782–4.
67. Lao, T.T., Halpern, S.H. and MacDonald, D. (1993) Spinal subdural haematoma in a parturient after attempted epidural anaesthesia. *Canadian Journal of Anaesthesia,* **40,** 340–5.
68. Roscoe, M.W.A. and Barrington, T.W. (1984) Acute spinal subdural hematoma: A case report and review of the literature. *Spine,* **9,** 672–5.
69. Martin, H.B., Gibbons, J.J. and Bucholz, R.D. (1992) An unusual presentation of spinal cord tumour after epidural anesthesia. *Anesthesia and Analgesia,* **75,** 844–6.
70. Bademosi, O., Osuntokun, B.O., Van de Werd, H.J. *et al.* (1980) Obstetric neurapraxia in the Nigerian African. *International Journal of Gynaecology and Obstetrics,* **17,** 611–14.
71. Bromage, P.R. (1993) Neurological complications of regional anesthesia for obstetrics, in *Anesthesia for Obstetrics,* 3rd edn (eds S.M. Shnider and G. Levinson), Williams and Wilkins, Baltimore, pp. 433–53.
72. Ackerman, W.E., Juneja, M.M. and Knapp, R.A.. (1990) Maternal paraparesis after epidural anesthesia and cesarean section. *Southern Medical Journal,* **83,** 695–7.
73. Tesio, L., Bassi, L. and Strada, L. (1992) Spinal cord lesion after penicillin gluteal injection. *Paraplegia,* **30,** 442–4.

C.C. Rout

MORTALITY

The confidential enquiries into maternal deaths from the UK have repeatedly identified emergency caesarean delivery [1] and emergency anaesthesia [2] as factors directly associated with maternal mortality. Factors contributing to death have been dominated by aspects of general anaesthesia, particularly problems of airway management and aspiration of gastric contents. The latest report is no exception, with general anaesthesia contributing to five of eight deaths associated with anaesthesia, six of which were emergencies. Airway problems occurred in four of the cases and aspiration in two [1].

Increasing use of regional anaesthesia for caesarean delivery is generally regarded as the reason for the decrease in mortality attributable to anaesthesia in the UK over the past twenty years. The growing popularity of spinal anaesthesia in particular may have contributed to a decline in the use of general anaesthesia for emergencies [3]. Wider application of regional techniques has led to concern that trainee anaesthetists are acquiring less experience of obstetric general anaesthesia. Lack of familiarity increases anxiety; add the frequent isolation of labour and delivery suites together with the predilection of the

unborn for the early hours of the morning, and the scene is set for a clinical disaster [4]. However, there are no data that directly link the elements of this argument. Maternal mortality reports generally lack accurate information on the number of caesarean deliveries performed or the type of anaesthesia used. It has been suggested that the number of general anaesthetics administered may have changed little over the years, and that the increasing use of regional anaesthesia has followed the increasing numbers of caesarean sections performed [5]. If the exposure of the average trainee to obstetric general anaesthesia has declined, it may well be a result of changes in training and work patterns, rather than a real reduction in the number of general anaesthetics. While changes in training and practice have been taking place, maternal mortality has been falling. Whether it is complacent to view apparently rising clinical standards as a sign that all is well, only time will tell. To summarize the trends:

- the numbers of caesarean sections are increasing;
- the numbers of regional anaesthetics are increasing;
- the numbers of general anaesthetics are stable;

Clinical Problems in Obstetric Anaesthesia
Edited by Ian F. Russell and Gordon Lyons. Published in 1997 by Chapman & Hall, London. ISBN 0 412 71600 3.

- the exposure of trainees to general anaesthesia is decreasing;
- mortality due to general anaesthesia is stable.

Although it is generally felt by anaesthetists that regional anaesthesia is inherently safer than general anaesthesia, there is little direct evidence for this view. Indirect evidence comes from sources such as mortality reports, closed claims studies [6] and surveys of intensive care admissions [7]; however comparable denominator data is lacking. Whilst studies such as OASIS [8] will provide much of what is required, the problem of comparability will remain. The bias towards the use of general anaesthesia in emergency cases and pre-existing morbidity has already been mentioned (Chapter 1) and this may have been partly responsible for the evil reputation of general anaesthesia. In the UK, regional anaesthesia for caesarean delivery has never been a direct cause of death. From an epidemiological point of view increased use of obstetric regional anaesthesia should be encouraged, but for the individual with a purely obstetric indication for elective caesarean delivery there is probably little to choose between general and regional anaesthesia in terms of maternal risk. As long as there are contraindications to regional anaesthesia, general anaesthesia will have its place. The risks associated with its use for emergency deliveries have been identified and are largely predictable. When underlying medical conditions dictate the need for emergency delivery, it is often these that will dominate the clinical picture and cause the major risks.

Whatever the circumstances, it is important that the anaesthetist can rely upon a familiar, well-practised protocol for general anaesthesia which will form the basis of safe operative delivery. Initial attention should focus on the problems of airway management and the prevention of aspiration, both clear hazards to the mother.

AIRWAY MANAGEMENT

Problems with intubation have been considered thoroughly elsewhere. The emphasis here is placed upon avoiding problems rather than solving them. When regional anaesthesia is a feasible option, and particularly where airway problems have been identified, general anaesthesia should be avoided altogether. Irrespective of the time constraints, the preoperative assessment and identification of potential airway problems should never be overlooked [9] and the possibility of a difficult laryngoscopy and intubation should be considered in every case. The available data concerning the risk of difficulty when securing the obstetric airway compared to non-obstetric anaesthesia do little to reassure the inexperienced trainee. Not only is a difficult laryngoscopy or failed intubation more likely in obstetric practice, but when they occur, a fatal outcome is also more likely [10]. The documented risk of failed intubation may vary from 1:300 [4,11] to 1:750 [12] obstetric general anaesthetics. Whilst it could be an annual event in a busy unit, it is sufficiently uncommon for an anaesthetist to work a lifetime without personal exposure to the problem. When it happens, it is likely to happen to an anaesthetist with no previous exposure, and successful management may well be dependent on familiarity and adherence to an intubation algorithm that involves a failed intubation drill.

Attention should be paid to patient position, obvious hazards such as large breasts and the availability of an adequate selection of equipment to ensure as easy a laryngoscopy and intubation as possible. Additional equipment should also be on hand if difficulty is encountered.

When dealing with a difficult intubation, the critical factor is maternal oxygenation. Pregnant women at term desaturate rapidly. Oxygen reserve is decreased and consumption increased. The role of preoxygenation is to replace pulmonary nitrogen with oxygen, thereby creating a reservoir, and to achieve this, preoxygenation should be as thorough as possible in the time available. Whilst four vital capacity breaths may speed up the process of preoxygenation they are no substitute for three to five minutes of normal tidal breathing of 100% oxygen [13]. Even then desaturation to below 95% can occur following 2.5–3 minutes of apnoea in the pregnant patient [14]. The best monitor of the effectiveness of preoxygenation is the measurement of end-tidal oxygen tension using a rapid response paramagnetic oxygen sensor. This monitors pulmonary de-nitrogenation and is a useful guide to the effectiveness of preoxygenation. It will detect the entry of room air into the circuit that occurs with ill-fitting masks [15, 16]. In a dire emergency it is best for the anaesthetist to accompany the patient to theatre. This provides an opportunity to complete the preoperative assessment before entry to theatre, when preoxygenation can be commenced immediately.

AVOIDING GENERAL ANAESTHESIA

Where absolute contraindications to regional anaesthesia exist this is impossible. In the absence of contraindications, the choice of anaesthesia is largely governed by the urgency of the situation. It is essential that the anaesthetist and the obstetrician communicate to establish the degree of urgency and how much time is available. The anaesthetic options should then be clear.

Current guidelines define an emergency caesarean section as one in which the requirement for the delivery of the baby is 30 minutes or less from the time of the decision to proceed to caesarean section. Given that it will take five minutes to transport the patient to the operating room following the decision to proceed, and at least five minutes to prepare and drape the patient upon the operating table and deliver the infant, this leaves the anaesthetist a maximum time of 20 minutes to anaesthetize the patient for surgery. This is insufficient time to guarantee a working epidural anaesthetic

from scratch but is ample time to allow spinal anaesthesia to be performed or to top up an existing epidural; increasingly both these methods are being used to provide anaesthesia for emergency caesarean delivery [17]. However, '30 minutes' is a generic recommendation and there will be circumstances when delivery of the infant is required in considerably less time. Whilst experienced obstetric anaesthetists exist who are capable of administering spinal anaesthesia within five minutes, few if any would guarantee it. If the delivery of the infant is required in less than 15 to 20 minutes from the time that the decision to proceed was taken, then general anaesthesia is really the only option [18].

When an anaesthetist is asked to perform emergency general anaesthesia in the presence of unseen clinical problems that add significantly to the hazard, it is reasonable to assume that there has been an error of judgement. Medical staff from both disciplines should appreciate the need to alert the other to potential problems before the situation becomes acute. One beneficial result of such exchanges is the formulation of strategies, one of which might be a move to operative delivery before the anticipated emergency arises. A regional anaesthetic that works is always preferable to a general anaesthetic that does not. The latter may carry a penalty for mother and baby. It is rare for a conflict of interests to develop between the mother and her foetus, but in these circumstances maternal survival should take priority.

AIRWAY ASSESSMENT

An airway assessment should consider

- previous intubations;
- teeth;
- Mallampati score;
- size of chin and neck;
- flexion and extension of head and neck.

Assessment requires a brief dental examination, a Mallampati score [19], a search for obvious features such as prominent maxillary incisors, receding chin and short neck and a test of head extension such as sternomental distance [20]. Unfortunately, whilst these tests can identify potential problems, they are not certain predictors. Even a combination of tests cannot predict difficulty with certainty, although it can be used to produce a probability of encountering difficulty [12]. This can be a useful exercise to incorporate into a difficult intubation protocol, with a view to alerting experienced help **before** getting into trouble. It is reassuring that a normal examination is associated with a very low probability of difficulty. What practical value these tests have remains to be seen [21]. It is likely that future refinement will involve a combination of tests which will improve their performance. The more attention paid to airway examination, the less frequently nasty surprises will occur.

PREVENTION OF ASPIRATION

Pulmonary aspiration of gastric contents is a predictable risk of emergency obstetric general anaesthesia. Circumstances surrounding emergency operative delivery combine to increase this risk and may confound prophylactic regimens. The onset of labour may follow a meal, and increase the likelihood of partly digested food remaining in the stomach when surgical intervention, often unpredictable, is required. Opiate analgesia during labour slows gastric emptying, increasing the volume of gastric contents which may already be high due to increased plasma gastrin levels [22]. Although aspiration has been the cause of many obstetric deaths, recent years have seen a marked reduction in mortality. The reason for this reassuring trend must surely be found in improved standards of anaesthetic management; which particular aspect of care is responsible, use of cricoid pressure or starvation, remains obscure.

CRICOID PRESSURE

Cricoid pressure has become an integral part of general anaesthetic technique for emergency

surgery and obstetrics, and whenever there is the risk of a full stomach. Introduced as a simple manoeuvre to prevent pulmonary aspiration of regurgitated gastric contents until intubation with a cuffed endotracheal tube, it was also recommended to prevent gastric inflation during bag and mask or mouth to mouth ventilation [23].

Despite the establishment of cricoid pressure as the 'linchpin' of mechanical prevention of pulmonary aspiration [24], its value as a routine part of general anaesthesia for obstetrics has recently been called into question [25]. Arguments against the need for cricoid pressure include the lack of direct evidence that cricoid pressure prevents deaths due to aspiration, the documented occurrence of aspiration deaths despite the use of cricoid pressure [2], and the low incidence of aspiration in France, where cricoid pressure is rarely used [26]. Additionally it is argued that as the majority of cases of aspiration occur either before anaesthetic induction or following extubation [27], cricoid pressure during induction is unlikely to be of benefit. There is also the possibility that cricoid pressure may distort the upper airway, increasing the difficulty of laryngoscopy and/or intubation [28].

Proponents of cricoid pressure argue that pregnant women are prone to gastro-oesophageal reflux, often asymptomatic, and point to the long history of deaths due to aspiration recorded in mortality reports, the documented incidence of intragastric contents of high volume and acidity, and the decline in incidence of deaths due to aspiration following introduction of the technique [29]. Animal and human cadaver studies demonstrate how cricoid pressure can easily prevent regurgitation and aspiration at intragastric pressures at least as high as might occur naturally [30].

It would be difficult to obtain a dispassionate view of the subject from an obstetric anaesthetist. However, some of the arguments against routine use of cricoid pressure are clearly spurious. The application of cricoid pressure might be the very reason why aspiration is less likely to occur during induction of anaesthesia. It could be easily argued that France's low incidence of aspiration might be further reduced if cricoid pressure were universally applied. Arguments either way on these issues are little more than speculative, and a national clinical trial is probably not feasible. Individual risk is variable. Measured volumes of gastric contents in controlled studies of aspiration risk can be sufficiently high to pose the threat of drowning, let alone acid pneumonitis [31].

Evidence that cricoid pressure prevents aspiration is more difficult to find, particularly in view of the number of documented maternal deaths due to aspiration despite its use. By the mid 1970s cricoid pressure was an established component of the rapid sequence induction of anaesthesia. Despite this the triennial reports on confidential enquiries into maternal deaths in England and Wales of 1976–1978, 1979–1981 and 1982–1984 [2, 32, 33] recorded 26 deaths out of a total of 70 due to aspiration of gastric contents, which were held to be directly resulting from anaesthesia. It might be assumed that all of these deaths occurred following cricoid pressure except in one case where it was specifically noted that cricoid pressure had not been applied. Assumptions aside, in 11 of the 19 cases in the reports from 1976 to 1981 it was specifically stated that cricoid pressure had been applied. These deaths can be interpreted as clear evidence that the 'simple and effective' technique of cricoid pressure is not as effective as might be wished. Proponents of cricoid pressure might argue that in these cases the cricoid pressure was applied incorrectly. Indeed, cricoid pressure often is applied incorrectly [34] and the importance of correct training in the technique has been stressed [35]. Mechanical devices have been designed to aid its correct application [36].

Although originally described as a simple technique, it may not be easy to master. Cricoid force sufficient to prevent regurgitation of material from the oesophagus requires the application of 40 N to the cartilage as consciousness is lost, as it is poorly tolerated in the awake patient. However, in some patients this may be too late as oesophageal tone has been demonstrated to decrease during thiopentone injection, before loss of consciousness [37]. It has therefore been recommended that a force of 20 N be applied initially, increasing to 40 N with loss of consciousness [37]. The introduction of a scientific approach means that the technique has lost some of its original simplicity, and now requires considerable training in its application. Whether it is possible to train anaesthetic assistants to consistently apply these forces remains to be seen. Recent evidence suggests that it may not be an easy task, and some subjects may even be untrainable [38].

Cricoid pressure is not the simple and effective technique originally proposed and has a high failure rate. The reduced mortality due to pulmonary aspiration seen in successive mortality reports is unlikely to have been directly due to the introduction of cricoid pressure over three decades ago. It is more likely that changes in anaesthetic staffing, more enlightened obstetric practices, shorter labours, less systemic opiate administration and increased use of regional analgesia have combined to produce the improvement. The exact role of cricoid pressure will likely remain unresolved. As an established part of our technique, it would be difficult ethically to withdraw it for research purposes. Perhaps a more balanced attitude to its importance should be taken. Whilst cricoid pressure often improves the view at laryngoscopy, it is possible that its application (or misapplication) might cause distortion of the airway and create difficulty with laryngoscopy and/or intubation. If this is suspected, it is reasonable to gradually release cricoid pressure under continuous laryngoscopy until intubation can be achieved. If it is still impossible to intubate then cricoid pressure should be reapplied and failed intubation procedure commenced.

CONTROL OF GASTRIC CONTENTS

Early investigators of the effects of aspiration of gastric contents upon the lungs suggested there was a critical combination of volume and acidity which led to pulmonary damage and the 'acid aspiration syndrome' [39]. Most investigators have used the combination of 25 ml or more of gastric contents at a pH of 2.5 or less to define risk of pulmonary aspiration. Cases of acid aspiration syndrome have been reported outside these limits however and it has been suggested that the threshold for acceptable gastric pH should be 3.5 [40]. However, it is possible that it is the hydrogen ion load that is important, and the more acidic the contents the less the volume required to produce damage, and vice versa [41, 42]. In any case, the principles of prevention remain the same, i.e. to reduce the volume and increase the pH of the gastric contents.

Since an outcome study based upon mortality would require vast numbers, the success of any particular regimen has to be assessed in terms of combination of pH and volume of gastric contents. If a drug designed to reduce hydrogen ion secretion is introduced into practice it is hardly surprising that the mean pH of a group of test subjects given the drug is found to be higher than the mean pH of a group of control subjects. What is more important is the number of subjects in whom the drug failed to increase the pH to above the critical value of 3.5 (or 2.5). Unfortunately, study groups are often not sufficiently large to achieve adequate statistical power.

Reducing the volume

Factors that increase gastric volume in labour are:

- increased plasma gastrin of pregnancy;
- feeding in labour;
- opioid analgesia.

Several methods have been used to decrease intragastric volumes prior to emergency cae-sarean delivery. These include preoperative orogastric intubation [43, 44], mechanical induction of vomiting [45], intravenous apomorphine [46], and intravenous metoclopramide [47, 48]. Of these methods the first three are unpleasant, and whichever method is used there is no guarantee that the stomach will be empty following its use. Wide-bore (28 French gauge) orogastric tubes have been shown to be effective for 15 to 20 minutes in reducing gastric fluid volume to less than 25 ml when used in conjunction with metoclopramide [49]. They might be useful in the situation of a patient presenting for emergency operative delivery with a contraindication to regional anaesthesia who has recently (within an hour or so) eaten a substantial meal. However, inserting the tube and draining the stomach takes time, so if there is no contraindication to regional anaesthesia, a spinal anaesthetic would be more appropriate. Quite often the effect of such a large tube is that of mechanical stimulation of vomiting rather than its intended use as a drain. Smaller tubes are ineffective in removing undigested food. Equally as effective [50] is the intravenous injection of apomorphine to induce vomiting, but this drug is seldom available. Intravenous metoclopramide is probably the least effective of any of these methods, particularly if opiates have been used [51], and it requires time to work. However, it will increase lower oesophageal sphincter tone within a few minutes of administration [52] which some might regard as important before induction. Care should be taken with intravenous injection of metoclopramide, which may cause transient hypotension and, rarely, supraventricular arrhythmias, in addition to extrapyramidal symptoms with large or repeated doses. Cisapride is the only agent that has been shown to overcome opiate-induced delay in gastric emptying but is available only as an oral preparation [53, 54].

Whilst attempts to empty the stomach before induction are rarely appropriate, it is reasonable practice to pass a gastric tube following induction and successful intubation, confirm its position in the stomach and leave it to drain throughout the procedure. This is particularly appropriate in view of the increasing proportion of incidents of aspiration occurring following extubation. Additional sodium citrate can be given through the tube before its removal.

One way of decreasing the volume of gastric contents is by withholding food and drink during labour. This policy was introduced following Mendelson's report on inhalation of gastric contents which included two deaths due to asphyxia [45]. Deaths from asphyxia were uncommon in the UK, but featured in reports up to the mid 1970s. The effects of 'nil by mouth' policies are however by no means clear [55] and considerable variation exists between policies for oral intake on different delivery suites. In general, policies in the UK [56, 57] tend to be more liberal than those in the USA and Canada [58, 59]. A considerable body of evidence has accumulated to justify the more liberal intake of clear fluids before elective surgery [60, 61] and this could be extrapolated to women in labour who have not received opiates. However, the issue of food has yet to be resolved.

Whilst nobody seems to be advocating a full diet, or permitting the intake of food after opiates, there is no consensus as to what diet should be given to whom [57]. Many units designate 'low risk' and 'high risk', and permit the former to eat and drink, while starving the latter. There are three criticisms of this approach. Firstly, the potential for ward confusion might lead to mistakes; secondly, while it might be possible to define high risk in terms of medical and obstetric history, outcome of labour cannot accurately be predicted; and finally, starving a high-risk group is in itself, an acknowledgement that feeding in labour could be a hazard. 'Low risk' would be better characterized as 'unknown risk' and all women should be managed with a single policy.

The introduction of liberal oral intake policies is largely motivated by a genuine concern for patient comfort, and a desire to incorporate 'consumer preference' into the management of labour. Many women find the withholding of food and drink during labour to be stressful [62]. With the increasing emphasis upon patient autonomy of recent years, it is not unreasonable for a woman to make an informed choice concerning oral intake during labour. However, how many women making this choice understand that it is a choice between comfort and safety, and how can they make a truly informed decision when those advising them do not have the benefit of results from controlled trials?

There has been only one prospective, randomized, controlled study of the risks and benefits of eating in labour. Scrutton and colleagues demonstrated a significant increase in β-hydroxybutyrate and non-esterified fatty acids and a decrease in glucose in the plasma of women permitted water only during labour compared to women permitted a light standardized low-fat diet [63]. However, patients allowed to eat demonstrated significantly greater mean gastric volumes (ultrasonographic antral cross-sectional area) and a significantly higher incidence of vomiting, with significantly greater volumes of vomitus than those allowed water only. The volume of vomitus (median 400 ml compared to 10 ml) was considerably in excess of the most generous view as to what might constiute a 'critical volume', and would have represented a threat in the event of general anaesthesia irrespective of pH. The significance of ketosis during labour has yet to be determined. Whilst an association has been demonstrated between ketosis and long labours [64] there has never been any direct evidence to show that ketosis impedes the progress of labour.

Reducing the acidity

Risk of maternal death at caesarean section, due to aspiration, has declined steadily since oral antacids were introduced in the 1970s. Magnesium trisilicate suspension became popular in the UK, and hydroxides in the USA. Frequent dosing regimes were required, and there is no doubt that distractions on the ward resulted in significant omissions. Continuing deaths despite the use of antacids provoked criticism, but this failed to take into account the increasing number of operative deliveries. When it was shown that the particulate nature of the hydroxides led to a pulmonary reaction in animals as severe as the condition it was supposed to prevent, the era of the 'white medicine' was over [65]. Despite the fuss, in the ten years that white oral antacids were given to all in labour, the incidence of death from aspiration at caesarean section fell. Subsequently non-particulate preparations such as 0.3 M sodium citrate have been introduced. However even the use of non-particulate antacids cannot guarantee stomach contents which will not place the patient at risk if aspirated.

Oral neutralizing antacids administered before the induction of anaesthesia have only a brief duration of action. Even following mechanical gastric emptying 30 ml 0.3 M sodium citrate can only ensure a 'safe' stomach for 15 to 20 minutes [49]. After this time, gastric emptying will remove it and continued acid secretion will counteract its effect. An inherent problem with oral neutralizing antacids is that their administration increases intragastric volume at a time when it is best reduced. However, the most important consideration is acidity and it is possible that aiming for a volume of less than 25 ml is not only unrealistic but also unnecessary. It is unlikely that gastric contents would be regurgitated and aspirated in their entirety. In the event of more than 20 minutes having elapsed since oral antacid administration, the wisest course is probably to repeat the dose. The best time to administer the antacid is immediately before transferring the patient to the operating table as the movement involved in transfer, particularly if the patient has to roll over, will help to mix the antacid more thoroughly in the stomach. Both 'layering' and 'pocketing' of

gastric contents can occur. Rebound acid secretion may follow the use of alkaline antacids.

Even when oral sodium citrate precedes anaesthetic induction, 1.8–6.7 % of patients may be at risk of acid aspiration at intubation [31]. In the elective case it is easy to supplement antacid therapy with an oral H_2 receptor antagonist the evening before and two to three hours before surgery, but in an emergency it is impossible to predict the timing of surgery. This has led to many units adopting a policy of repeated antacid administration to all labouring patients. This is costly and time-consuming, and difficult to oversee. It has been estimated that in order to prevent four deaths, 800 000 women would have to receive treatment, 700 000 of whom would never have been placed at risk in the first place [66]. Also, there is no guarantee that such an H_2 receptor regimen will be successful, and deaths have been reported despite their use.

A more economical approach is to target those patients who will be requiring surgery by either applying the regimen to 'high risk' cases, or even more selectively using an intravenous preparation as soon as the decision to proceed with surgery has been taken. The first course of action is subject to the same criticisms levelled at a two tier policy for feeding in labour. The use of intravenous ranitidine (50 mg) has been shown to be capable of eliminating the risk of acid aspiration (when used in combination with oral sodium citrate) provided that at least 30 minutes have elapsed between its injection and the subsequent induction of anaesthesia [31]. Clearly, this is inadequate for dire emergencies, but it is still worth using because of the reduced risk at extubation. Proton pump inhibitors are a possible alternative to H_2 receptor antagonists but omeprazole (40 mg), in combination with intravenous metoclopramide and oral sodium citrate, does not seem to be as successful, although a higher dose might be required [67]. In view of the extensive investigation of ranitidine in labouring women and its observed safety to the neonate, it is probably the agent of choice if this type of prophylaxis is to be used [68]. Ranitidine also may have some beneficial effect on lower oesophageal sphincter tone [69].

SPECIAL PROBLEMS ASSOCIATED WITH CAESAREAN DELIVERY

AWARENESS

General anaesthesia for caesarean delivery is of necessity unbalanced. Concern to reduce foetal exposure to depressant drugs by administering ultralight anaesthesia to the mother, heavily reliant upon neuromuscular blockade, inevitably increases the risk of either amnesic wakefulness or awareness with recall. The latter may lead to litigation and adverse publicity. There is a high level of public concern about the problem, although such cases are fortunately rare. There are degrees of awareness, and almost certainly underreporting occurs. The use of the isolated forearm technique has demonstrated that amnesic wakefulness may accompany a typical obstetric general anaesthetic [70].

Unfortunately, despite the many advances in physiological monitoring, there is as yet no clinically practical monitor to consistently and accurately register the depth of anaesthesia. The best results have been achieved using electronically processed electroencephalogram (EEG) signals, either spontaneous or evoked. Increase in latency and decrease in amplitude of the mid-latency auditory evoked response may presently provide the best guide to awareness [71]. Other electronic signals (e.g. oesophageal contraction, frontalis electromyelogram (EMG)) have not proved particularly useful, and deductions based upon clinical signs may be worthless [72]. The isolated forearm technique (IFT) is a valuable research tool but is not a particularly useful clinical monitor. Interpretation of IFT responses can be problematic. If a positive response indicates conscious awareness, then this is the very state we are trying to avoid, and the information has come too late. On the other hand, it is possible that positive responses may be elicited at a stage of 'subconscious awareness' without any explicit memory, in which case the technique may be too sensitive. Also, much depends upon the patient's understanding and co-operation; absence of a response cannot guarantee lack of conscious awareness. In emergency cases, time for adequate explanation of the technique is lacking.

If awareness is to be avoided, some balance must be restored to the anaesthetic technique. A volatile agent must be used in addition to nitrous oxide. There will inevitably be an increase in blood loss associated with uterine relaxation but this is seldom of clinical importance [73]. The use of any agent is probably more important than which agent to choose. In general terms an agent with the most rapid uptake and elimination characteristics will be the most desirable. Thus isoflurane has largely supplanted halothane and, in the same way, the newer agents sevoflurane [74] and desflurane are likely to supplant isoflurane. Although the more rapid recovery characteristics of the newer agents might be of value to the mother immediately following caesarean section, in practice the agents are not used in high enough concentrations or for long enough to show any advantage over isoflurane. The main advantage of these agents will be in the rapid achievement of the necessary minimum anaesthetic concentration (MAC) value, with or without the use of overpressure [75]. Of the available monitors, the most useful for guarding against patient awareness is currently the anaesthetic agent monitor. A combined MAC value of end-expired nitrous oxide and volatile agent known to be associated with an adequate depth of anaesthesia must reduce the risk of wakefulness. Agent monitors should now be regarded as essential equipment in any theatre where obstetric general anaesthesia is administered.

Following uterine incision, increasing maternal inspired oxygen concentration is of no benefit to the baby and may increase the risk of maternal awareness [76]. Following delivery, opiate analgesia (e.g. morphine 10–15 mg or fentanyl 150 g) may be administered to the mother and the inspired concentration of nitrous oxide may be increased to 67%, although it is doubtful whether the latter increase of 17% would have much impact on the incidence of maternal awareness. It is usual to administer a synthetic oxytocic following delivery to cause prompt uterine contraction and limit blood loss. Oxytocin is usually the agent of choice (initial bolus of 2–10 units followed by an infusion) as ergometrine is associated with a high incidence of postoperative vomiting and also may cause unacceptable hypertension. Oxytocin on the other hand usually causes hypotension and in situations where cardiovascular stability is of importance the bolus should be curtailed or omitted and only the infusion used.

One point to remember is that more rapid maternal uptake of anaesthetics inevitably means higher foetal blood values at delivery [77]. Whilst this is unlikely to be clinically relevant in the concentrations used for caesarean section with a full-term infant, growth retarded and premature infants might be affected. Provided sound neonatal support is available, this will not influence the outcome.

The most important consideration in preventing awareness immediately following induction, before adequate MAC levels of volatile agent can be achieved, is to ensure that the patient becomes unresponsive before administering suxamethonium. The almost simultaneous administration of a fixed dose of thiopentone and 1–1.5 mg/kg of suxamethonium is not necessary. Safe and rapid induction can be accomplished using 4–7 mg/kg thiopentone, checking for loss of response to command and then injecting the suxamethonium. Although circumstances may dictate the choice of agent (for example, ketamine in the hypotensive patient), thiopentone remains the induction agent of choice for caesarean section [78]. Both midazolam and propofol can be

associated with an intermediate plane of anaesthesia that carries a high risk of awareness. Midazolam has a particularly slow onset time which either places the patient at risk for aspiration or increases the chance of consciousness during the onset of action of suxamethonium. This can also be a problem with propofol. The only potential advantage of propofol is that it might help suppress the haemodynamic response to intubation and skin incision, which might be of value in hypertensive subjects. However, both propofol and midazolam are associated with lower Apgar and neonatal neurobehavioural scores than thiopentone. Etomidate is an additional choice where cardiovascular stability is desirable.

HYPERTENSIVE RESPONSE TO INTUBATION

The same factors which increase the risk of maternal awareness also contribute to the adrenergic response to intubation. Tachycardia and hypotension are so common following induction and intubation that they are accepted as the normal pattern. Such haemodynamic instability is well tolerated by healthy young women but may pose a serious threat to those with heart disease or pre-existing hypertension [79, 80]. In such cases the anaesthetic induction sequence may have to be modified. Modifications include the administration of a short acting opiate (such as alfentanil) [81] just before induction or magnesium sulphate [82], or a combination of the two [83]. Use of alfentanil will invariably necessitate the administration of naloxone to the neonate. If magnesium sulphate is used the bolus should be given following the induction agent and before the suxamethonium as it is a very painful injection. More potent hypotensive agents such as nitroglycerine and labetalol have also been used. Beta adrenergic blocking agents may be contraindicated by the underlying heart condition and as a rule hypertensive patients do not respond well to a decrease in cardiac output, which may cause foetal bradycardia. The exception would be the use of labetalol in the preoperative management of hypertensive crisis, which has been shown to reduce the incidence of malignant ventricular arrhythmias [84]. Lignocaine is not an effective agent and large intravenous doses are ill advised due to the risk of ion-trapping in acidotic neonates.

Reversal and extubation can be associated with cardiovascular effects as severe as those seen at intubation [79]. If it is felt important to suppress these then the agent used should not suppress consciousness or respiration. Here agents such as nitroglycerine or labetalol may be of more value.

NEONATAL OUTCOME

Despite a desire to limit the exposure of the foetus to the pharmacology of general anaesthesia, some drug-induced depression is inevitable [85]. The normal term foetus is tolerant of a wide variety of anaesthetic techniques [86] but few studies have been conducted on the premature or compromised foetus. It is the latter which often provides the indication for emergency general anaesthesia. While, in principle, drug-induced depression should be minimized, it should be appreciated that minimalism can be counterproductive. Catecholamine production associated with awareness or light anaesthesia could theoretically lead to reduced placental blood flow and asphyxia. Early clinical compromise (reduced Apgar and neurobehavioural scores) can reflect either pharmacological or asphyxial effects. Neonatal support that permits recovery from anaesthesia should mean that pharmacological effects have only a transient effect on Apgar scores. Asphyxia, relative foetal hypoxia, produces neonatal acidosis. This can be measured by analysis of umbilical arterial and venous blood gases in a length of cord double clamped at delivery.

Studies of singleton pregnancies at term generally demonstrate an association between general anaesthesia and depressed Apgar scores [87] which may increase the need for active resuscitation. Poorer performance is also seen with neurobehavioural testing in the early post-delivery period [88]. These effects are transient however and the biochemical status is not affected. In fact, there are claims that spinal anaesthesia might produce a greater degree of acidosis [86]. Logistic regression of the effect of anaesthetic technique for caesarean delivery on premature infants demonstrates a clear influence of general anaesthesia on poor clinical performance, independent of confounding variables such as malpresentation, primiparity, low gestational age and maternal diabetes [89]. Neonatal status following caesarean section for foetal distress also demonstrates poor clinical performance associated with general anaesthesia, but again biochemical status is preserved.

With pre-existing foetal compromise however, concentrations of inhalational agents higher than those usually used may aggravate both the clinical and biochemical condition of the neonate [90]. Prolonged uterine incision to delivery times (greater than 90 s) tend to adversely affect neonatal outcome under general anaesthesia but are less important under epidural anaesthesia [91, 92]. It is also better to avoid a very short interval (less than five minutes) or prolonged interval (over 15 minutes) between general anaesthesia induction and delivery [92].

Circumspection is required in the interpretation of the commonly used parameters of neonatal outcome. In clinical terms, Apgar scores are still the most useful in determining the need for and response to active resuscitation, but as a research tool they are not particularly sensitive to changes in anaesthetic technique. They will demonstrate gross differences such as between general and regional anaesthesia.

Umbilical blood gas and acid–base analysis on the other hand may be useful in comparing different techniques (particularly with regional anaesthesia) but unless grossly deranged are of dubious clinical value. Despite

Table 12.1 Indications for unscheduled caesarean delivery

Emergency (less than 20 minutes)	Urgent	Planned emergencies
Abruptio placentae with a viable foetus	Meconium-stained liquor	Pregnancy-induced hypertension
Bleeding placenta praevia	Non-reassuring pattern of foetal heart rate	Booked caesarean delivery presenting in labour
Ruptured uterus	Obstructed labour	
Foetal distress	Operative delivery of second twin	
Cord prolapse		
Uterine scar dehiscence		

a wide range of values, the clinical condition of the baby at birth is often excellent. Neurobehavioural testing will detect much more subtle changes in clinical status and is a valuable research tool, but it is not of much practical clinical value to the anaesthetist and is of questionable significance. In general, any statistical comparison of group means or medians is not as valuable as non-parametric comparison of outlying values (for example, the number of neonates with an Apgar score less than six at five minutes, or an umbilical arterial pH less than 7.00).

THE PLACE OF GENERAL ANAESTHESIA IN OBSTETRICS

The data obtained from maternal mortality reports and evidence of impaired neonatal performance (albeit transient) suggests that general anaesthesia should be avoided for operative delivery, particularly in the emergency case. Yet this is precisely the moment when general anaesthesia excels, particularly when haemorrhage occurs, or when imminent foetal demise is anticipated (Table 12.1). Much can be done to reduce the need for emergency general anaesthesia by intelligent ward management. For example, breech or twin deliveries should never result in emergency general anaesthesia. However, the truly unanticipated obstetric emergencies will always remain a problem.

VAGINAL BIRTH AFTER CAESAREAN DELIVERY

Concerns have been expressed about the increasing rates of operative delivery [93, 94]. To a certain extent efforts have been successful in limiting the number of caesarean sections by encouraging vaginal birth after previous caesarean delivery. Whilst this policy results in a global reduction of operative deliveries, every failed trial of labour will add to the number of emergency caesarean sections, with all the attendant risks. It makes no sense to transfer a woman from the relatively low-risk procedure of elective caesarean delivery under regional anaesthesia to the higher risk of emergency caesarean delivery under general anaesthesia. It is important that patients undergoing trials of labour are screened by the anaesthetist for obvious airway abnormalities, and the use of epidural analgesia for labour strongly encouraged.

FOETAL DISTRESS

In the long term more benefit might be derived from avoiding unnecessary operative deliveries in first labours. A common cause of emergency caesarean delivery is the diagnosis of intrapartum foetal asphyxia. The decreasing maternal mortality and morbidity associated with operative delivery over the years, and the increasing litigation associated with poor neonatal outcome have led to an increased readiness to resort to caesarean delivery at the first signs of impending foetal asphyxia. Unfortunately both foetal heart rate monitoring and meconium-stained liquor are very poor prognosticators of neonatal outcome. By far the commonest outcome of emergency caesarean delivery is an infant in good clinical condition and in retrospect it may be felt that the operative delivery was unnecessary. When this happens it has become fashionable to call the indication for surgery 'obstetrician's distress'. This is probably unfair. The aim of intervention is to prevent irreversible asphyxia, therefore a good neonatal outcome implies a successful policy. There are, however, problems both with the diagnosis of intrapartum asphyxia and its implications for long-term neonatal outcome.

It has been suggested that intrapartum asphyxial events may not be as important in the aetiology of neonatal encephalopathy as previously believed. Retrospective analysis of full-term singleton neonates suggest that long term antepartum factors are much more important, and intrapartum foetal heart abnormalities may be the first sign of a pre-existing abnormality which will not be prevented by caesarean delivery [95]. However, when the only identifiable problem has been an intrapartum one, argument must be expected. Also such data are derived from units in which modern obstetric principles are applied to prevent encephalopathic outcome.

Whilst the search continues for more accurate predictors of neonatal outcome such as computerized foetal heart rate analysis, S–T segment analysis, intrapartum oximetry and umbilical arterial blood velocity waveforms, cardiotocography remains the ubiquitous monitor of foetal well-being in labour. If foetal asphyxia is being misdiagnosed and caesarean deliveries performed unnecessarily, the likeliest reason is misinterpretation of the foetal heart rate patterns, combined with omission of foetal scalp sampling. Cardiotocography should only be regarded as a screening test, and non-reassuring foetal heart rate patterns must always be backed up by foetal scalp sampling before a diagnosis of foetal asphyxia is made.

Maternal mortality associated with anaesthesia has probably decreased to the lowest figure that can be achieved. Improvements have been credited to the increasing use of regional anaesthesia and the increasing safety of general anaesthesia. Audits of maternal mortality have also been of value in directing attention towards areas of greatest concern and in identifying substandard care. Although maternal anaesthetic mortality has declined, reports will continue to be of value. It should be remembered that the reports are a collation of anecdotes, and while they provide a useful pointer, they are not a substitute for a scientifically designed assessment. Wherever possible, clinical practice should be based on the evidence of properly conducted studies. The advocates of liberalization of feeding policies in labour or the abandonment of cricoid pressure must first prove that such action is safe before widespread introduction into practice. It is possible that the use of cricoid pressure and starvation in labour has equally contributed to the reduction in mortality associated with emergency general anaesthesia. If so, then it is astonishing that anaesthetists who would never consider inducing a general obstetric anaesthetic without cricoid pressure would allow the intake of solids during labour.

One explanation might be the perception that the anaesthetist should only influence the course of events in the operating room. When anaesthetists are increasingly involved in labour analgesia, maternal resuscitation, invasive monitoring and post-delivery intensive care, this perception is clearly inappropriate. There will always be the occasional need for emergency general anaesthesia in obstetrics. To ensure that this is a safe procedure the anaesthetist must be confident that the identifiable risk factors have been controlled or corrected where possible. This can only be achieved if obstetric anaesthetists involve themselves in the evolution of labour ward protocols.

REFERENCES

1. Department of Health, Welsh Office, Scottish Office Home and Health Department, Department of Health and Social Security, Northern Ireland (1996) *Report on Confidential Enquiries into Maternal Death in the United Kingdom. 1991–1993*, HMSO, London.
2. Department of Health (1987) *Report on Confidential Enquiries into Maternal Death in England and Wales 1982–1984*, HMSO, London.
3. Madej, T.H., Jackson, I.J.B., Wheatley, R.G. and Wilson, J. (1992) Assessing introduction of spinal anaesthesia for obstetric procedures. *Quality in Health Care*, **2**, 31–34.
4. Hawthorne, L.A., Wilson, R.C., Lyons, G. and Dresner, M. (1996) Failed intubation revisited: 17 year experience in a teaching maternity unit. *British Journal of Anaesthesia*, **76**, 680–4.
5. Brown, G.W. and Russell, I.F. (1995) A survey of anaesthesia for Caesarean section. *International Journal of Obstetric Anaesthesia*, **4**, 214–8.
6. Chadwick, H.S., Posner, K., Caplan, R.A. et al. (1991) A comparison of obstetric and nonobstetric anesthesia malpractice claims. *Anesthesiology*, **74**, 242–9.
7. Stephens, I.D. (1991) ICU admissions from an obstetrical hospital. *Canadian Journal of Anaesthesia*, **38**, 677–81.
8. Zucker-Pinchoff, B. (1996) Obstetric Anesthesia Safety Improvement Study (OASIS): Results of a survey of 320 hospitals (abstract). 28th Annual Meeting, Society for Obstetric Anesthesia and Perinatology, Tucson.
9. Samsoon, G.L.T. and Young, J.R.B. (1987) Difficult tracheal intubation: a retrospective study. *Anaesthesia*, **42**, 487–90.
10. Glassenberg, R. (1991) General anesthesia and maternal mortality. *Seminars in Perinatology*, **15**, 386–96.
11. Lyons, G. (1985) Failed intubation: Six year's experience in a teaching maternity unit. *Anaesthesia*, **42**, 487–90.
12. Rocke, D.A., Murray, W.B., Rout, C.C. and Gouws, E. (1992) Relative risk analysis of factors associated with difficult intubation in obstetric anesthesia. *Anesthesiology*, **77**, 67–73.
13. Chong, J.L., Chin, E.Y., Chan, S.Y. et al. (1990) Denitrogenation in pregnant women. *Singapore Medical Journal*, **31**, 327–30.
14. Baraka, A.S., Hanna, M.T., Jabbour, S.I. et al. (1992) Preoxygenation of pregnant and nonpregnant women in the head-up versus supine position. *Anesthesia and Analgesia*, **75**, 757–9.
15. Campbell, I.T. and Beatty, P.C.W. (1994) Monitoring preoxygenation (editorial). *British Journal of Anaesthesia*, **72**, 3–4.
16. Berry, C.B. and Myles, P.S. (1994) Preoxygenation in healthy volunteers: a graph of oxygen 'washing' using end-tidal oxygraphy. *British Journal of Anaesthesia*, **72**, 116–8.
17. Marx, G.F., Luyx, W.M. and Cohen, S. (1984) Fetal–neonatal status following caesarean section for fetal distress. *British Journal of Anaesthesia*, **56**, 1009–13.
18. Quinn, A.J. and Kilpatrick, A. (1994) Emergency caesarean section during labour: response times and type of anaesthesia. *European Journal of Obstetrics, Gynaecology and Reproductive Biology*, **54**, 25–9.
19. Mallampati, S.R., Gatt, S.P., Gugino, L.D. et al. (1985) A clinical sign to predict difficult tracheal intubation: a prospective study. *Canadian Anaesthetists' Society Journal*, **32**, 429– 34.
20. Ramadhani, S.A., Mohamed, L.A., Rocke, D.A. and Gouws, E. (1996) Sternomental distance as the sole predictor of difficult laryngoscopy in obstetric anaesthesia. *British Journal of Anaesthesia*, **77**, 312–6.
21. Charles, P. (1996) What future is there for predicting difficult intubation? *British Journal of Anaesthesia*, **77**, 309–11.
22. Attia, R.R., Ebeid, A.M., Fischer, J.E. and Goudsouzian, N.G. (1982) Maternal fetal and placental gastrin concentrations. *Anaesthesia*, **37**, 8–21.
23. Sellick, B.A. (1961) Cricoid pressure to control regurgitation of stomach contents during induction of anaesthesia. *Lancet*, 404–6.
24. Rosen, M. (1981) Editorial. *Anaesthesia*, **36**, 145–6.
25. Benhamou, D. (1993) Controversies in obstetric anaesthesia: cricoid pressure is unnecessary in obstetric general anaesthesia. *International Journal of Obstetric Anaesthesia*, **4**, 30–1.
26. Benhamou, D. (1993) French obstetric anaesthesia and acid aspiration prophylaxis. *European Journal of Anaesthesiology*, **10**, 27–32.
27. Warner, M.A., Warner, M.E. and Weber, J.G. (1993) Clinical significance of pulmonary aspiration during the perioperative period. *Anesthesiology*, **78**, 56–62.
28. Morgan, M. (1986) The confidential enquiry into maternal deaths (editorial). *Anaesthesia*, **41**, 689–91.
29. Vanner, R. (1995) Controversies in obstetric anaesthesia: cricoid pressure is unnecessary in obstetric general anaesthesia. *International Journal of Obstetric Anaesthesia*, **4**, 32–3.

30. Fanning, G.L. (1970) The efficacy of cricoid pressure in preventing regurgitation of gastric contents. *Anesthesiology*, **32**, 553–5.

31. Rout, C.C., Rocke, D.A. and Gouws, E. (1993) Intravenous ranitidine reduces the risk of acid aspiration of gastric contents at emergency cesarean section. *Anesthesia and Analgesia*, **76**, 156–61.

32. Department of Health (1982) *Report on Confidential Enquiries into Maternal Deaths in England and Wales 1976–1978*. HMSO, London.

33. Department of Health (1986) *Report on Confidential Enquiries into Maternal Deaths in England and Wales 1979–1981*. HMSO, London.

34. Howells, T.H., Chamney, A.R., Wraight, W.J. and Simons, R.S. (1983) The application of cricoid pressure. An assessment and survey of its practice. *Anaesthesia*, **38**, 457–60.

35. Wraight, W.J., Chamney, A.R. and Howells, T.H. (1983) The determination of an effective cricoid pressure. *Anaesthesia*, **38**, 461–6.

36. Lawes, E.G., Duncan, P.W., Bland, B. *et al.* (1986) The cricoid yoke – a device for providing consistent and reproducible cricoid pressure. *British Journal of Anaesthesia*, **58**, 925–31.

37. Vanner, R.G., Pryle, B.J., O'Dwyer, J.P. and Reynolds, F. (1992) Upper oesophageal sphincter pressure and the intravenous induction of anaesthesia. *Anaesthesia*, **47**, 371–5.

38. Ashurst, N., Rout, C.C., Rocke, D.A. and Gouws, E. (1996) Use of a mechanical simulator for training in applying cricoid pressure. *British Journal of Anaesthesia*, **77**, 468–72.

39. Roberts, R.B. and Shirley, M.A. (1974) Reducing the risk of acid aspiration during caesarean section. *Anaesthesia and Analgesia*, **53**, 859–68.

40. Rocke, D.A., Brock-Utne, J.G. and Rout, C.C. (1993) At risk for aspiration: new critical values of volume and pH? *Anaesthesia and Analgesia*, **76**, 666.

41. James, C.F., Modell, J.H., Gibbs, C.P. *et al.* (1984) Pulmonary aspiration: effects of volume and pH in the rat. *Anaesthesia and Analgesia*, **63**, 650–68.

42. Raidoo, D.M., Rocke, D.A., Brock-Utne, J.G. *et al.* (1990) Critical volume for pulmonary acid aspiration: reappraisal in a primate model. *British Journal of Anaesthesia*, **65**, 248–50.

43. Brock-Utne, J.G., Barclay, A.J. and Houton, P.J.C. (1977) Gastric volume and acidity at caesarean section. *South African Medical Journal*, **52**, 182–3.

44. Vandam, L.D. (1965) Aspiration of gastric contents in the operative period. *New England Journal of Medicine*, **273**, 1206–8.

45. Mendelson, C.L. (1946) The aspiration of stomach contents into the lungs during obstetric anesthesia. *American Journal of Obstetric Gynecology*, **52**, 191–205.

46. Bannister, W.K. and Sattilaro, A.J. (1962) Vomiting and aspiration during anesthesia. *Anesthesiology*, **23**, 251–4.

47. Howard, F.A. and Sharp, D.S. (1973) Effects of metoclopramide on gastric emptying during labour. *British Medical Journal*, **1**, 446–8.

48. Adelhoj, B., Petring, O.U., Pedersen, N.O. *et al.* (1985) Metoclopramide given preoperatively empties the stomach. *Acta Anaesthesiologica Scandinavica*, **29**, 322–5.

49. Brock-Utne, J.G., Rout, C., Moodley, J. and Mayat, N. (1989) Influence of preoperative gastric aspiration on the volume and pH of gastric contents in obstetric patients undergoing caesarean section. *British Journal of Anaesthesia*, **62**, 397–401.

50. Holdsworth, J.D., Furness, R.M.B. and Roulston, R.G. (1989) A comparison of apomorphine and stomach tubes for emptying the stomach before general anaesthesia in obstetrics. *British Journal of Anaesthesia*, **46**, 526–9.

51. Nimmo, W.S., Wilson, J. and Prescott, L.F. (1975) Narcotic analgesics and delayed gastric emptying during labour. *Lancet*, **1**, 890–3.

52. Brock-Utne, J.G., Rubin, J., Welman, S. *et al.* (1978) The action of commonly used antiemetics on the lower oesophageal sphincter. *British Journal of Anaesthesia*, **50**, 295–8.

53. Rowbotham, D.J. and Nimmo, S. (1987) Effect of cisapride on morphine-induced delay in gastric emptying. *British Journal of Anaesthesia*, **59**, 536–9.

54. Grange, C.S., Adams, T.J., Kliffer, A.P. and Douglas, M.J. (1996) Effect of cisapride on gastric emptying following caesarean section (abstract). 28th Annual Meeting, Society for Obstetric Anesthesia and Perinatology, Tucson, p. 66.

55. O'Sullivan, G. (1995) The stomach – fact and fantasy: eating and drinking during labor, in *International Anesthesiology Clinics* (ed. D.A. Rocke) pp. 31–44.

56. Garcia, J. and Garforth, S. (1989) Labour and delivery routines in English consultant maternity units. *Midwifery*, **5**, 155–62.

57. Michael, S., Reilly, C.S. and Caunt, J.A. (1991) Policies for oral intake during labour. A survey of maternity units in England and Wales. *Anaesthesia*, **46**, 1071–3.

58. McKay, S. and Mahan, C. (1988) How can aspiration of vomitus in obstetrics best be prevented? *Birth*, **15**, 222–9.

59. Douglas, M.J. and McMorland, G.H.(1984) Food and fluids during labour. *Society for Obstetric Anesthesia and Perinatology Newsletter*, **14**, 4.

60. Maltby, J.R., Lewis, P., Martin, A. and Sutherland, L.R. (1991) Gastric fluid volume and pH in elective patients following unrestricted oral fluid until three hours before surgery. *Canadian Journal of Anaesthesia*, **38**, 425–9.

61. Maltby, J.R. (1993) New guidelines for preoperative fasting. *Canadian Journal of Anaesthesia*, **40**, R113–R117.

62. Simpkin, P. (1986) Stress, pain and catecholamines in labor; part 2. Stress associated with childbirth events: a pilot survey of new mothers. *Birth*, **13**, 234–40.

63. Scrutton, M., Lowry, C. and O'Sullivan, G. (1996) Eating in labor: an assessment of the risks and benefits (abstract). 28th Annual Meeting, Society for Obstetric Anesthesia and Perinatology, Tucson, p. 37.

64. Dumoulin, J.G. and Foulkes, J. (1984) Ketonuria during labour. *British Journal of Obstetric Gynaecology*, **91**, 97–8.

65. Gibbs, C.P., Schwartz, D.J., Wynne, J.W. *et al.* (1975) Antacid pulmonary aspiration in the dog. *Anesthesiology*, **51**, 380–5.

66. Thorburn, J. and Moir, D.D. (1987) Antacid therapy for emergency caesarean section. *Anaesthesia*, **42**, 352–5.

67. Rocke, D.A., Rout, C.C. and Gouws, E. (1994) Intravenous administration of the proton pump inhibitor omeprazole reduces the risk of acid aspiration at emergency cesarean section. *Anesthesia and Analgesia*, **78**, 1093–8.

68. Rocke, D.A. and Rout, C.C. (1995) Intravenous omeprazole before emergency cesarean section. In response. *Anesthesia and Analgesia*, **80**, 848–57.

69. Brock-Utne, J.G., Downing, J.W. and Humphrey, D. (1984) Effect of ranitidine given before atropine sulphate on lower oesophageal sphincter tone. *Anaesthesia and Intensive Care*, **12**, 140–2.

70. King, H., Ashby, S., Brathwaite, D. *et al.* (1993) Adequacy of general anesthesia for cesarean section. *Anesthesia and Analgesia*, **77**, 84–8.

71. Schwender, D., Madler, C., Klasing, S. *et al.* (1995) Mid-latency auditory evoked potentials and wakefulness during caesarean section. *European Journal of Anaesthesiology*, **12**, 171–9.

72. Moerman, N., Bonke, B. and Oosting, J. (1993) Awareness and recall during general anaesthesia; Facts and feelings. *Anesthesiology*, **79**, 454–6.

73. Andrews, W.W., Ramin, S.M., Maberry, M.C. *et al.* (1992) Effect of type of anesthesia on blood loss at elective repeat cesarean section. *American Journal of Perinatology*, **9**, 197–200.

74. Gambling, D.R., Sharma, S.K., White, P.F. *et al.* Use of sevoflurane during elective cesarean birth: a comparison with isoflurane and spinal anesthesia. *Anesthesia and Analgesia*, **81**, 90–5.

75. McCrirrick, A., Evans, G.H. and Thomas, T.A. (1994) Overpressure isoflurane at caesarean section: a study of arterial isoflurane concentrations. *British Journal of Anaesthesia*, **72**, 122–4.

76. Perreault, C., Blaise, G.A. and Meloche, R. (1992) Maternal inspired oxygen concentration and fetal oxygenation during caesarean section. *Canadian Journal of Anaesthesia*, **39**, 155–7.

77. Dwyer, R., Fee, J.P. and Moore, J. (1995) Uptake of halothane and isoflurane by mother and baby during caesarean section. *British Journal of Anaesthesia*, **74**, 379–83.

78. Celleno, D., Capogna, G., Emanuelli, M. *et al.* (1993) Which induction drug for cesarean section? A comparison of thiopental sodium, propofol and midazolam. *Journal of Clinical Anesthesia*, **5**, 284–8.

79. Hodgkinson, R., Husain, R.F. and Hayashi, R.H. (1980) Systemic and pulmonary blood pressure during cesarean section in parturients with gestational hypertension. *Canadian Anaesthetists' Society Journal*, **27**, 389–93.

80. Connell, H., Dalgleish, J.G. and Downing, J.W. (1987) General anaesthesia in mothers with severe pre-eclampsia/eclampsia. *British Journal of Anaesthesia*, **59**, 1375–80.

81. Rout, C.C. and Rocke, D.A. (1990) Effects of alfentanil and fentanyl on induction of anaesthesia in patients with severe pregnancy-induced hypertension. *British Journal of Anaesthesia*, **65**, 468–74.

82. Cork, R.C. and James, M.F.M. (1985) Magnesium pretreatment at c-section for pregnancy induced hypertension. *Anesthesia and Analgesia*, **64**, 202–5.

83. Allen, R.W., James, M.F.M. and Uys, P.C. (1991) Attenuation of the pressor response to tracheal intubation in hypertensive proteinuric pregnant patients by lignocaine, alfentanil and magnesium sulphate. *British Journal of Anaesthesia*, **66**, 216–23.

84. Bhorat, I.E., Naidoo, D.P., Rout, C.C. and Moodley, J. (1993) Malignant ventricular arrhythmias in eclampsia: a comparison of

labetalol with dihydralazine. *American Journal Obstetric Gynecology*, **168**, 1292–6.

85. Gin, T. (1993) Pharmacokinetic optimisation of general anaesthesia in pregnancy. *Clinical Pharmacokinetics*, **25**, 59–70.

86. Ratcliffe, F.M. and Evans, J.M. (1983) Neonatal well-being after elective caesarean delivery with general, spinal and epidural anaesthesia. *European Journal of Anaesthesiology*, **10**, 175–81.

87. Ng, P.C., Woug, M.Y., Nelson, E.A. (1995) Paediatrician attendances at caesarean section. *European Journal of Paediatrics*, **154**, 672–5.

88. Abboud, T.K., Nagappala, S. and Murakawak *et al*. (1985) Comparison of the effects of general and regional anaesthesia for cesarean section on neonatal neurologic and adaptive capacity scores. *Anesthesia and Analgesia*, **64**, 996–1000.

89. Rolbin, S.M., Cohen, M.M., Levinton, C.M. *et al*. (1994) The premature infant: anaesthesia for cesarean delivery. *Anesthesia and Analgesia*, **78**, 912–17.

90. Pedersen, J.E., Fernandes, A. and Christiansen, M. (1992) Halothane 2% for caesarean section. *European Journal of Anaesthesiology*, **9**, 319–24.

91. Dick, W., Traub, E., Kraus, H. *et al*. (1992) General anaesthesia versus epidural anaesthesia for primary caesarean section – a comparative study. *European Journal of Anaesthesiology*, **9**, 15–21.

92. Kamat, S.K., Shah, M.V., Chaudary, L.S. *et al*. (1991) Effect of induction-delivery and uterine-delivery on Apgar scoring of the newborn. *Journal of Postgraduate Medicine*, **37**, 125–7.

93. Macfarlane, A. and Chamberlain, G. (1993) What is happening to caesarean section rates? *Lancet*, **342**, 1005–6.

94. Treffers, P.E. and Pel, M. (1993) The rising trend for caesarean birth. *British Medical Journal*, **307**, 1017–8.

95. Adamson, S.J., Alessandri, L.M., Badawi, N. *et al*. (1995) Predictors of neonatal encephalopathy in full term infants. *British Medical Journal*, **311**, 598–602.

CONSENT FOR OBSTETRIC ANAESTHESIA AND ANALGESIA

D.J. Bush

INTRODUCTION

There are sound moral and legal arguments for obtaining consent before all medical treatment [1, 2]. In practice there is considerable confusion and disagreement amongst clinicians: exactly what should patients be told? Is written consent necessary? Is consent from a distressed patient valid? This chapter explores such issues in relation to obstetric anaesthesia.

ETHICAL AND PHILOSOPHICAL PERSPECTIVES

AUTONOMY

The right to give or withdraw consent for medical treatment derives from the fundamental entitlement of an autonomous individual to determine his own fate [2]. Ethically valid consent requires that the autonomous patient has:

- sufficient relevant information to make a decision;
- the opportunity to express this decision;
- the assurance that their decision will be respected and implemented.

Some authorities propose that the truly autonomous patient would not be asked to give passive consent at all but would actively request treatment after considering the relevant information [3]. Such a policy would be somewhat impractical in the context of emergency obstetric anaesthesia during labour. While promotion of patient autonomy is very worthwhile it is not practically helpful in guiding discussion with a particular patient before treatment.

BENEFICENCE

The primary duty of any physician is to benefit his patient, to 'help, or at least do no harm' [2]. Some physicians feel that fully involving the patient in the choice of treatment may conflict with this duty. For example, a mother might choose general rather than regional anaesthesia for caesarean section even though the anaesthetist would recommend regional anaesthesia. One approach to resolving such conflict is to present the evidence for each option fairly and openly such that the patient also reaches the 'correct' conclusion. The practical difficulty is that supporting evidence is often lacking; most anaesthetists believe regional anaesthesia is safer than general anaesthesia for caesarean section [4] but the mortality solely from anaesthesia is too small to be dogmatic [5]. Ultimately, guidelines from

Clinical Problems in Obstetric Anaesthesia
Edited by Ian F. Russell and Gordon Lyons. Published in 1997 by Chapman & Hall, London. ISBN 0 412 71600 3.

the UK Department of Health are quite clear: where safe and reasonable alternatives exist all must be discussed and the patient's decision respected [6].

THERAPEUTIC PRIVILEGE

Therapeutic privilege is the term used to describe the practice of withholding particular information in order to benefit the patient. Many physicians believe that complete discussion may cause distress [7] or generate anxiety, which might increase morbidity from anaesthesia [8]. There is little evidence that providing more detailed information before treatment increases anxiety and indeed the reverse may be true [9, 10]. It would be difficult to prove excess morbidity from anaesthesia specifically resulting from anxiety in the obstetric population. For these reasons therapeutic privilege might be difficult to justify in this group.

LEGAL PERSPECTIVES

Litigation relating exclusively to consent for medical treatment is relatively rare but may be more common in some disciplines such as obstetric anaesthesia [11]. In fact most medico-legal problems arise from the actual performance of medical treatment: witness the periodic interest in awareness during general anaesthesia for caesarean section but problems have arisen after the failure to warn of the possibility of post-dural puncture headache [11]. Obviously disclosing the risk of a complication does not automatically protect the doctor against all actions for breach of duty to care if such an event actually occurs.

EVIDENCE OF CONSENT

Obstetric anaesthesia involves significant risk so formal, express consent is more appropriate than implied consent [12]. Oral consent is legally and ethically valid but can be difficult to prove later so some form of written evidence

of consent would seem advisable even if this is just an entry in the case notes [6]. Anaesthetists must obtain and document valid consent from patients themselves rather than relying on the reference to anaesthesia found in the generic consent form administered by the surgeon, who is often lacking in detailed knowledge of anaesthesia. Most obstetric anaesthetists do not obtain written consent even before epidural analgesia for labour when there is no corresponding surgical consent form [13].

There is no more justification for introducing a separate specific consent form for obstetric anaesthesia than for any other discipline. Presumably separate forms would be needed for elective and emergency work, regional and general techniques and the whole exercise would be greatly complicated. All that is required is to record the topics discussed in the case notes or on the generic consent form. (Table 13.1). Indeed, such an individualised record might well be more convincing than a printed proforma in demonstrating that proper discussion occurred.

Many patients do not recall reliably specific information discussed during the consent process [14] but in obstetric anaesthetic practice patient recall (and presumably understanding) can be improved when written information supplements the oral discussion [15]. Such written information is already used in many units and examples may be found in the literature [16].

HISTORICAL DEVELOPMENT OF CONSENT LAW

Treatment without any consent, even implied, is unusual and risks an action in battery. In recent times courts have resisted claims of battery on this basis, preferring actions in negligence for inadequately informed consent [12]. The major medico-legal issue has therefore become the quality and quantity of information provided to the patient and in particular who should set the standard. Two standards prevail in the English-speaking

Table 13.1 Information always discussed with parturients by author (and indicated as such in patient record)

Epidural analgesia	Elective general anaesthesia
Effectiveness	Aspiration
Potential for operative use	Awareness
Post-dural puncture headache	Dental trauma
Backache	Adverse effects of drugs
Any further details required	Sore throat

world, representing either end of a spectrum of patient autonomy. They are the **professional standard** and the **patient need standard**.

PROFESSIONAL STANDARD

In the UK there is no constitutional or statutory law defining the standard of information necessary for valid consent, so the 'professional standard' has evolved from the influential Bolam judgment on the standard of care required in ordinary medical practice. The standard should be consistent with the contemporary practice of a responsible body of medical opinion but need not necessarily represent majority practice [17]. The second clause encourages clinical freedom and many would argue that this puts physicians in a favoured position compared to other professions. The Bolam principle was first applied to determine validity of consent in the Sidaway case. Judgment stated that the standard of information provided must 'allow a patient to understand the nature, consequences and any substantial risks of the treatment proposed' [18]. Disclosure of all information is not required but the court did reserve the right to intervene if 'disclosure of a risk was so obviously necessary to an informed choice on the part of the patient that no reasonably prudent medical man could fail to make it'. Therefore, in the UK less than fully informed consent is still valid.

Sectionalized consent

The UK courts have not required separate 'sectionalized' consent for component parts of an anaesthetic, for example performing regional block during general anaesthesia [19]. However the General Medical Council has recently implied that component parts of an anaesthetic might have to be specifically discussed if they are unusual or potentially distressing to the patient, such as placement of a suppository during general anaesthesia [20]. Such professional regulatory bodies are likely to influence practice at least as much as the courts.

Current practice

The professional standard is effectively defined by current practice. Lanigan surveyed 523 members of the Obstetric Anaesthetists Association regarding the risk information they would supply to an obese mother presenting for elective caesarean section for breech [4]. The results surely represent the contemporary practice of a responsible body of medical opinion and so can be used as guidance in clinical practice. (Figure 13.1). Consensus for regional blockade was good: most doctors would mention intra-operative discomfort, conversion to general anaesthesia and accidental dural puncture but not rare neurological sequelae. There was less agreement when considering general anaesthesia; while most would mention postoperative pain and the relative safety of the alternative regional techniques not all doctors would mention aspiration or awareness. General comments suggested that respondents used therapeutic privilege when deciding what to discuss with patients. Concordant results

Table 13.2 Discussion of risk benefit information by UK anaesthetists before epidural analgesia for labour. Reproduced by permission from reference [13]; published by Churchill Livingstone, 1995

Benefit or complication of epidural analgesia	Percentage of anaesthetists discussing this item
Effectiveness of analgesia	96
Benefit to foetus	80
Immobility in labour	78
Use for potential operative delivery	77
Risk of headache	66
Post-operative backache	53
Incidence of instrumental delivery	52
Urinary catheterization	41
Neurological sequelae	21
Total spinal	16

were reported by Bush who also showed that before epidural analgesia for labour the majority of UK anaesthetists discussed benefits and common complications but often ignored rare problems such as total spinal or neurological problems (Table 13.2) [13]. Individual practitioners also influence practice if they are experts in their field: Aitkenhead has recommended that both awareness and discomfort under regional blockade should usually be discussed before caesarean section [21].

PATIENT NEED STANDARD

The **patient need standard** for valid consent emphasizes the autonomy of the patient and is often misinterpreted as requiring full disclosure of all information to the patient, viz. the doctrine of fully informed consent. This standard is accepted in a minority of the states of the USA (and in Canada and Australia) and follows the US judgment of Canterbury versus Spence [22]. This case ruled that discussion should be of 'a reasonable standard of what is material to the patient's decision rather than a professional standard based on customary practice'. The original judgment and subsequent legal opinion acknowledged that a physician could not always know what an individual patient might find relevant or 'material' to his decision and accepted the principle of therapeutic privilege so that full disclosure might not always be necessary [2].

Materiality

When deciding what risks to discuss the anaesthetist must consider the interaction of severity and incidence, the 'materiality', of a complication to the patient. Unfortunately there is no satisfactory legal measure of materiality but the UK courts have indicated that a risk of 10% for a complication such as stroke would warrant automatic disclosure to a patient [18]. Few risks of obstetric anaesthesia approach this level of materiality but recently a Canadian court has ruled that even the 1 in 14 000 risk of total blindness following ophthalmic surgery should have been disclosed to a patient who had asked general questions about complications [23].

The anaesthetist must decide if a risk is material to a particular patient. For example it is likely that most women planning to leave hospital a few hours after delivery would regard even the small risk of post-dural puncture headache and the resulting inpatient stay as very relevant when considering epidural analgesia so this risk should be disclosed even although it is of the order of 0.5%. The prudent obstetric anaesthetist would be wise to discuss even more remote risks such as neurological sequelae after regional techniques when asked for complete information about safety by the patient. A practical difficulty is that the benefits and risks of our techniques are often not well quantified nor are they familiar to all anaesthetists practising in obstetrics. Ultimately there are no infallible rules regarding materiality so clinical experience must guide discussion before consent.

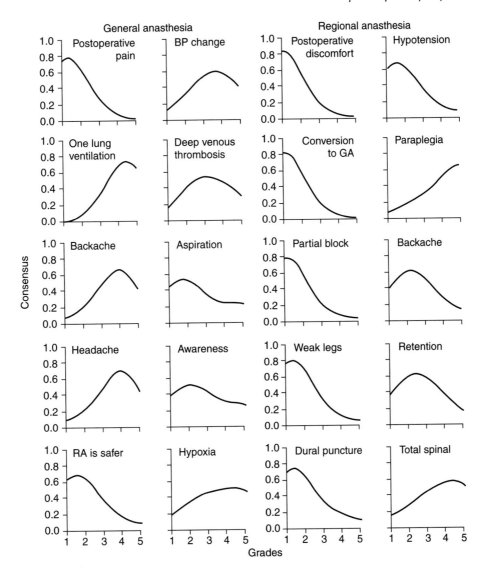

Figure 13.1. Consensus agreement on the delivery of risk information on anaesthesia for elective caesarean section. Grades: 1 = must be told; 2 = worth mentioning; 3 = optional; 4 = not worth mentioning; 5 = must not be mentioned unless specifically asked. Consensus: 1.0 = full agreement. GA = general anaesthesia and RA = regional anaesthesia. Reproduced with permission from reference [4]; published by Churchill Livingstone, 1995.

Patients' views

Patients views on what they should be told about their treatment are relevant to the **patient need standard** and so can guide practice. The views of obstetric patients have not been directly reported but studies of other patient groups have revealed that they wanted to know most about 'everyday' aspects of their management such as pain relief and return to normal diet and least about details of anaesthesia such as drips and dangerous

Table 13.3 Information about treatment desired by Australian surgical patients. Reproduced with permission from reference [25]; published by W.B. Saunders Ltd, 1993

Information category	Percentage of patients wanting this information
When allowed to eat/drink	97
Details of pain/pain relief	92
Common complications	92
Drip or bladder catheter upon waking	89
Alternative methods of anaesthesia	87
Dangerous complications	82
Details of drips/needles used	82

complications [24] (Table 13.3). However younger patients wanted to know the most and the more recent surveys show an increasing expectation for information [25]. It would seem that the majority of patients do want to be well informed about their treatment.

COMPETENCY

Many anaesthetists obtain consent for epidural analgesia from labouring women whose judgement may be impaired by pain or analgesic drugs [13]. The validity of such consent is debatable [26] but the alternative of routinely obtaining consent antenatally for all possible interventions is inefficient and so obviously contrived that it is of dubious value anyway. This does not detract from the value of anaesthetists providing more general education antenatally [27].

The individual anaesthetist must assess the labouring mother's competency and if she cannot give valid consent he is obliged to act in her best interest [6]. Unfortunately there is no satisfactory means to determine competency in the presence of pain or drugs apart from clinical judgement. Grice showed that information provided to labouring women could be

recalled months later and so was by implication understood during labour [15]. Even the US courts have not been unduly demanding when considering competency for consent in labour, requiring only that there is evidence that a discussion occurred, that the patient did not object and co-operated during the treatment [28].

Consent for research from labouring patients causes similar problems when assessing competency. For this reason some research ethics committees feel that more stringent standards are required than for consent for treatment, sometimes including obtaining antenatal consent. This is presumably because the patient does not benefit directly.

ADVANCE DIRECTIVES

Should the anaesthetist provide epidural analgesia for the distressed, labouring mother now requesting help but who has previously made a deliberate decision to forgo an epidural, a kind of 'advance directive'? Thornton would argue that this woman should be actively encouraged to manage without an epidural because her new decision is temporary and will revert after delivery whatever happens [26]. Nevertheless she is entitled to change her mind [6, 27]. The anaesthetist concerned must use clinical judgement to assess her competency and act accordingly. The prudent anaesthetist will take account of any previously documented wishes of the patient and the opinion of a partner but neither is likely to be legally binding during a temporary state such as labour, unlike a true advance directive for terminal care. The anaesthetist is ultimately obligated to act in the patient's best interest if she is judged incompetent to give consent.

CONCLUSION

Obtaining valid consent is more than a medicolegal exercise. The underlying purpose is to respect and benefit the patient and this should guide clinical practice. We must recognize that patients increasingly expect to be involved actively in their own care and we should respect this. When obtaining consent anaesthetists must volunteer material information such as the chance of success and failure of blocks, the risk of awareness and post-dural puncture headache. Questions about rare complications such as paralysis must be answered honestly. A more detailed consideration of the content of informed consent could be specified in the *de facto* national guidelines for obstetric anaesthesia care, published by the Obstetric Anaesthesia Association [27]. In the meantime local guidelines should be developed.

REFERENCES

1. Kessel, A.S. (1994) On failing to understand informed consent. *British Journal of Hospital Medicine*, **52**, 235–8.
2. Gild, W.M. (1989) Informed consent: A review. *Anesthesia and Analgesia*, **68**, 649–53.
3. Lawson, A. and Cohen, J. (1993) Informed consent. *British Medical Journal*, **306**, 927.
4. Lanigan, C. and Reynolds, F. (1995) Risk information supplied by obstetric anaesthetists in Britain and Ireland to mothers awaiting elective caesarean section. *International Journal of Obstetric Anaesthesia*, **4**, 7–13.
5. Department of Health, Welsh Office, Scottish Office Home and Health Department, Department of Health and Social Security, Northern Ireland (1994) *Report on Confidential Enquiry into Maternal Deaths in the United Kingdom 1988–1990*, London, HMSO.
6. NHS Management Executive (1990) *A Guide to Consent for Examination or Treatment*, HC9022, London.
7. Tobias, J.S. and Souhami, R.L. (1993) Fully informed consent can be needlessly cruel. *British Medical Journal*, **307**, 1199–201.
8. Lyons, S.M. and Saunders, D.S. (1995) A fundamental problem of consent: Nothing is inherently remiss in obtaining consent. *British Medical Journal*, **310**, 935.
9. Lankton, J.W., Batchelder, B.M. and Ominsky, A.J. (1977) Emotional responses to detailed risk disclosure for anaesthesia, a prospective randomised study. *Anesthesiology*, **46**, 294–6.
10. Kerrigan, D.D., Thevasagaym, R.S., Woods, T.O. *et al.* (1993) Who's afraid of informed consent? *British Medical Journal*, **306**, 298–300.
11. Aitkenhead, A.R. (1994) The pattern of litigation against anaesthetists. *British Journal Anaesthesia*, **73**, 10–21.
12. Mason, J.K. and McCall Smith, R.A. (1994) *Law and Medical Ethics*, 4th edn, Butterworths, London.
13. Bush, D. (1995) A comparison of informed consent for obstetric anaesthesia in the US and the UK. *International Journal of Obstetric Anaesthesia*, **4**, 1–7.
14. Wade, T.C. (1990) Patients may not recall risk of death: Implications for informed consent. *Medicine Science and Law*, **30**, 259–61.
15. Grice, S.C., Eisenach, J.C., Dewan, D.M. *et al.* (1988) Evaluation of informed consent for anesthesia for labor and delivery. *Anesthesiology*, **69**, A664.
16. Price, J. (1986) Consent for epidural anaesthesia. *Canadian Anaesthetic Society Journal*, **33**, 534–5.
17. Bolam versus Friern Barnet Hospital Management Committee, 1957 **1**, WLR 582.
18. Sidaway versus Board of Governors of Bethlem Royal Hospital, 1985 AC 871.
19. Davis versus Barking, Havering and Brentwood Health Authority, 1993 4 Med LR 85.
20. Mitchell, J. (1995) A fundamental problem of consent. *British Medical Journal*, **310;** 43– 6.
21. Aitkenhead, A.R. (1990) Awareness during anaesthesia: what should the patient be told? *Anaesthesia*, **45**, 351–3.
22. Canterbury versus Spence, 464 F.2d783,784d.c. Circuit 1972.
23. Ottley, R. (1993) Duty to warn. *Australasian Journal of the Medical Defence Union*, **7**, 43–4.
24. Lonsdale, M. and Hutchinson, G.L. (1991) Patients' desire for information about anaesthesia. *Anaesthesia*, **46**, 410–412.
25. Farnill, D. and Inglis, S. (1993) Patients' desire for information about anaesthesia: Australian attitudes. *Anaesthesia*, **48**, 162–4.
26. Thornton, J. and Moore, M. (1995) Controversies: Women who request epidural analgesia should always be given it. *International Journal of Obstetric Anaesthesia*, **4,** 40–3.
27. Obstetric Anaesthetists Association (1995) *Recommended Minimum Standards for Obstetric Anaesthesia Services*. Obstetric Anaesthetists Association, OAA Secretariat, P.O. Box 3219, London.
28. Knapp, R.M. (1990) Legal view of informed consent for anesthesia during labor. *Anesthesiology*, **72**, 211.

POST-DURAL PUNCTURE HEADACHE 14

G. Capogna and D. Celleno

INTRODUCTION

Cerebrospinal fluid (CSF) acts as a hydraulic cushion, supporting and protecting the brain. Leakage of CSF from the subarachnoid space, through a dural breach, can lead to loss of support, and the resulting traction on the innervated tissues around the brain can be responsible for headache. A relationship exists between headache, rate of CSF loss, size of dural breach, and diameter of the needle involved. This headache, called post-dural puncture (PDPH) or low-pressure headache (LPH), is typically fronto-occipital and worse in the upright position. It is usually self-limiting, appearing on the first or on the second day after dural puncture and lasting less than seven days.

SYMPTOMS

Usually patients feel pain in the fronto-occipital region, occasionally with radiation to both temples, forehead and behind the eyes. In 50% of the patients the pain in localized to the frontal area, in 25% to the occipital area and in the remaining 25% the pain is diffuse and radiates to the neck [1]. The most important feature to distinguish PDPH is its postural character. The pain is maximal in the sitting or upright position and diminishes or disappears in the horizontal position. Some women have a mild headache that allow full ambulation, while in others the pain may be more severe and may interfere with eating, walking and breast-feeding. The magnitude and rapidity of CSF loss and the rate at which it is restored affect the incidence, rapidity of onset and severity of headache.

PDPH may be associated with auditory (dizziness, tinnitus, hearing impairment) or visual (blurred or double vision, photophobia, spots before the eyes) symptoms, both explained by a low CSF pressure [2]. Sixth cranial nerve palsy occurs occasionally (1 in 5–8000) after puncture with large-gauge needles [3]. The frequency of associated symptoms is low (<1%); however, recently a transient hearing loss following spinal anaesthesia for caesarean section has been reported in 20% of patients without headache, even using an atraumatic needle [4]. Unfortunately, PDPH is not necessarily benign: permanent neurologic damage (persistent visual loss) and death have been reported [5].

AETIOLOGY

The dural breach produced by needle puncture of the dura causes CSF leakage that decreases

Clinical Problems in Obstetric Anaesthesia
Edited by Ian F. Russell and Gordon Lyons. Published in 1997 by Chapman & Hall, London. ISBN 0 412 71600 3.

Table 14.1 Influence of size and needle bevel on the incidence of PDPH in obstetric patients

Author and reference	Gauge and bevel of the needle	% PDPH	Type of study	Sample size	Statistical significance
Crawford [9]	18 G Tuohy	77	review	27 000	
Barker [10]	26 G Quincke	2	random.	49	S
	25 G Quincke	17.6		51	
Cesarini [11]	25 G Quincke	14.5	random.	55	S
	24 G Sprotte	0		55	
Leeman [12]	24 G Sprotte	3.6	random.	55	NS
	22 G Sprotte	1.7		57	
Devcic [13]	25 G Quincke	19.6	?	46	S
	24 G Sprotte	5.6		71	
Mayer [14]	27 G Quincke	3.5	random.	147	NS
	24 G Sprotte	0.7		151	
Shutt [15]	25 G Whitacre	0	random.	49	NS
	22 G Whitacre	2		49	
	26 G Quincke	10.4		48	
Ross [16]	25 G Quincke	9	review	74	S
	26 G Quincke	8		160	
	24 G Sprotte	1.5		132	
Hurley [17]	26 G Quincke	5.2	retrospect.	2256	S
	27 G Quincke	2.5		852	
	25 G Whitacre	1.1		1000	
Campbell [18]	25 G Whitacre	0.7	random.	150	
	24 G Sprotte	4		150	
Wiesel [19]	24 G Sprotte	15.2	random.	46	NS
	27 G Quincke	12.8		47	
Amuzu [20]	25 G Whitacre	1.9	random.	106	NS
	26 G Atraucan	4.9		102	

the cushioning effect on the brain, producing traction on nerves and blood vessels when the patient assumes the upright position. Headache follows this traction on pain-sensitive cranial structures. Pain is referred above the tentorium via the trigeminal nerve to the frontal region, and below the tentorium, via the glossopharyngeal and vagal nerves to the occipital region and via the upper cervical nerves (C1–C3) to the neck and shoulders. Associated symptoms may be due to traction of cranial nerve six. Headache may be also due, in part, to cerebrovasodilation which is a compensatory mechanism to restore the intracranial volume.

Modern non-invasive diagnostic techniques have clearly confirmed the aetiology of PDPH. Magnetic resonance imaging has been used to demonstrate the reduction of intracranial volume of CSF [6, 7] and Doppler ultrasound revealed higher flow velocities in cerebral vessels in patients with PDPH [8].

Psychological factors may also affect the patient's response to headache.

INCIDENCE AND EPIDEMIOLOGY

The incidence and the severity of headache is directly related to the size and the design of the needle used (Table 14.1) [9–20]. The majority of parturients suffering inadvertent dural puncture with a Tuohy needle will develop a PDPH. The introduction of small-gauge needles with pencil points has greatly reduced the incidence of headaches after spinal anaesthesia and created new enthusiasm for this technique in obstetrics. However, even in a reduced percentage, the problem still exists. The choice of the needle and of the anaesthetic technique may have medico-legal importance. The anaesthetist who chooses an epidural technique, and inadvertently punctures the dura, can argue in defence that this is an accepted complication of the technique, whereas failure to use an appropriate needle for spinal anaesthesia is likely to attract criticism of the anaesthetist himself. In fact in a review of closed claims in the American Society of Anesthesiologists database, headaches are in the third place for claims against anaesthetists in obstetrics [21].

The incidence of PDPH is higher in the puerpera and is multifactorial. Increased incidence can be due to

- stress of labour and delivery;
- dehydration;
- increased loss of CSF due to increased CSF pressure;
- gender and age at greater risk for PDPH;
- hormonal factors.

The incidence of PDPH with the 24 gauge Sprotte needle ranges from 0 to 15.2%, and the greatest single study difference (Cesarini) is of the same magnitude, 0 to 14.5%. Interpretation of this data may not be as simple as it seems. The most important factors affecting the incidence of headaches are age, gender and pregnancy.

Several theories have been suggested to explain this age-related finding. With increasing age, the routes for the escape of CSF from the epidural space narrow significantly and therefore the pressure in the epidural space remains high and may tamponade the leak. The pain threshold may be increased in the aged, the elasticity of blood vessels is reduced and less stretching of the pain-sensitive structures may occur. Young females generally have an increased incidence and severity of headache [2]. Women may have enhanced vascular reactivity (migraine is more frequent in females) and cerebral blood flow changes are

more likely to produce pain in women than in men. This cerebrovascular reactivity may also increase with hormonal changes in the postpartum period. The rapid falling levels of oestrogen and progesterone or alteration in serotonin metabolism may increase the incidence of headache. Reduction of intra-abdominal pressure may lead to a reduction of epidural pressure, facilitating CSF leakage. It is unclear if maternal pushing during delivery may increase CSF leak, but it may certainly be influenced by the size of the hole in the dura due to the size of the needle used. In addition, relative dehydration may frequently occur in parturients, due to withholding of fluids, diaphoresis and blood losses.

Other factors are

- history of previous PDPH;
- multiple dural punctures;
- continuous spinal anaesthesia;
- antiseptics;
- hyperbaric local anaesthetics.

A history of previous headache after spinal anaesthesia may predispose to development of PDPH after another dural puncture. Multiple dural punctures may most likely result in a higher incidence of PDPH, but studies have reported conflicting results [22].

Some studies suggested that the presence of a spinal catheter may cause an inflammatory response which may promote a more rapid closure of the dural hole, but clinical studies on continuous spinal anaesthesia in obstetric patients do not support this hypothesis [23].

Possible aggravating factors may be the antiseptic and the local anaesthetic agents used for the block. An increased incidence of PDPH has been reported with patients who did not have povidone-iodine removed from the skin [24]. Like skin cleansers, anaesthetic agents may represent an aggravating factor in PDPH. In particular an acute, postural, transient headache, influenced by the local anaesthetic selected, has been described. Amide local anaesthetics may be more irritant than esters, and also glucose, contained in the hyperbaric solution, may have an osmotic or irritant effect on cerebral or meningeal structures [25].

ANATOMICAL FINDINGS

Anatomical features of dural puncture have been studied *in vitro* [26]. The size of the hole depends on the size of the needle. The gross morphology of the hole depends on the type of the needle: the Quincke needle produces an oval or ellipsoidal shaped hole, whereas pencil-point needles (Sprotte or Whitacre) produce more rounded holes. Microscopic examination of the dural samples punctured with the Quincke needles reveal an irregular border with sectioned and compressed fibres, while pencil-point needles produce a pattern of compressed but not sectioned fibres.

DIFFERENTIAL DIAGNOSIS

Diagnosis of PDPH is based on the onset, duration and characteristics of headache, in particular on the postural contribution to the symptoms. Exacerbation of symptoms with the upright position does not occur with other forms of postpartum headache, with the exception of pneumoencephalus. There are many conditions that may lead to postpartum headache:

- non-specific;
- migraine;
- hypertension;
- meningitis;
- cortical vein thrombosis;
- intra-, extra-, sub-dural haematoma;
- pneumoencephalus.

During the first week after delivery women may suffer from headache. This postpartum headache is unrelated to anaesthesia and has been reported in approximately 12% of puerperae [27]. Common causes include sinusitis and migraine. The latter presents with typical symptoms (unilateral, pulsatile headache, associated with vasomotor signs).

Manifestations of hypertensive disorders of pregnancy may include headache as a premonitory sign of seizures. Septic and aseptic meningitis are extremely rare but are reported complications of current anaesthetic practice [28]. Symptoms of meningeal headache are increasing, non-postural headache, nausea, vomiting and neck stiffness.

Cortical vein thrombosis is a rare complication of pregnancy (1:6000 pregnancies); symptoms include a headache of increasing intensity with sweating, nausea and vomiting. Diagnosis is difficult and should be confirmed by computed tomography, angiography and magnetic resonance imaging [29]. Another rare cause requiring radiological confirmation is Chiari I malformation [30].

Although extremely rare, a subdural haematoma can occur after a significant loss of CSF: risk factors are previous history of head trauma or overlooked anticoagulant therapy [31, 32] (Figure 14.1).

Pneumoencephalus may occur after the injection of air in the subdural or subarachnoid space in association with epidural loss of resistance techniques that use air. It is accompanied with a sudden onset of headache, perhaps with neck and back pain. Symptoms worsen in the sitting position and are relieved by lying down. The headache disappears after few hours.

TREATMENT

The PDPH is usually self-limiting and lasts only few days (although chronic post-dural puncture headache in one non-obstetric patient had been described 19 months after the initial insult [33]). However, the development of a severe headache in an otherwise healthy parturient requires an effective solution to avoid pain, anxiety, difficulties in ambulation, breast-feeding and infant-bonding, and an extended hospital stay. For these reasons the headache must be treated as soon as possible, starting with conservative measures and becoming more aggressive as the headache persists to avoid the vicious cycle of 'immobility–weakness–depression'.

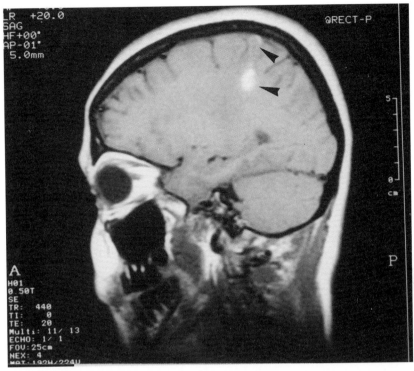

Figure 14.1 Axial and sagittal T1 weighted MR images of cerebral (pre-rolandic) haematoma 30 days after inadvertent dural puncture with a Tuohy needle for epidural analgesia in labour. Courtesy of G. Cannelli, Department of Anaesthesia, Catholic University of Sacred Heart, Rome, Italy.

Treatment of PDPH involves:

- symptomatic relief:
  psychological support
  bed rest
  analgesics
  caffeine
- increase CSF production:
  hydration
- increase epidural pressure:
  abdominal binder
  epidural saline, dextran and albumin
- obliterate epidural rent:
  epidural blood patch.

PSYCHOLOGICAL SUPPORT

During the postpartum period, parturients are at risk for depression, and the occurrence of severe headache which may interfere with patient's care for her baby and other relatives may make this patient depressed. In addition, parturients are usually healthy and do not expect to feel ill after childbirth. Therefore it is very important to give the patient complaining of PDPH psychological support and offer detailed therapeutic options.

BED REST

Bed rest is effective in that it avoids the upright position, which exacerbates the headache.

ANALGESICS

Simple analgesics, such as non-steroid anti-inflammatory drugs (NSAIDS), given orally may bring some relief. Theophylline, acting as a cerebral vasoconstrictor, has been demonstrated to be more effective than placebo [34].

CAFFEINE

Since PDPH results in part from dilation of the intracranial veins, caffeine (oral or intravenous), a cerebral vasoconstrictor, has been demonstrated to be effective in approximately 70% of cases, with permanent relief in 50% of cases [35, 36]. However caffeine is also a potent stimulant of the central nervous system and there are reports of seizure after intravenous administration of caffeine for PDPH treatment [37].

HYDRATION

It is believed that hyperhydration may increase CSF production. Hydration may require the intravenous administration of fluids in patients who are unable or unwilling to take fluids orally. Although there is no evidence of the therapeutic effect of vigorous hydration, no patient with PDPH should allowed to become dehydrated.

ABDOMINAL BINDER

A tight abdominal binder as well as the prone position causes increased intra-abdominal pressure which may result in an increase in CSF. This method may be uncomfortable and is rarely used.

EPIDURAL PLACEMENT OF FLUIDS

Since 40 years ago, epidural administration of saline has been used to relieve headache after dural puncture [38]. Lumbar injection of 20 ml of saline may temporarily relieve the pain, due to increased lumbar CSF pressure and therefore decreased intracranial traction. The benefit of a single bolus of saline is only transient and continuous infusion has been proposed [39]. However the rate of infusion (15–20 ml/h) is limited by the occurrence of side-effects such as pain in the back, legs and eyes. Intra-ocular haemorrhage has been reported after an injection of 120 ml of epidural saline [40].

Dextran 40 may be also effective for headache relief. The epidural administration of 20–30 ml produced a permanent relief of pain in all patients treated [41]. Animal studies failed to demonstrate anatomical microscopic changes after epidural administration of dextran [42]. The high molecular weight of dextran 40 may delay the reabsorption from the epidural space and lead to a more prolonged mass effect than saline, enabling closure of the dural puncture without the inflammation and fibrosis observed with an epidural blood patch. Dextran has been proposed as an alternative to a blood patch when there are reasons to question the safety of introducing autologous blood into the epidural space (bacteraemia and human immunodeficiency virus infection) or when patients are unwilling to use their own blood (Jehovah's Witnesses) [43].

There are few case reports that describe the efficacy of epidural administration of gelatin [44] or albumin (20 ml) [45]. In the first case complete and permanent relief of pain was obtained; in the second case only transient relief was observed. Further information on the possible neurologic effects of such agents is needed. In addition, the possible risk of anaphylactic reactions should be also considered.

EPIDURAL BLOOD PATCH

Blood patching is a procedure where a sample of the patient's blood is injected into the epidural space to seal the leak of CSF. This is an invasive technique and should be used only to treat the most severe, incapacitating headaches or when the most conservative measures have failed. The procedure is illustrated below.

- Inform the patient and obtain her consent for the procedure.
- Insert a Tuohy epidural needle at one level below the original puncture.
- At the same time an assistant takes aseptically 20 ml of venous blood from the antecubital fossa and hands it to the colleague performing the blood patching.

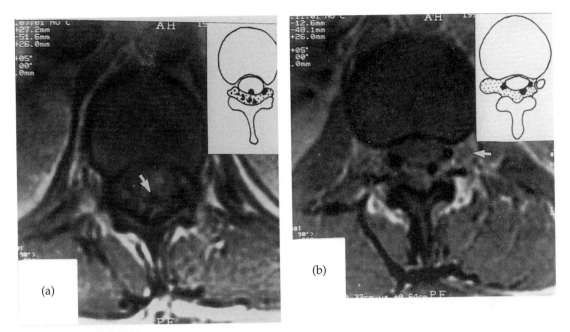

Figure 14.2 MRI of epidural blood patch: axial T1 weighted gadolinium-enhanced images (three hours after blood patch). (a) The arrow indicates a small focus of clot lying within and adherent to the thecal sac. (b) The arrow indicates the dorsal root ganglion displaced downwards and anteriorly by the extradural clot. Adapted from reference [47]; published by the British Medical Journal Publishing Group, 1993.

- A further sample of venous blood is taken for bacteriological culture and for a white cell count.
- Inject the 20 ml of blood slowly into the epidural space via the needle. If pain or paraesthesia is complained of by the patient during the injection, it must be temporarily stopped and then continued.
- Remove epidural needle.
- Keep the patient in the supine position for 30 minutes.
- Assess the success of the procedure (the patient should be able to get up with complete pain relief).
- Discharge the patient after 24 hours.

The blood clot acts as a gelatinous tamponade which prevents the leak of CSF and allows the dural rent to undergo a normal reparative process [46]. The success rate is approximately 90% of all cases and the method seems to be well established, but controversies exist concerning timing (whether or not blood patching should be carried out early or even prophylactically) and dosing (the adequate volume of blood to inject into the epidural space).

Mechanism of action

Two mechanisms may explain the therapeutic effect of blood patching. Magnetic resonance imaging (MRI) [47], radioactively labelled red blood cell injections [48] and animal studies [49] have contributed to the comprehension of these two mechanisms. The blood exerts a mass effect in the epidural space, compressing the dural sac and displacing the conus medullaris, cauda equina and sometimes also the nerve roots nearby (Figure 14.2). This mass effect lasts up to three hours and produces a compression that increases the CSF pressure

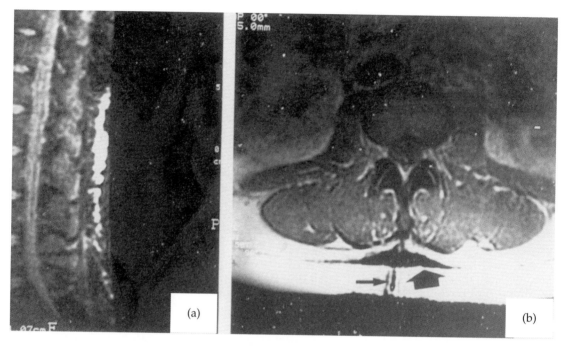

Figure 14.3 (a) MRI of epidural blood patch: sagittal STIR image (18 hours after blood patch): thin residual layer of epidural blood and extensive subcutaneous spread (blood appears white). (b) MRI of epidural blood patch: axial T1 image showing blood spread into the subcutaneous fat (large arrow: blood appears dark) and at the level of needle track (small arrow). Adapted from reference [47]; published by the British Medical Journal Publishing Group, 1993.

and corresponds, clinically, to the immediate relief of the symptoms. From seven hours onwards the mass effect disappears and the blood forms a thin layer, adherent to the dural sac, extending more cephalad than caudad, and acting as a gelatinous tampon (Figure 14.3). After 8–18 hours a significant leakage of blood into the dorsal fascial planes and between the subcutaneous fat may be observed [47] and after approximately 30 hours no blood may be observed with MRI in either the epidural space or dorsal fascial planes (personal observation). Interestingly laboratory studies reported that an accelerated coagulation may occur in the presence of CSF [50], and MRI investigation [47] clearly demonstrated a clot extending through the puncture site into the subarachnoid space.

Anatomical findings

Animal studies have tended to reassure the clinical anaesthetist [51]. Clot organization, with intense fibroblastic activity, has been described four days after patching. Collagen deposition had commenced by two weeks and fibroblastic activity was most marked at three weeks, at which time the patch was five times thicker than the dura to which it was adherent and by three months it was as thick as the underlying dura. The eventual tissue reaction did not differ from control animals [46]. Many separate clots adherent to the dura have been demonstrated by postmortem examination, and myelography [52] has demonstrated that blood may be still present as a space-occupying mass one week after injection.

Timing and dosing

It is commonly believed that the success of blood patching increases significantly when the blood patch is performed more than 24 hours after the dural puncture [53, 54]. However, there are some reports that claimed good results with an early blood patch, stating that the essential for the success was to use an adequate volume of blood (15–20 ml) [55–57]. The ideal volume of blood to be injected is not established, ranging from 5 to 20 ml [58–60]. It is more likely that to exert a double action (mass and clotting effects), and therefore a prompt, immediate clinical effect, at least 10 ml of blood are necessary. In addition, there is a close relationship between the injection volume and the success of blood patching. However the injection of 18–20 ml of blood has been demonstrated to produce a significant leakage of blood into the fascial planes between the subcutaneous fat [47]. This feature may be due to the insertion of the Tuohy needle into the epidural space during the injection of blood or to the leakage of injected blood back through the ligamenta flava. This observation may also explain the backache following epidural patching.

The blood injected spreads extensively into the epidural space, to the extent of about 1.6 ml per spinal segment [48]; however the majority of clot and the mass effect are restricted to three to five segments around the injection site and the spread of the blood is mainly upwards from the injection site. For this reason it seems appropriate to perform the blood patch at the level below the original puncture.

Efficacy and failure

The success rate for the first epidural blood patch is 68–90%, [59, 61, 62] and after the second it is even greater (97%) [59, 61]. Failure of epidural blood patching may be due to inadequate injection volume or the introduction of blood at the wrong level. In all cases the diagnosis should be always re-evaluated.

Side-effects

Transient side-effects include back pain, neckache, paraesthesia in the legs and toes, dizziness, radicular pain, abdominal cramping, cranial nerve palsy and epidural haematoma. If large volumes of blood are injected rapidly the transdural gradient pressure may be inverted and blood may penetrate into the subarachnoid space, where it may form a clot if the entry rate is rapid [49].

Risks and complications

The most frequent minor complication is backache which may occur in approximately 16% of patients and may last for up to three months [63]. It is probably due to infiltration of blood in the fascial planes of the back [47]. Severe, immobilizating lumbovertebral syndrome has been also reported [64].

It is unclear whether blood patching may affect the efficacy of subsequent epidural anaesthesia, due to possible adhesion between the dura and ligamenta flava [63]. However there are studies that indicate a reduction of success rate with epidural anaesthesia in patients who previously received epidural blood patches [65]. Radiculitis with severe back pain radiating down the legs has been also infrequently reported [63, 66]. More serious complications, such as infection and adhesive arachnoiditis, are rare. A subdural epiarachnoid haematoma, diagnosed at lumbar laminectomy, has been reported after six repeated blood patches [67].

Contraindications

Contraindications of blood patching are similar to those of regional anaesthesia, and include local or systemic infection, patient refusal and coagulation disorders. The presence of high fever or other evidence of sepsis contraindicates the performance of a blood patch but there are no reports of epidural abscess after autologous blood patch.

The risk of epidural injection of blood in the presence of human immunodeficiency virus infection is unknown, although there are reports of successful blood patches with no complications in seropositive patients followed as long as two years [68].

PREVENTION

The prevention of PDPH consists in minimizing the post-puncture leakage of CSF. Methods to prevent PDPH are:

- controversial methods:
  bed rest
  hydration
  abdominal binder
  spinal opioids
  epidural patch with saline, dextran or blood
  paramedian approach
  choice of local anaesthetic solution
- effective methods:
  altered regional anaesthesia technique
  needle size
  needle design
  direction of bevel insertion.

BED REST

Traditional methods such as restricting the patient to a supine position or applying an abdominal binder are not helpful. However, in the case of severe headache, while awaiting blood patching, bed rest may help to prevent the rare, but severe complications, such as cerebral haematoma and cranial nerve palsy.

HYDRATION

There is no evidence that excess hydration will increase CSF production, since CSF production is relatively constant. For this reason the traditional advice to drink copious volumes of fluids has no place in the prevention of PDPH [69].

SPINAL OPIOIDS

It is controversial whether the addition of opioids to spinal local anaesthetic solution may decrease the incidence of PDPH [70–72].

EPIDURAL PATCH OF SALINE

Conflicting results have been also reported with prophylactic epidural saline. Some reduction in the incidence of PDPH has been obtained with a continuous infusion of epidural saline or Ringer's lactate but the merits of prophylactic saline in the management of PDPH cannot be quantified easily since it is a treatment that cannot be divorced readily from bed rest. We are reluctant to recommend a procedure that immobilizes the mother and disrupts child care, as the treatment will be unnecessary in a number of cases [73, 74].

EPIDURAL PATCH WITH DEXTRAN 40

Epidural administration, via the epidural catheter, of 20 ml of dextran 40 has been used successfully in young patients to prevent PDPH resulting from unintentional puncture with a Tuohy needle with no adverse effects.

EPIDURAL BLOOD PATCH

The prophylactic epidural blood patch has its advocates [58] and critics [54]. In one study the prophylactic blood patch (15 ml) [75] reduced the incidence of PDPH from 80 to 21% in obstetric patients who had received an unintentional dural puncture during epidural block. However, at least 20% of patients will receive unnecessary treatment.

PARAMEDIAN APPROACH

The insertion of the needle at an oblique angle may result in decreased leakage of CSF, but the clinical benefits are uncertain [76, 77].

CHOICE OF LOCAL ANAESTHETIC SOLUTION

In one study [25] the use of hyperbaric solutions of local anaesthetic was associated with higher incidence of early, moderate headache in the first 36 hours post-puncture, but this did not translate into a greater percentage of patients requiring blood patching for the control of PDPH. The osmotic, cerebral irritant effect of glucose has been postulated to be responsible for these findings.

NEEDLE SIZE, NEEDLE DESIGN, ORIENTATION OF THE BEVEL

In general, the relative risk of post-puncture headache decreases with each successive reduction in needle diameter [9–20]. This clinical observation is also supported by *in vitro* studies that have demonstrated a direct relation between needle diameter and residual dural hole diameter and CSF flow [78, 79]. Many clinical trials investigated the relation between the size and the design of the spinal needle and the incidence of PDPH [11–20]. The conclusion from these studies is that needle size is of primary importance in preventing headache, but given two needles of the same size, an atraumatic, Whitacre, Sprotte or Atraucan type needle will produce fewer cases of PDPH than the equivalent Quincke needle. Published experience reveals a low incidence in obstetric patients with 24 gauge Sprotte, 25–26 gauge Whitacre and 27 gauge Quincke needles, but there are no studies large enough to demonstrate significant differences among these needles. In fact the mean incidence of PDPH is about 7% and to achieve a statistical power of 0.8, with $\alpha = 0.05$, the sample size should be 700 patients per group in order to detect a 50% difference in incidence of this complication. In a study which used meta-analysis [80], 450 articles were examined and only 16 were accepted for analysis. There was a reduction in the incidence of PDPH when the use of non-cutting spinal needles and small needles were compared with a large needle of the same type. This study confirms that a non-cutting needle or/and the smallest gauge needle available should be used. The disadvantage of smaller needles is the increased technical difficulty of dural puncture, especially when very small needles, such as 29 gauge, are used [81]. The costs increase as needles become smaller and non-cutting.

The dura consists of multidirectional collagen fibres and transverse and longitudinal elastic fibres. The insertion of Tuohy and Quincke point needles with the bevel parallel to the longitudinal axis of the spine may cut fewer fibres and leave a smaller dural breach [82].

SUMMARY

1. Prevention of dural puncture
- Adequate teaching of junior doctors
- Correct choice of regional anaesthesia technique if your choice is subarachnoid anaesthesia use small gauge, atraumatic needles (25–27 gauge)
2. Management of dural puncture
- Simple non-invasive treatments are often successful in headaches after small atraumatic needles
- More invasive methods may be needed after inadvertent dural puncture with a large Tuohy needle
- The benefits of invasive treatments should be carefully evaluated against the side-effects and possible complications for each patient
- With any doubtful headache, a differential diagnosis should be carefully evaluated with the help of a neurologist, if necessary.

In all cases recognize that the occurrence of severe headache may interfere with the patient's care for her baby and other dependants, and this may make the patient anxious or depressed. Most mothers are healthy and do not expect to feel ill after childbirth. Severe headache may interfere with feeding, walking, breast-feeding and hospital discharge.

Therefore it is very important to give the patient psychological, reassuring support and offer detailed therapeutic options.

REFERENCES

1. Jones, R.J.R.(1974) The role of recumbency in the prevention and treatment of postspinal headache. *Anesthesia and Analgesia*, **53**, 788–96.
2. Vandam, L.D. and Dripps, R.D. (1955) A long-term follow-up of 10,098 spinal anesthetics: incidence and analysis of minor sensory neurological defects. *Surgery*, **38**, 463–9.
3. Greene, N.M. (1961) Neurologic sequelae of spinal anesthesia. *Anesthesiology*, **22**, 682–95.
4. Hussain, S.S.M., Heard, C.M.B. and Bembridge, J.L. (1994) An evaluation of the incidence of transient hearing loss following spinal anaesthesia for elective caesarean section. *Proceedings of the Scientific Meeting of the Obstetric Anaesthetist' Association*, Derby, 29 April.
5. Newrick, P. and Read, D. (1982) Subdural haematoma as a complication of spinal anaesthetic. *British Medical Journal*, **285**, 341–2.
6. Grant, R., Condon, B., Hart, I. *et al.* (1991) Changes in intracranial CSF volume after lumbar puncture and their relationship to post-LP headache. *Journal of Neurology, Neurosurgery and Psychiatry*, **54**, 440–2.
7. Lybecker, H., Mathiesen, F.K. and Helbo-Hansen, H.S. (1995) Change in intracranial CSF volume after extradural blood patch in patients with severe postdural puncture headache (PDPH). *British Journal of Anaesthesia*, **74** (supplement), A245.
8. Gobel, H., Klostermann, H., Linder, V. *et al.* (1990) Changes in cerebral haemodynamics in cases of post-lumbar puncture headache: a prospective transcranial Doppler ultrasound study. *Cephalgia*, **10**, 117–22.
9. Crawford, J.S. (1972) Lumbar epidural block in labour: a clinical analysis. *British Journal of Anaesthesia*, **44**, 66–74.
10. Barker, P. (1990) Are obstetric spinal headaches avoidable? *Anaesthesia and Intensive Care*, **18**, 553–4.
11. Cesarini, M., Torrielli, R., Lahaye, F. *et al.* (1990) Sprotte needle for intrathecal anaesthesia for Caesarean section: incidence of postdural puncture headache. *Anaesthesia*, **54**, 656–8.
12. Leeman, M.I., Sears, D.H., O'Donnell, L. *et al.* (1991) The incidence of PDPH in obstetrical patients comparing the 24-gauge and 22-gauge Sprotte needle. *Anesthesiology*, **75**, A853.
13. Devcic, A., Sprung, J., Maitra-D'Cruze, A. *et al.* (1992) Post-dural puncture headache in an obstetric population: comparison of 24-gauge Sprotte and 25-gauge Quincke needles. *Regional Anesthesia*, **17**, S69.
14. Mayer, D.C., Quance, D. and Weeks, S.K. (1992) Headache after spinal anesthesia for caesarean section: a comparison of the 27-gauge Quincke and 24-gauge Sprotte needles. *Anesthesia and Analgesia*, **75**, 377–80.
15. Shutt, E.L., Valentine, S.D.I., Wee, M.Y. *et al.* (1992) Spinal anaesthesia for caesarean section: comparison of 22-gauge and 25-gauge Whitacre needles with 26-gauge Quincke needles. *British Journal of Anaesthesia*, **69**, 589–94.
16. Ross, B.K., Chadwick, H.S., Mancuso, J.J. *et al.* (1992) Sprotte needle for obstetric anaesthesia: decreased incidence of post dural puncture headache. *Regional Anesthesia*, **17**, 29--33.
17. Hurley, R.J., Lambert, D., Hertwig, L. *et al.* (1992) Postdural puncture headache in the obstetric patient: spinal vs epidural anesthesia. *Anesthesiology*, **77**, A1018.
18. Campbell, D.C., Douglas, M.J., Pavy, T.J.C. *et al.* (1993) Comparison of 25G Whitacre vs 24G Sprotte spinal needle for elective caesarean section. Cost implications. *Canadian Journal of Anaesthesia*, **40**, 1131–5.
19. Wiesel, S., Tessler, M.J. and Eastdown, L.J. (1993) Postdural puncture headache: a randomized prospective comparison of the 24 gauge Sprotte and the 27 gauge Quincke needles in young patients. *Canadian Journal of Anaesthesia*, **40**, 607–11.
20. Amuzu, J., Patel, S. and Maitra-D'Cruze, A. (1995) Incidence of postdural puncture after cesarean section: comparison of 26G Atraucan and 25G Whitacre spinal needles. *Regional Anesthesia*, **20**, 2S 150.
21. Chadwick, H, Postner, K, Caplan, R *et al.* (1991) A comparison of obstetric and nonobstetric anesthesia malpractice claims. *Anesthesiology*, **74**, 242–9.
22. Lybeker, H., Moller, J.T., May, O. *et al.* (1990) Incidence and prediction of postdural puncture headache: a prospective study of 1,021 spinal anesthesias. *Anesthesia and Analgesia*, **70**, 389–94.
23. Norris, M.C. and Leighton, B.L. (1990) Continuous spinal anesthesia after unintentional dural puncture in parturients. *Regional Anesthesia*, **15**, 285–7.
24. Gurmarnik, S. (1988) Skin preparation and spinal headache. *Anaesthesia*, **43**, 1057–8.
25. Naulty, J.S., Hertwig, L., Hunt, C.O. *et al.* (1990) Influence of local anesthetic solution on postdural puncture headache. *Anesthesiology*, **72**, 450–4.

26. Celleno, D., Capogna, G., Costantino, P. *et al.* (1993) An anatomic study of the effects of dural puncture with different spinal needles. *Regional Anesthesia*, **18**, 218–21.

27. Benhamou, D., Hamza, J. and Ducot, B. (1995) Post partum headache after epidural analgesia without dural puncture. *International Journal of Obstetric Anaesthesia*, **4**, 17–20.

28. Harding, S.A., Collis, R.E. and Morgan, B.M. (1994) Meningitis after combined spinal–extradural anaesthesia in obstetrics. *British Journal of Anaesthesia*, **73**, 545–7.

29. Gewirtz, E.C., Costin, M. and Marx, G.F. (1987) Cortical vein thrombosis may mimic postdural puncture headache. *Regional Anesthesia*, **12**, 188–90.

30. Hullander, R.M., Bogard, T.O., Leivers, D. *et al.* (1992) Chiari I malformation presenting as recurrent spinal headache. *Anesthesia and Analgesia*, **75**, 1025–6.

31. Mantia, A.M. (1981) Clinical report of the occurrence of an intracerebral hemorrhage following post-lumbar puncture headache. *Anesthesiology*, **55**, 684–5.

32. Campbell, D.A. and Varma, T.R.K. (1993) Chronic subdural haematoma following epidural anaesthesia, presenting as puerperal psychosis. *British Journal of Obstetrics and Gynaecology*, **100**, 782–4.

33. Wilton, N.T.C. and Globerson, J.H. (1986) Epidural blood patch for postdural puncture headache: it's never too late. *Anesthesia and Analgesia*, **65**, 895–6.

34. Schwalbe, S.S., Schiffmiller, M.W. and Marx, G.F. (1990) Theophilline for post-dural puncture headache *Anesthesiology*, **75**, A1082.

35. Camann, W.R., Murray, R.S., Mushlin, P.S. *et al.* (1990) Effects of oral caffeine on postdural puncture headache: a double-blind placebo-controlled trial. *Anesthesia and Analgesia*, **70**, 181–4.

36. Sechzer, P.H. and Able, L. (1978) Post-spinal anesthesia headache treated with caffeine. Evaluation with demand method. Part I. *Current Therapeutic Research*, **24**, 307–12.

37. Cohen, S.M., Laurito, C.E. and Curran, M.J. (1992) Grand mal seizure in a post-partum patient following intravenous caffeine sodium benzoate to treat persistent headache. *Journal of Clinical Anesthesia*, **4**, 48–51.

38. Rice, G.G. and Dabbs, C.H. (1950) The use of peridural and subarachnoid injections of saline solution in the treatment of severe postspinal headache. *Anesthesiology*, **11**, 7–23.

39. Bart, A.J. and Wheeler, A.S. (1978) Comparison of epidural saline placement and epidural blood placement in the treatment of post-lumbar puncture headache. *Anesthesiology*, **48**, 221--3.

40. Clark, C.J. and Whitwell, J. (1961) Intraocular haemorrhage after epidural injection. *British Medical Journal*, **ii**, 1612–3.

41. Barrios-Alarcon, J., Aldrete, J.A. and Paragas-Tapia, D. (1989) Relief of post-dural puncture headache with epidural dextran 40: a preliminary report. *Regional Anesthesia*, **14**, 78–80.

42. Lander, C.J. and Korbon, G.A. (1988) Histopathologic consequences of epidural blood patch and epidurally administered Dextran 40. *Anesthesiology*, **69**, A410.

43. Stevens, D.S. and Peeters-Asdourian, C. (1993) Treatment of postdural puncture headache with epidural dextran patch. *Regional Anesthesia*, **18**, 324–25.

44. Ambesh, S.P., Kumar, A. and Bajaj, A. (1991) Epidural gelatin (Gelfoam) patch treatment for post dural puncture headache. *Anaesthesia and Intensive Care*, **19**, 444–53.

45. Stuart-Taylor, M.E., Lawes, E.G. and Goodrum, D.T. (1994) Epidural albumin for the treatment of post dural puncture headache. *Proceedings of the Scientific Meeting of the Obstetric Anaesthetist' Association*, Derby, 29 April.

46. Di Giovanni, A.J., Galbert, M.W. and Wahle, W.M. (1972) Epidural injection of autologous blood for postlumbar puncture headache. II. Additional clinical experiences and laboratory investigation. *Anesthesia and Analgesia*, **51**, 226–32.

47. Beards, S.C., Jackson, A., Griffiths, A.G. *et al.* (1993) Magnetic resonance imaging of extradural blood patches: appearances from 30 min to 18 h. *British Journal of Anaesthesia*, **71**, 182–8.

48. Szeinfeld, M., Ihmeidan, I.H., Moser, M.M. *et al.* (1986) Epidural blood patch: evaluation of the volume and spread of blood injected into epidural space. *Anesthesiology*, **64**, 820–2.

49. Rosenberg, P.H. and Heavner, J.E. (1985) *In vitro* study of the effect of epidural blood patch on leakage through a dural puncture. *Anesthesia and Analgesia*, **64**, 501–4.

50. Cook, M.A. and Watkins-Pitchford, J.M. (1990) Epidural blood patch: a rapid coagulation response. *Anesthesia and Analgesia*, **70**, 567–8.

51. Brownridge, P. (1983) The management of headache after accidental dural puncture in obstetric patients. *Anaesthesia and Intensive Care*, **11**, 4–15.

52. Hardy, P.A.J. (1988) Extradural blood patch after an intradural injection. *Anaesthesia*, **43**, 251.

53. Loeser, E.A., Hill, G.E., Bennett, G.M. *et al.* (1978) Time vs success rate for epidural blood patch. *Anesthesiology*, **49**, 147–8.

54. Palhaniuk, R.J. and Cumming, M. (1979) Prophylactic blood patch does not prevent post lumbar puncture headache. *Canadian Journal of Anaesthesia*, **26**, 132–3.

55. Quaynor, H. and Corbey, M. (1985) Extradural blood patch – why delay? *British Journal of Anaesthesia*, **57**, 538–40.

56. Cheek, T.G., Banner, R., Sauter, J. *et al.* (1988) Prophylactic extradural blood patch is effective. *British Journal of Anaesthesia*, **61**, 340–2.

57. Cristensen, F.R. and Lund, J. (1983) Accidental dural puncture: immediate or delayed blood patch. *British Journal of Anaesthesia*, **55**, 89–90.

58. Di Giovanni, A.J. and Dunbar, B.S. (1960) Epidural injections of autologous blood for postlumbar puncture headache. *Anesthesia and Analgesia*, **49**, 268–71.

59. Ostheimer, G.W., Palhaniuk, R.J. and Shnider, S.M. (1974) Epidural blood patch for post-lumbar puncture headache. *Anesthesiology*, **41**, 307–8.

60. Crawford, J.S., Taivainen, T., Pitkanen, M. *et al.* (1993) Efficacy of epidural blood patch for postdural puncture headache. *Acta Anaesthesiologica Scandinavica*, **37**, 702–5.

61. Crawford, J.S. (1980) Experiences with epidural blood patch. *Anaesthesia*, **61**, 340–2.

62. Stride, P.C, Coper, G.M. (1993) Dural taps revisited. *Anaesthesia*, **48**, 247–55.

63. Abouleish, E., de la Vega, S., Blendinger, I. *et al.* (1975) Long-term follow-up of epidural blood patch. *Anesthesia and Analgesia*, **54**, 459–63.

64. Seeberger, M.D. and Urwyler, A. (1992) Lumbovertebral syndrome after extradural blood patch. *British Journal of Anaesthesia*, **69**, 414–6.

65. Ong, B.Y., Graham, C.R., Ringaert, K.R. *et al.* (1975) Impaired epidural analgesia after dural puncture with or without subsequent blood patch. *Anesthesia and Analgesia*, **70**, 76–9.

66. Shanta, T.R., McWhirter, W.R. and Dunbar, R.W. (1973) Complications following epidural blood patch for postlumbar puncture headache. *Anesthesia and Analgesia*, **52**, 67–72.

67. Reynolds, A.F. Jr, Hameroff, S.R., Blitt, C.D. *et al.* (1980) Spinal subdural epiarachnoid hematoma: a complication of a novel epidural blood patch technique. *Anesthesia and Analgesia*, **59**, 702–3.

68. Tom, D.J., Gulevich, S.J., Shapiro, H.M. *et al.* (1992) Epidural blood patch in the HIV- positive patient. *Anesthesiology*, **76**, 943–7.

69. Dieterich, M. and Brandt, T.(1988) Incidence of post-lumbar puncture headache is independent of daily fluid intake. *European Archives of Psychiatry and Neurological Sciences*, **237**, 194–6.

70. Abboud, T,K., Miller, H., Afrasiabi, A. *et al.* (1992) Effect of subarachnoid morphine on the incidence of spinal headache. *Regional Anesthesia*, **17**, 34–6.

71. Devcic, A., Sprung, J., Patel, S. *et al.* (1993) PDPH in obstetric anesthesia: comparison of 24-gauge Sprotte and 25-gauge Quincke needles and effect of subarachnoid administration of fentanyl. *Regional Anesthesia*, **18**, 222–5.

72. Johnson, M.D., Hertwig, L., Vehring, P.H. *et al.* (1989) Intrathecal fentanyl may reduce the incidence of spinal headache. *Anesthesiology*, **71**, A911.

73. Crawford, J.S. (1972) The prevention of headache consequent upon dural puncture. *British Journal of Anaesthesia*, **44**, 598–9.

74. Thomas, D.I., Suresh, M.S., Stride, P.C. *et al.* (1992) Prophylaxis of dural headache: epidural saline bolus versus infusion. *Anesthesia and Analgesia*, **74**, S319.

75. Colonna-Romano, P. and Shapiro, B.E. (1989) Unintentional dural puncture and prophylactic epidural blood patch in obstetrics. *Anesthesia and Analgesia*, **69**, 522–3.

76. Hatfalvi, B.I. (1990) The dynamics of post-spinal headache. *Headache*, **17**, 64–6.

77. Jorgensen, N.H. (1991) Postdural puncture headache is more common with the paramedian approach. *Anesthesia and Analgesia*, **72**, S131.

78. Cruickshank, R.H. and Hopkinson, J.M. (1989) Fluid flow through dural puncture sites. An *in vitro* comparison of needle point types. *Anaesthesia*, **44**, 415–8.

79. Holst, D., Mollman, M., Hausmann, R. *et al.* (1995) Evaluation of cerebro spinal fluid loss after dural puncture: which type and size of needle shows the minimal leak rate? *Regional Anesthesia*, **20**, 2S, 84.

80. Halpern, S. and Preston, R. (1994) Postdural puncture headache and spinal needle design. *Anesthesiology*, **81**, 1376–83.

81. Flaatten, H., Rodt, S.A., Vammes, J. *et al.* (1989) Postdural puncture headache. A comparison between 26- and 29-gauge needles in young patients. *Anaesthesia*, **44**, 147–9.

82. Fink, B.R. and Walker, S. (1989) Orientation of fibers in human dorsal lumbar dura mater in relation to lumbar puncture. *Anesthesia and Analgesia*, **69**, 768–72.

MUSCULOSKELETAL DISORDERS

15

D. Celleno and G. Capogna

INTRODUCTION

The choice of anaesthetic technique for pregnant women with musculoskeletal disorders requires knowledge both of the pathophysiology of the disorder and the associated issues. In addition, pre-existing musculoskeletal disorders may be exacerbated during pregnancy to a varying degree.

BACKACHE

GESTATIONAL BACKACHE

Backache occurs frequently during pregnancy and is regarded as a normal concomitant. As the uterus enlarges anteriorly, progressive lordosis is the common compensatory posture. In addition, because of increased secretion of the hormone relaxin, there is increased mobility of the sacroiliac, sacrococcygeal and pubic joints. Protrusion of the lumbar disc, which may be asymptomatic, has been reported to be a common feature in pregnancy [1] but is usually well compensated by the mother's posture. A study using magnetic resonance imaging [2] found that tissue damage following labour and delivery was apparent in the dorsolumbar region, but was superficial rather than involving muscles or ligaments and did not appear to be related to the occurrence of back pain. Severe backache associated with a herniated lumbar disc and sciatic radiculopathy is relatively rare, with an incidence estimated to be in 1 in 10 000 pregnant women [3].

Mild backache is treated by avoiding aggravating stress and strain. Treatment of severe, acute backache varies from analgesics to complete bed rest depending on the aetiology, and occasionally requires orthopaedic consultation.

Anaesthetic management

Regional anaesthesia is not contraindicated in women with back pain. Patients with severe backache however, should be visited by an anaesthetist before the expected date of delivery, and examined to determine the source and type of pain. Sensory and motor deficits should be documented. These patients need particular care when positioned in the lithotomy position, due to the associated stresses on the lumbar region.

CHRONIC BACKACHE

Approximately one half of pregnant women with a previous history of low back pain

Clinical Problems in Obstetric Anaesthesia
Edited by Ian F. Russell and Gordon Lyons. Published in 1997 by Chapman & Hall, London. ISBN 0 412 71600 3.

experience an exacerbation of symptoms during pregnancy. Prolapse of an interverte-bral disc occurs in 1% of patients with acute back pain. Nerve root compression most commonly occurs at the L4, L5 or S1 segments, and may result in sciatica.

A herniated lumbar disc in association with severe backache can be an indication for cae-sarean section. This avoids the exacerbation of lumbar symptoms associated with the effects of labour and vaginal delivery.

Anaesthetic management

Regional anaesthesia is rarely contraindicated in these patients [4]. In the presence of a herni-ated lumbar disc, there is the possibility of delayed onset of epidural blockade or the occurrence of a 'missed segment' at the site of the damaged intervertebral disc [5]. This may be related to abnormal spread of local anaes-thetic in the epidural space. 'One-shot' spinal or continuous spinal anaesthesia using micro-catheters may be used. The onset of backache after delivery can have medico-legal conse-quences and, as such, may affect the choice of technique.

POSTPARTUM BACKACHE

Postpartum backache is a common complaint of parturients. Retrospective [6] and prospec-tive [7] studies have suggested that epidural anaesthesia is a risk factor but it is difficult to differentiate the effects of gestation, labour and delivery, and inappropriate positioning, from those of epidural blockade. A large, retrospec-tive survey [8] reported a high incidence (26%) one year after delivery, of new long-term back-ache in mothers who had received epidural analgesia. (Long-term backache was defined as back pain which began within three months of delivery and lasted more than six weeks.) One of the problems with this retrospective analy-sis was that it tended to underestimate antena-tal backache. Russell's prospective study showed that when pre-existing backache was

taken into account, the incidence of new back-ache was 7%, and this was not influenced by the choice of pain relief in labour [9].

A possible preventative measure is the use of a field block into the interspinous space, near the lamina, prior to spinal or epidural anaes-thesia [10]. A proposed mechanism of action of the field block is the production of profound and prolonged regional sympathetic and sensory block, which in turn causes local vasodilatation, promoting tissue healing from needle injury. However, the use of field anaes-thesia before epidural block did not influence the incidence of long-term backache when compared to the incidence in non-obstetric patients [10].

One question remains unanswered: can epidural analgesia influence the course of severe pre-existing back problems in the post-partum period, adversely or otherwise? While awaiting an answer to this question, it might be considered prudent to instigate preventa-tive measures. Suggested methods of avoiding backache are:

1. minimize trauma to the back:

- avoid the periosteum
- keep attempts to a minimum
- do not use force
- try field block

2. position carefully since postpartum back-ache is believed to be caused by faulty litho-tomy position and the lordosis of pregnancy.

What women should be told about the risk of backache

When insufficient information is given, there is the risk of legal action against the anaesthetist. In a study comparing the process of informed consent for obstetric anaesthesia in the USA and in the UK, backache was discussed in 45–65% of cases [11]. In a report of the risk information supplied by the obstetric anaes-thetist to mothers before elective caesarean section, only 6% of the anaesthetists interviewed discussed back problems with their patients. Most would mention it only to dismiss the possibility of an increased incidence with regional anaesthesia [12]. The practice of anaesthetists in other European countries is unknown, but the general impression is that doctors tailor information to what they feel the mother needs and wants to know. If given adequate information, the well-informed mother is in a position to make a choice of anaesthetic alternatives. European anaesthetists do not necessarily use the consultation to ensure that women are well versed in all the possible risks, such as happens in USA, where legal opinion recommends that anaesthesia and its potential complications are described in detail [13].

Whilst a consensus is emerging amongst anaesthetists that long-term postpartum backache is not related to regional analgesia, this is unlikely to filter into the magazines and books read by expectant mothers for some years, and it is likely to remain a contentious issue for the present. Other reasons for keeping a watching brief exist. In a report of anaesthesia malpractice claims in the USA [14], more claims involving relatively minor injuries, such as backache, occurred in obstetric cases compared to non-obstetric cases. Financial settlements were made in two out of three claims for backache, which suggests that in legal minds there is a link between backache and malpractice. European practice is under no obligation to take its lead from North America, but while scientific support of regional anaesthesia is gathering momentum, it is advisable that information about backache is provided, especially to those already suffering from back pain.

SCOLIOSIS

Scoliosis is a skeletal deformity associated with lateral curvature of the spine and rotation of the vertebrae. It may have idiopathic, congenital, neuromuscular, connective tissue or traumatic causes. Its overall incidence varies from 1.8 to 4 per 1000 general population [15, 16] depending on the diagnostic source, and it is approximately eight times more frequent in females than in males. Whether the risk of progression of the scoliotic curve increases during pregnancy is of critical importance. A few reports with small numbers suggest that the angle of the curvature of the scoliosis may increase if it is already greater than 25% and the spine is unstable [17, 18]. A large retrospective survey [19] confirmed that scoliosis may progress in adults, but pregnancy does not increase the risk of progression of the curve. Depending on the site of the vertebral curvature, mechanical deformity of the pelvis may occur with consequent implications for foetal presentation, labour and delivery. There are controversial reports concerning this issue. Scoliosis patients may have more premature births than expected, but their rates of other adverse reproductive events do not differ from expected [20]. Higher caesarean section rate has been reported with patients affected by thoracolumbar scoliosis [21]; and although scoliosis of a mild to moderate degree does not have an adverse effect on pregnancy, more than one half suffer from backache during their pregnancy [20].

The physiological changes to the cardiovascular and respiratory systems that occur with pregnancy may encroach on the limited reserve of the kyphoscoliotic [22]. In these patients pulmonary function is already compromised with a reduction in vital capacity and total lung capacity. The increased demands of gas exchange in pregnancy can impose an impossible burden, as a rising respiratory rate with a reduced tidal volume tries to meet the minute volume requirement. The work of breathing can rise disproportionately to the minute ventilation, and respiratory failure may ensue. In addition, in the later stages of pregnancy uterine enlargement may decrease mechanical efficiency of the chest wall. Chronic maternal hypoxia can result, which may lead to premature labour. Compensatory changes in cardiac output, with further demands from labour and delivery, may precipitate cardiorespiratory failure. It is important that this is not confused with the signs of preeclampsia. Access to an intensive care unit is a mandatory safeguard, and negative pressure ventilation can provide effective relief for those in cardiorespiratory failure [22].

Anaesthetic management

Regional anaesthesia is not contraindicated in patients with scoliosis. Patients with severe kyphoscoliosis should have an early anaesthetic consultation including a complete assessment of their cardiorespiratory status. Epidural or spinal anaesthesia in obstetric patients with kyphoscoliosis may be difficult to perform. Since distortion of the spinal column and epidural space can prevent placement of an epidural catheter or may interfere with the distribution of local anaesthetic, women should be informed of the possibility that regional anaesthesia will fail. Spinal anaesthesia with hyperbaric solutions may also result in a patchy or inadequate block, because of altered spinal anatomy. Continuous subarachnoid anaesthesia with an intrathecal catheter may be an option in such patients. The level of anaesthesia may be reached gradually, using local anaesthetics with varying baricity [23]. When kyphoscoliosis is severe, however, the woman with cardiorespiratory problems may not tolerate lying supine and general anaesthesia will be necessary. The usual precautions for airway management, together with particular care of cardiac and ventilatory parameters, with comprehensive monitoring, should be observed. Effective postoperative pain relief, which might include epidural or spinal opioids, should not be overlooked.

SURGICALLY CORRECTED BACK PROBLEMS

SCOLIOSIS

The aim of surgical correction of kyphoscoliosis is to arrest the natural progression of the

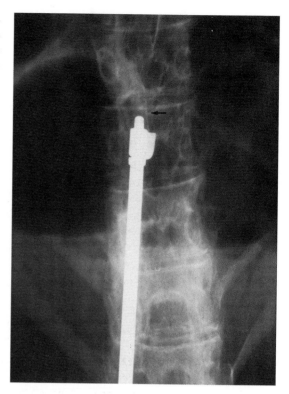

Figure 15.1 Properly sited epidural catheter in a patient with Harrington rod instrumentation, undergoing caesarean section with successful epidural analgesia.

disease and improve the deformity. Among various surgical techniques for the correction of scoliosis, posterior spinal fusion is the most relevant to the anaesthetist. Posterior spinal fusion or arthrodesis is indicated in patients with a scoliotic curvature greater than 40% and creates a bony fusion of all rotated vertebrae. Harrington or Roycamille rods are usually inserted to produce internal stabilization of the fused mass. Parturients with corrected surgical scoliosis do not usually have any problems during pregnancy [19].

Anaesthetic management

Epidural blockade for labour, delivery or caesarean section is not contraindicated (Figure 15.1), but some associated problems can arise.

- Insertion of the needle in the fused area may be difficult or impossible.
- Adhesions or obliteration of epidural space may alter the spread of local anaesthetic solutions (surgical injury of ligamentum flavum may result in scar tissue).
- Obliteration of epidural space may increase the incidence of inadvertent dural puncture or subdural catheterization.
- Regional anaesthesia in patients with residual back pain may result in litigation if persistent back pain occurs after the block.

The rate of successful epidural placement varies widely [24], depending on the level of fusion. Failure to enter the vertebral canal occurs only if fusion extends to L3 or lower. No short or long-term (up to eight years) complications have been observed in patients requiring lumbar epidural analgesia for labour [25]. Alternatively, subarachnoid block at the L5–S1 interspace may offer some advantages. If the subarachnoid approach has been chosen, a microcatheter technique should be considered, in order to optimize the local anaesthetic dose and provide adequate postoperative analgesia [19, 26].

The potential advantages of using continuous spinal anaesthesia in parturients with surgically corrected scoliosis are:

- the point of entry to the subarachnoid space is of lesser importance;
- both iso- and hyperbaric local anaesthetics and opiates can be given incrementally, to minimize cardiorespiratory disturbance;
- intelligent positioning of the patient in conjunction with the above can overcome problems with spread.

LAMINECTOMY–DISCECTOMY

Surgical treatments for severe lumbar disc disease include laminectomy, with or without the removal of extruded or degenerated portions of intervertebral discs. After laminectomy, organized scar tissue may be present around the dura and can obliterate the epidural space at that level. Post-laminectomy spinal stenosis may also occur, usually immediately above the fusion mass.

Anaesthetic management

Although possibly less successful, epidural anaesthesia is not contraindicated. Spinal blockade may be more reliable. A careful neurological examination should always be performed, and findings recorded, in order to avoid medico-legal problems arising from postpartum backache.

CONGENITAL DISORDERS

MARFAN'S SYNDROME

Marfan's syndrome is an uncommon, hereditary disease of the connective tissue with an occurrence rate of 4–6 cases per 100 000 population. The skeletal, ocular and cardiovascular systems are mainly involved. Skeletal features include long tubular bones with excessive length relative to the trunk, hyperextensible joints and kyphoscoliosis. Ocular symptoms include bilateral dislocation of the lens, myopia and detached retina. The cardiovascular system may be affected, the commonest finding being degeneration of the elastic lamina in the media of the aorta (cystic medial necrosis). The risk of aortic valvular incompetence and dissecting aneurysm is increased during pregnancy. This is due to increased cardiac output on the one hand, and hormonally related connective tissue changes on the other. Stress and pain during labour and delivery will potentiate the risk [27]. In this case, caesarean section should be considered to avoid maternal expulsive efforts during delivery.

Anaesthetic management

The management consists of strict blood pressure control and minimization of vascular shear stresses. When beta- and/or calcium-channel blockers are prescribed antenatally, they should be continued in the puerperium. Continuous epidural analgesia is the anaesthetic of choice and blood pressure should be controlled by carefully titrated intravascular volume expansion. Drugs such as ephedrine, adrenaline, calcium chloride, dopamine, digoxin and ergot alkaloids should be avoided, and tachycardia should be treated promptly. Continuous cardiovascular monitoring (arterial and central venous pressure lines) should be available during labour, delivery and in the postoperative period, since the cardiac output continues to increase postpartum, with the attendant risk of aortic dissection.

ACHONDROPLASIA

Achondroplasia is the most common form of dwarfism. It is an autosomal dominant condition (but 80% of cases result from spontaneous mutation) with an incidence of one in 200 000, and is more common in women. Achondroplastic dwarfs have low fertility rates and full-term pregnancy almost always results in caesarean section because of cephalopelvic disproportion. Craniofacial and spinal abnormalities are always present.

Anaesthetic management

Both general and regional anaesthesia pose problems in these patients. The shape of the head and mandible may make intubation difficult, and a small endotracheal tube is required. Because stenosis of the foramen magnum is common, hyperextension of the neck should be avoided during intubation in order to prevent cervical cord compression. Cardiorespiratory function may be compromised by a narrow rib cage and the presence of kyphoscoliosis. Higher intra-abdominal pressure can increase the risk of maternal aspiration. Kyphosis, scoliosis, lumbar lordosis, spinal stenosis, osteophytes, short pedicles and a

narrow epidural space all combine to make landmarks difficult, and regional anaesthesia a challenge. Difficulties in locating the epidural space and insertion of the epidural catheter, increased risk of dural puncture and poor spread of local anaesthetic have been commonly reported [28–30]. Although neurological sequelae have not been reported after regional anaesthesia, it might be judicious to avoid it if spinal pathology is present, due to possible litigation in the case of mishaps.

If subarachnoid anaesthesia is chosen, the narrower spinal canal and the exaggerated spinal curves may result in unpredictable spread and it would seem more prudent to use epidural blockade. The optimal dose in achondroplastic patients is uncertain and careful titration of local anaesthetic solution via the epidural catheter is required.

Other factors to be considered include excess skin and subcutaneous fat which may make intravenous access difficult, and gross anatomical deformities may hamper monitoring and increase the risk of positional trauma.

SPINA BIFIDA

Spina bifida is defined as failed fusion of the neural arch without (spina bifida occulta) or with (spina bifida cystica) herniation of the meninges or neural elements. In the former, the defect is limited to a single vertebra and may be considered an anatomical variant (occurring in 5–30% of population). An overlying lipoma or tuft of hair may suggest an underlying lesion. In attempting to identify the epidural space at the level of the lesion, accidental dural puncture may result. Spina bifida cystica is very rare (1–3 per 1000 births). Neurological deficits, hydrocephalus and kyphoscoliosis are often present and early surgical treatment is usually needed. Because the abnormal epidural space is not continuous, spread of local anaesthetic may be inadequate. Subarachnoid injection, if used, should be performed in the lower spine because the terminal portion of the spinal cord lies at a lower level.

General anaesthesia is preferred in these patients.

OSTEOGENESIS IMPERFECTA

This is a rare, hereditary, connective tissue disorder which involves various organ systems, and its clinical manifestations depend on the organs involved. Dwarfism, kyphoscoliosis and pectum excavatum may be associated. Ocular changes (blue discoloration of the sclera) and deafness (due to otosclerosis) may also be present. Platelet aggregation and adhesion may be impaired, and represent an important problem for the anaesthetist [31].

KLIPPEL–FEIL SYNDROME

Klippel–Feil syndrome is an inherited autosomal dominant condition in which cervical spine abnormalities may be associated with kyphoscoliosis, genitourinary and cardiac anomalies. This syndrome has been classified into three morphological types. In type I several cervical and thoracic vertebrae are incorporated into a single block. In type II patients have fusion at only one or two interspaces, although hemivertebrae, occipito-atlantal fusion and other abnormalities may be also present. Type III includes those with both cervical and thoracic, or lumbar fusion.

Anaesthetic management

Spinal deformities may cause difficulties with both tracheal intubation and regional techniques. Epidural anaesthesia may prove technically difficult with an increased risk of dural puncture; severe kyphoscoliosis can interfere with the spread of local anaesthetic. In the case of spinal anaesthesia, the appropriate dose of local anaesthetic must be estimated. Type II abnormalities are frequently asymptomatic and are incidental findings [32]. General anaesthesia, using awake fibreoptic intubation, and microspinal catheter techniques have been reported in these patients [33, 34]

MUSCULAR DYSTROPHY

Muscular dystrophies comprise a variety of inherited conditions each characterized by progressive degeneration of the skeletal muscle with intact innervation. The most common dystrophies affecting females are facioscapulohumeral dystrophy, an autosomal dominant condition with a slow progression, and limb–girdle dystrophy, also an autosomal dominant which is a regressive disease. In patients with facioscapulohumeral dystrophy, facial weakness and atrophy of the neck and shoulder are the most important features. Limb–girdle dystrophy is characterized by progressive weakness of the hip and shoulder.

Anaesthetic management

Regional anaesthesia is recommended in these patients as they are at increased risk of malignant hyperthermia. If general anaesthesia is required, triggering agents should be avoided [35].

MYOTONIC DYSTROPHY

Myotonic dystrophy is a relatively common, inherited, autosomal dominant disorder with a prevalence of 5 per 100 000 population. Myotonia is the prolonged contraction of muscles after stimulation, with delayed relaxation. Muscles that are particularly susceptible include the hand, facial, masseter and pretibials. The disease is slowly progressive and has a wide range of severity. With time, pharyngeal, laryngeal, proximal limb muscles and diaphragm become involved. In the more severe form (congenital myotonic dystrophy), smooth muscle is also affected and cardiac muscle is involved, leading to conduction abnormalities or cardiomyopathy. Pulmonary or cardiac failure represent fatal events in these patients. Drugs such as quinine and procainamide are often used to improve myotonic symptoms. Weakness and myotonia remain unchanged or may worsen during pregnancy

Table 15.1 Equivalent doses (mg) of commonly used anticholinesterase drugs

	Duration (h)	Intravenous	Subcutaneous	Intramuscular	Oral
Neostigmine	2–3	0.5	1.5	0.7	15
Pyridostigmine	4–6	2		3	60

and can result in a prolonged second stage with an increased incidence of instrumental delivery, uterine atony and haemorrhage. The affected neonate may have respiratory distress and/or feeding problems.

Anaesthetic management

Weak intestinal motility can delay gastric emptying, resulting in a greater risk of aspiration. These patients are very sensitive to opioid analgesics and general anaesthetics, which may precipitate apnoea in the postoperative period [36]. Regional anaesthesia is preferred for labour and delivery analgesia although this does not relieve the myotonia. Since shivering and cold may trigger a myotonic crisis, particular care should be taken to avoid them. If general anaesthesia is required, succinylcholine should be avoided as this is also a trigger agent. There is no contraindication to the use of non-depolarizing agents, and volatile agents are also safe. Acute myotonic crises may be treated with quinidine 300–600 mg intravenously, steroids, dantrolene or direct injections of local anaesthetics into the contracted muscle. Patients receiving quinidine may require a reduced dose of non-depolarizing muscle relaxants

MYASTHENIA GRAVIS

Myasthenia gravis is a rare autoimmune disorder with a prevalence of 1 in 10–50 000. It can occur at any age but is seen more frequently in females. It is characterized by weakness and fatigue, and most commonly affects the facial, oculomotor, laryngeal, pharyngeal and respiratory muscles. Partial recovery with rest and after the administration of anticholinesterase

drugs is an important feature of this disease. Immunoglobulin G antibodies against the acetylcholine (ach) receptor, which can be detected in 85–90% of patients, result in a decrease in the number of ach receptors on the neuromuscular junction. There is a common association with thymic hyperplasia and other autoimmune disorders such as rheumatoid arthritis and polymyositis. Treatment includes thymectomy, medical treatment with anticholinesterase drugs (neostigmine, pyridostigmine) (Table 15.1), immunosuppresssive agents and plasmapheresis.

Myasthenic patients may present with cholinergic or myasthenic crises (abdominal cramps, diarrhoea, nausea, vomiting, increased salivary and tear duct secretions, muscle weakness and respiratory failure). Cholinergic crisis results from an excess of the muscarinic effects of anticholinesterase drugs following a poor response to therapy. Myasthenic crisis results from a worsening of the disease. The two may be distinguished by administration of 10 mg of i.v. edrophonium (the symptoms will not improve in the case of a cholinergic crisis). All these patients are very sensitive to drugs that may potentiate muscular weakness:

* aminoglycoside antibiotics;
* cardiac drugs: quinidine, propranolol;
* beta-mimetics: ritodrine, terbutaline;
* tocolytics: magnesium sulphate;
* others: quinine, penicillamine, lithium salts.

The course of the disease in pregnancy is variable: approximately 40% worsen, 30% experience a relapse and 30% have no changes [37]. After delivery, 30% of patients have a serious exacerbation of their disease. Maternal mortality is also increased. The incidence of preterm labour is approximately 40%, which may be due to the oxytocic effects of ach inhibitors. Transient myasthenia in 10–20% of neonates may result from the transplacental passage of maternal antibodies. Neonatal myasthenia, which responds well to anticholinesterase therapy, usually presents within the first two days after delivery and is characterized by a weak cry, poor sucking and hypotonia.

Anaesthetic management

All patients should undergo an antepartum anaesthetic consultation which includes an assessment of the degree of bulbar and respiratory function, and a review of medication that may have a significant anaesthetic interaction. Plasma cholinesterase activity is decreased in patients taking anticholinesterase drugs. As ester local anaesthetics generally have a longer half-life, amide local anaesthetic agents are preferred. Patients with some degree of respiratory or bulbar compromise are at greater risk of respiratory depression associated with opioids. Since uterine muscle is not involved in the myasthenic process, vaginal delivery is possible and regional analgesia is indicated. This is also true for caesarean section provided there is no significant degree of bulbar or respiratory involvement [38]. In the case of general anaesthesia, muscle relaxant drugs may have an exaggerated effect [39] and the duration of depolarizing agents can be unpredictably prolonged. The use of inhalation agents may also potentiate muscle relaxation. Neuromuscular blockade should be monitored with a nerve stimulator and small doses of neostigmine may be given for neuromuscular blockade reversal. Factors which may merit the need for postoperative mechanical ventilation are shown below [40]:

- duration of myasthenia > six years;
- chronic respiratory disease;
- pyridostigmine dosage > 750 mg/day;
- vital capacity < 2.9 l.

Rheumatoid arthritis

Rheumatoid arthritis is the most common chronic, systemic rheumatic disease and complicates 1 in 1–2000 pregnancies [41]. The origin of this disease is not fully understood but may be due to an abnormal immune response that produces synovial proliferation leading to joint destruction and deformity. Chronic complex abnormalities such as atlanto-axial subluxation in association with deformation of the trachea and larynx occur primarily in patients with long-standing disease, and rarely affect young patients. Extra-articular features are common in patients with higher titres of autoantibodies (rheumatoid factor). Approximately 75% of patients see an improvement in their symptoms during pregnancy, but many suffer an exacerbation of their disease in the postpartum period [42].

Anaesthetic management

Anaesthetic management of the parturient with rheumatoid arthritis depends on the degree of multiorgan involvement. Extra-articular features of rheumatoid arthritis include:

- cardiovascular: pericarditis, cardiac granulomas, arteritis/vasculitis;
- airway: mandibular hypoplasia, mandibular joint disfunction, deviation of larynx;
- pulmonary: pleural/pulmonary nodules, pulmonary fibrosis;
- neurological: peripheral nerve compression;
- haematological: anaemia, Felty's syndrome (lymphadenopathy keratoconjunctivitis sicca).

Young patients do not usually present with cervical and mandibular dysfunction, or extra-articular complications (such as cardiovascular, pulmonary or neurological involvement). Patients with severe airway abnormalities may be very difficult to intubate and require regional anaesthesia. If peripheral neuropathies are present regional anaesthesia is not contraindicated, but neurological deficits need to be documented in advance. Aspirin and steroids are the mainstay of treatment for rheumatoid arthritis and this should be considered when regional anaesthesia is performed. Aspirin can result in interference with platelet function for up 10 days, and some authorities would recommend that bleeding time should be assessed if regional anaesthesia is contemplated. Steroid use may result in adrenal suppression and supplementation should be considered. A more detailed account can be found in the section dealing with immunological problems.

REFERENCES

1. Weinreb, J.C., Wolbarst, L.B., Cohen, J.M. et al. (1989) Prevalence of lumbosacral intervertebral disc abnormalities on MR images in pregnant and asymptomatic nonpregnant women. *Radiology*, **170**, 125–8.
2. Samsoon, G., Badouin, C. and Holdcroft, A. (1990) Relation of lumbar tissue damage and backache after delivery. *British Journal of Anaesthesia*, **65**, 577P.
3. Le Ban, M.M., Perrin, J.C.S. and Latimer, F.R. (1983) Pregnancy and the herniated lumbar disc. *Archives of Physical Medicine and Rehabilitation*, **64**,319–21.
4. Ong, B.Y. (1987) Paresthesias and motor dysfunction after labor and delivery. *Anesthesia and Analgesia*, **66**,18–22.
5. Benzon, H.T., Braunschweig, R. and Molloy, R.E. (1981) Delayed onset of epidural anesthesia in patients with back pain. *Anesthesia and Analgesia*, **60**, 874–7.
6. MacArthur, C., Lewis, M., Knox, E.G. et al. (1990) Epidural anaesthesia and long term backache after childbirth. *British Medical Journal*, **301**,9–12.
7. Jullien, P., Hamza, J., Troche, G. et al. (1990) Pathologie lombaire et anesthésie péridurale en obstétrique. *Annale Françaises d'Anesthésie et de Réanimation*, **10**, R 134.
8. Mac Leod, J., Macintyre, C., McClure, J.H. et al. (1995) Backache and epidural analgesia. A retrospective survey of mothers 1 year after childbirth. *International Journal of Obstetric Anaesthesia*, **4**, 21–5.
9. Russell, R., Dundas, R. and Reynolds, F. (1996) Long term backache after childbirth: prospective search for causative factors. *British Medical Journal*, **312**,1384–8.
10. Peng, A.T.C., Behar, S. and Blancato, L.S. (1985) Reduction of postlumbar puncture backache by the use of field block anesthesia prior to lumbar puncture (letter) *Anesthesiology*, **63**, 227–8.
11. Bush, D.J. (1995) A comparison of informed consent for obstetric anaesthesia in the USA and the UK. *International Journal of Obstetric Anaesthesia*, **4**, 1–6.
12. Lanigan, C. and Reynolds, F. (1995) Risk information supplied by obstetric anaesthetists in Britain and Ireland to mothers awaiting elective caesarean section. *International Journal of Obstetric Anaesthesia*, **4**, 7–13.
13. Knapp, R.M. (1990) Legal view of informed consent for anaesthesia during labor. *Anesthesiology*, **72**, 211.
14. Chadwick, H.S., Posner, K., Caplan, R. et al. (1991) A comparison of obstetric and nonobstetric anesthesia malpractice claims. *Anesthesiology*, **74**, 242–9.
15. Wynne-Davies, R. (1968) Familial (idiopathic) scoliosis: A family survey. *Journal of Bone and Joint Surgery (British Volume)*, **50**, 24–30.
16. Shands, A.R. and Eisberg, H.B. (1955) The incidence of scoliosis in the state of Delaware. *Journal of Bone and Joint Surgery (American Volume)*, **37**, 1243.
17. Blount, W.P. and Mellencamp, D. (1980) The effect of pregnancy in idiopathic scoliosis. *Journal of Bone and Joint Surgery (British Volume)*, **62** A, 1083–7.
18. Berman, A.T., Cohen, D.L. and Schwentker, E.P. (1982) The effects of pregnancy on idiopathic scoliosis. A preliminary report of eight cases and a review of the literature. *Spine*, **7**, 76–7.
19. Betz, R.R., Bunnell, W.P., Lambrecht-Mulier, E. et al. (1987) Scoliosis and pregnancy. *Journal of Bone and Joint Surgery (British Volume)*, **69**, 90–6.
20. Visscher, W., Lonstein, J.E., Hoffman, D.A. et al. (1988) Reproductive outcomes in scoliosis patients. *Spine*, **13**, 1096–8.
21. Phelan, J.D., Dainer, M.J. and Cowherd, D.W. (1978) Pregnancy complicated by thoracolumbar scoliosis. *Southern Medical Journal*, **71**, 76–8.
22. Sawicka, E.H., Spencer, G.T. and Branthwaite, M.A. (1986) Management of respiratory failure complicating pregnancy in severe kyphoscoliosis: a new use for an old technique? *British Journal of Diseases of the Chest*, **80**, 191–6.

23. Moran, D.H. and Johnson, M.D. (1990) Continuous spinal anesthesia with combined hyperbaric and isobaric bupivacaine in a patient with scoliosis. *Anesthesia and Analgesia*, **70**, 445–7.

24. Daley, M.D., Robbin, S.M., Hew, E.M. *et al.* (1990) Epidural anaesthesia for obstetrics after spinal surgery. *Regional Anesthesia*, **15**, 280–4.

25. Daley, M.D., Rolbin, S., Hew, E. *et al.* (1990) Continuous epidural anaesthesia for obstetrics after major spinal surgery. *Canadian Journal of Anaesthesia*, **37**, S112.

26. Kardash, K., King, B.W. and Datta, S. (1993) Spinal anaesthesia for caesarean section after Harrington instrumentation. *Canadian Journal of Anaesthesia*, **40**, 667–9.

27. Kitchen, D.H. (1974) Dissecting aneurysm of the aorta in pregnancy. *British Journal of Obstetrics and Gynaecology*, **81**, 410.

28. Wardall, G.J. and Frame, W.T. (1990) Extradural anaesthesia for caesarean section in achondroplasia. *British Journal of Anaesthesia*, **64**, 367–70.

29. Carstoniu, J., Yee, I. and Halpern, S. (1992) Epidural anaesthesia for caesarean section in an achondroplastic dwarf. *Canadian Journal of Anaesthesia*, **39**, 708–11.

30. Brimacombe, J.R. and Caunt, J.A. (1990) Anaesthesia in a gravid achondroplastic dwarf. *Anaesthesia*, **45**, 132–4.

31. Rocke, D.A. and Moodley, J. (1996) Trauma and orthopaedic problems, in *Anesthetic and Obstetric Management of High Risk Pregnancy*, 2nd edn (ed. S. Datta), Mosby Year Book, St Louis, p. 307.

32. Lyons, G. (1985) Failed intubation. Six years' experience in a teaching maternity unit. *Anaesthesia*, **40**, 759–62.

33. Daum, R.E. and Jones, D.J. (1988) Fibreoptic intubation in Kippel–Feil syndrome. *Anaesthesia*, **43**, 18–21.

34. Dresner, M.R. and Maclean, A.R. (1995) Anaesthesia for caesarean section in a patient with Klippel–Feil syndrome. *Anaesthesia*, **50**, 807–9.

35. Smith, C.L. and Bush, G.H. (1985) Anaesthesia and progressive muscular dystrophy. *British Journal of Anaesthesia*, **57**, 1113–8.

36. Ravin, M., Newmark, Z. and Saviello, G. (1975) Myotonic dystrophy: an anesthetic hazard: two cases report. *Anesthesia and Analgesia*, **54**, 216–8.

37. Plauché, W.C. (1983) Myasthenia gravis. *Clinical Obstetrics and Gynecology*, **26**, 592– 604.

38. Mitchell, P.J. and Bebbington, M. Myasthenia gravis in pregnancy. (1992) *Obstetrics and Gynecology*, **80**, 178–81.

39. Foldes, F.F. and McNall, P.G. (1962) Myasthenia gravis: a guide for anesthesiologists. *Anesthesiology*, **23**, 837–72.

40. Leventhal, S.R., Orkin, F.K. and Hirsh, R.A. (1980) Prediction of the need for postoperative mechanical ventilation in myasthenia gravis. *Anesthesiology*, **53**, 26–30.

41. O'Sullivan, J.B. and Cathcart, S.E. (1972) The prevalence of rheumatoid arthritis: followup evaluation of the effect of criteria on rates in Sudbury Massachusetts. *Annals of Internal Medicine*, **76**, 573–7.

42. Klippe, G.L. and Cecere, F.A. (1989) Rheumatoid arthritis and pregnancy. *Rheumatology Clinics of North America*, **15**, 213–39.

16

PROBLEMS WITH COMBINED SPINAL–EPIDURAL ANAESTHESIA

N. Rawal

INTRODUCTION

Epidural and spinal blocks have a long history of safe use for a variety of surgical procedures and pain relief. Both techniques are used extensively world-wide. Nevertheless both techniques have well-recognized drawbacks which are particularly prominent in obstetric and high-risk patients. For example it is generally recognized that a S5–T4 block is necessary for adequate analgesia during caesarean section. Epidural technique for such an extensive block may be associated with a relatively high incidence of hypotension [1] and a potential risk of toxic complications because of the requirement for large doses of local anaesthetic drugs [2, 3]. Furthermore, in spite of these large doses the block may be inadequate in 10 to 25% of patients, mainly because of difficulty in blocking sacral roots or because the block is not high enough [4]. Spinal anaesthesia is more reliable than epidural anaesthesia and produces a denser block but the upper level of spinal block is unpredictable and the technique may be associated with a high risk of precipitous maternal hypotension which may be harmful for the neonate [5, 6]. Since spinal block is usually a 'single-shot' technique there is no possibility of improving an inadequate block or providing extended postoperative pain relief.

The combined spinal–epidural (CSE) technique can reduce or eliminate some of the disadvantages of spinal and epidural anaesthesia while preserving their advantages. CSE offers the speed of onset, efficacy and minimal toxicity of a spinal block combined with the possibility of improving an inadequate block or prolonging the duration of anaesthesia with epidural supplements and extending the analgesia well into the postoperative period. For labour pain the CSE technique offers the possibility of combining almost instantaneous intrathecal opioid analgesia with the flexibility of epidural analgesia; this approach allows ambulation throughout labour. These advantages are making CSE blocks increasingly popular especially in obstetrics and for orthopaedic surgery [7] (Table 16.1). In recent years an array of special CSE packaged combination sets and sophisticated needles designed to reduce risks of complications have been introduced.

PROBLEMS WITH CSE TECHNIQUE

RISK OF CATHETER PENETRATION THROUGH DURAL PUNCTURE

Epidural catheter migration into the subarachnoid space is potentially very serious because

Clinical Problems in Obstetric Anaesthesia
Edited by Ian F. Russell and Gordon Lyons. Published in 1997 by Chapman & Hall, London. ISBN 0 412 71600 3.

Table 16.1 Reported indications for the CSE technique

- Orthopaedic surgery (major hip and knee surgery)
- Obstetrics (caesarean section, walking CSE for labour pain)
- Major vascular surgery*
- Urologic surgery*
- Gynaecologic surgery*
- Paediatric surgery (hernia)
- Ambulatory surgery (knee arthroscopy)
- Research tool for controlled comparison between epidural and intrathecal techniques

---

*CSE block alone or in combination with light general anaesthesia.

failure to recognize misplacement of the catheter and injection of the usual epidural dose would result in total spinal anaesthesia. Although CSE block has been performed in tens of thousands of patients in Europe in the last decade there are few published reports of epidural catheter penetration through the dural hole or any other serious complications [8]. At our institution we have not seen any epidural catheter migration or any other major complication in over 3500 patients. However, at the time of performing CSE block we have seen two cases of epidural catheter penetration into the subarachnoid space. Dural damage by Tuohy needle could not be ruled out in either case. In both cases malposition of the epidural catheter was easily identified by an aspiration test. At the Queen Charlotte's Hospital in London, where CSE is routinely used for vaginal and caesarean deliveries, no catheter migrations were noted during a three-year period [9]. In a recent 17-nation European survey no major complications were noted in any of the 5347 patients who received CSE block during a period of one year [10].

Our studies on isolated human dura showed that it was impossible to force an 18 gauge Portex epidural catheter through dural holes made by 26 or 27 gauge spinal needles. Also, it was quite difficult to force the catheter through holes made by spinal needles of 22 to 25 gauge diameter. Twenty-two gauge or larger diameter spinal needles made holes large enough to permit the passage of the catheter [11]. These results were confirmed by our epiduroscopic studies with video recording in fresh cadavers. In these studies epidural catheters were directed to single and multiple holes made by 25 gauge spinal needles and single holes made by 18 gauge Tuohy needles. It was impossible to force 16 or 18 gauge epidural catheters through dural holes made by a single dural puncture with a 25 gauge spinal needle. Even when five holes were made in the same area of the dura by a 25 gauge spinal needle epidural catheter penetration into the subarachnoid space occurred in only one out of 20 recordings (5%) (Figure 16.1). After intentional dural puncture with Tuohy needle epidural catheter penetration into the subarachnoid space occurred in 45% of cases [12].

It is also emphasized that the possibility of subarachnoid or intravenous placement exists with any epidural catheter and that the danger of massive inadvertent intrathecal injection is not unique to the CSE technique. Total spinal blocks are a rare but recognized complication of 'top-ups' of previously normally functioning epidural catheters [13, 14]. Epidural catheters that have functioned normally at previous injection have also been documented to erode into epidural blood vessels [15, 16]. Clearly, the risk of catheter migration can be expected to be greater if there is a hole in the dura. It is therefore important that the routine for 'top-up' doses in the epidural catheter should be clearly defined at all institutions where the CSE technique is practised. However, the routine is not different from that for standard epidural technique and consists of

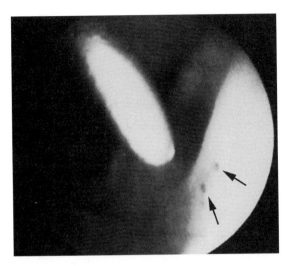

Figure 16.1 Epiduroscopy study to evaluate the risk of epidural catheter penetration through dural hole made by spinal needle. The multiple dural holes made by the spinal needle were visible at the 4 and 5 o'clock positions. The tip of the Tuohy needle is seen coming into the epidural space from the top of the picture. Reproduced with permission from Holmström *et al.* (1995) *Anesthesia and Analgesia*, **80**, 747—53.

confirmation of the catheter position by aspiration as well as frequent assessment of the block following injection of fractionated doses of local anaesthetics. Continuous epidural infusion of low concentration local anaesthetic may be safer than high concentration bolus injection. Every reinjection should be considered a test dose.

EXTENSION OF SPINAL BLOCK FOLLOWING EPIDURAL INJECTION OF LOCAL ANAESTHETIC

Ensuring a satisfactory upper level of spinal block and adequate analgesia has prompted the use of relatively large intrathecal doses of local anaesthetic for caesarean section. With the CSE technique the presence of an epidural catheter permits the anaesthesiologist to use smaller doses for spinal block thereby decreasing the incidence and severity of maternal

hypotension. Doses of subarachnoid bupivacaine in the range of 7.5–10 mg have been shown to provide effective analgesia for most patients undergoing caesarean section [11, 17, 18]. These doses are considerably less than those reported by others [3]. However, in some patients additional doses of epidural local anaesthetic will be necessary to extend the spinal block [11,17–19].

It is unclear how relatively small doses of epidural local anaesthetic can rapidly elevate the level of spinal block. The following hypotheses have been proposed: (1) leakage of epidural local anaesthetic through the dural hole into the subarachnoid space; (2) continuing spread of initial subarachnoid block (unrelated to epidural injection); (3) existence of 'subclinical' analgesia at a higher level which is enhanced and becomes evident by perineural or transdural spread of epidural local anaesthetic; (4) change in epidural pressure (the pressure becomes atmospheric which may result in better spread of local anaesthetic through an effect on volume and circulation of CSF [17]); and (5) compression of the subarachnoid space by the presence of the epidural catheter and by the volume of local anaesthetic resulting in a 'squeezing' of CSF and more extensive upward spread of local anaesthetic [11, 20].

Although leakage of epidural local anaesthetic into the subarachnoid space is theoretically possible the rapidity with which extension occurs suggests some other mechanism. Furthermore our knowledge of pressures within the epidural and subarachnoid spaces and of the role of CSF leakage in post-dural puncture headache suggest that the flow of fluids is more likely to be away from the subarachnoid space rather than towards it. Data from numerous studies have not shown any clinically significant increased spread of sensory block with the combined technique, suggesting that there is no substantial passage of epidurally injected local anaesthetic through the dural opening left by the spinal needle. However, caution is in order when large volumes of drugs are injected over short periods as epidural pressure may become positive. The main reason for the rapid extension of subarachnoid block by epidural local anaesthetics appears to be related to increased volume within the epidural space causing a decrease in CSF volume and a cephalad shift of local anaesthetic within the CSF [20].

RISK OF HIGH SPINAL BLOCK

Theoretically the meningeal hole made by the spinal needle may allow dangerously high concentrations of subsequently administered epidural drugs to reach the subarachnoid space [21]. The possibility of this risk is supported by reports of high or total spinal block during epidural anaesthesia after inadvertent dural perforation [22, 23].

Bernards *et al.* investigated the risk of epidural drug reaching the subarachnoid space through the meningeal perforation left by the spinal needle. The authors measured the flux of morphine and lidocaine through the spinal meninges of the monkey *in vitro* after puncture with 27 gauge Whitacre, 24 gauge Sprotte and 18 gauge Tuohy needles. The flux of drugs through the meningeal tissue was significantly increased by puncture with the study needles. The magnitude of this flux was dependent on hole size and not on any physicochemical properties of the drugs because the flux was similar for both drugs and because there is a difference between the drugs when meningeal tissue is intact, i.e. the flux of morphine is less than that of lidocaine. The authors concluded that the amount of drug reaching the subarachnoid space is not significant if the hole is made by a small-diameter spinal needle and the volume of epidural solution is large [21]. However, Suzuki *et al.* have recently shown that the spread of an epidural block was influenced by the existence of a prior dural puncture with a 26 gauge spinal needle [24]. The net amount of epidural drug in the subarachnoid space can be expected to increase considerably if a small volume of concentrated

epidural solution is injected close to the dural hole made by a large diameter needle [21].

ROTATION OF EPIDURAL NEEDLE

It has been advocated that the Tuohy needle be rotated 180% between the subarachnoid injection and epidural catheter insertion so that the site of dural puncture is at some distance from the point at which the catheter impinges [25, 26]. This would presumably decrease the risk of catheter migration into the subarachnoid space. However, at our institution we have stopped this procedure since 1988. It has been demonstrated that rotating the epidural needle may cause dural tear or puncture [27, 28]. In one study a failure rate of 3% increased to 17% when rotation of the epidural needle was introduced [29].

FAILURE

In one study of caesarean section patients the technical aspects of 'needle-through-needle' versus double space technique were compared. A high technical failure rate (13%) was noted with the former technique. This was mainly due to difficulty in establishing a spinal block [30]. No other study has reported such high technical failure rates [3, 6, 11, 31, 32]. Indeed the spinal block is easier to perform because the Tuohy needle serves as an introducer. Since this 'introducer' needle is in the epidural space the spinal needle does not have to go through different anatomical structures, it has only to penetrate the dura. A majority of anaesthetists perform CSE blocks using long spinal needles (11–12 cm) of varying diameters that are introduced through 16 or 18 gauge regular Tuohy needles. As mentioned earlier there is a risk of spinal needle displacement at the time of syringe connection, aspiration of CSF or injection of local anaesthetic. Special devices to fix the spinal needle in place while it is in the Tuohy needle have been described [33]. The use of special kits and matching needles with locking mechanisms can be expected to improve the

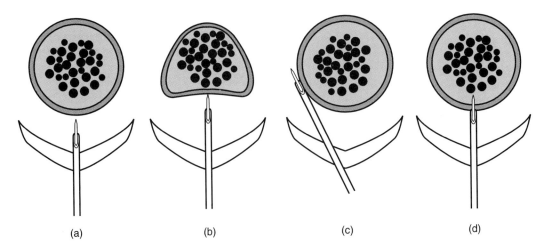

(a)   (b)   (c)   (d)

Figure 16.2 Various possibilities for CSE block failure due to incorrect technique (a, b and c) and correct position of epidural and spinal needles (d). (a) Length of spinal needle protruding from tip of epidural needle is too short (or epidural needle is not introduced far enough into epidural space). (b) Tip of spinal needle 'tents' the dura but fails to pierce it (greater risk with 'pencil-point' needle). (c) Malposition of epidural needle. (d) Ideal positioning.

success rate. Thus in a recent study of 150 caesarean section patients the failure rate with 'Portex' CSE needles was 0.67% [34]. This is considerably lower than the failure rate for spinal block reported in recent literature [35, 36].

BEST PROTRUDING LENGTH OF SPINAL NEEDLE BEYOND THE TIP OF THE TUOHY NEEDLE

The distance from the tip of the epidural needle to the posterior wall of the dural sac in the midline varies considerably between patients (0.3–1.05 cm) [37]. Further, the antero-posterior diameter of the dural sac varies considerably during extension and flexion of the spinal column. At L3–4 the diameter increases from a range of 9 to 20 mm in extension to 11 to 25 mm in flexion [38]. Additionally, this is only valid when the epidural puncture is performed in the midline. This is because the dural sac is triangular with its base resting on the vertebral body and the triangle top points posteriorly to the ligamentum flavum [39]. The point of dural contact by the spinal needle will clearly depend on the direction of the Tuohy needle

[38]. In some special CSE kits the hub of the spinal needle locks into the hub of the Tuohy needle and a fixed length of spinal needle protrudes from the tip of the Tuohy needle. This length of protrusion may vary from 10 mm (Vygon CSE set) to 13 mm (Braun CSE set). In a recent study, when these sets were compared, the authors concluded that the length of protrusion should be more than 13 mm because a failure rate of 15% with the Vygon set was noted [40]. Vandermeersch considers that a protrusion of at least 17 mm is best; he also recommends selection of separate long spinal needles of sufficient length for maximal flexibility rather than needles with locking hubs and fixed protrusion [38]. The type of spinal needle may also influence the success rate of CSE block; because of needle design the length of protrusion for pencil point needles should be greater than that for Quincke point needles (Figure 16.2).

EQUIPMENT-RELATED PROBLEMS

In recent years several modifications of the CSE technique or needle design have been

Table 16.2 Various options for combined spinal–epidural technique

- Double needle – separate interspaces*
- Double needle (needle-through-needle) – single interspace
- Double catheter (catheters in epidural and subarachnoid space)
- Double needle (needle beside needle) – single interspace†
  (a) spinal needle guide fixed alongside outer wall of epidural needle
  (b) spinal needle guide incorporated within epidural needle wall‡

*Epidural catheter insertion followed by spinal block at a lower interspace.
†Allows epidural catheter insertion before spinal block
‡E-SP needle. This device is FDA approved, but no clinical data are available so far.

reported. Disposable CSE sets have been commercially available since 1986. At present there are at least 12 medical companies that distribute special CSE kits. Furthermore, as shown in Table 16.2, there are several modifications of the CSE technique. Since the tip of the spinal needle may scrape against the inner wall of the Tuohy needle concern has been expressed about possible metal particles in the epidural or subarachnoid space [41]. However, there is no report of any neurological problem in any of the thousands of patients who have received CSE block by such needles. Indeed, such needles are still used for the majority of CSE blocks performed world-wide. The risk of damage to the bevel of the spinal needle can be eliminated by the Espocan system which contains a spinal needle with a plastic sleeve that keeps it centrally in the epidural needle and guides it through the 'back' eye in the curve of the epidural needle tip. The spinal needle enters this hole easily and can be introduced into the dura without coming in contact with the internal wall of the epidural needle.

There are no reports of any major problems with the Braun (Espocan), Portex or B-D CSE needles so far. Although the E-SP needle is FDA approved there are no clinical data at present; similarly the safety of other CSE needles remains to be established.

SUMMARY

Although epidural and spinal blocks are well-accepted regional techniques they have several disadvantages. A combined spinal–epidural technique reduces or eliminates the risks of these disadvantages. CSE block combines the rapidity, density and reliability of spinal block with the flexibility of continuous epidural to extend the duration of analgesia. The technique is used routinely at many institutions particularly for major orthopaedic surgery and in obstetrics. It has been used in tens of thousands of patients without any reports of major problems. Catheter penetration through the dural hole, though unlikely, is not impossible. Before any injection in the epidural catheter its position should always be confirmed by the aspiration test. The risk of leakage of epidural local anaesthetic into the subarachnoid space to cause high spinal block appears to be low. It seems prudent to avoid rotation of the epidural needle. The technique should be used only by those who are experienced in spinal and epidural blocks. CSE is an important addition to the armamentarium of the anaesthetist.

ACKNOWLEDGEMENT

The authors wish to thank Ing-Marie Dimgren for excellent secretarial help.

REFERENCES

1. Lewis, M., Thomas, P. and Wilkes, R.G. (1983) Hypotension during epidural analgesia for caesarean section. *Anaesthesia*, **38**, 250.
2. Thorburn, J. and Moir, D.D. (1984) Bupivacaine toxicity in association with extra-dural

analgesia for caesarean section. *Br. J. Anaesth.*, **56**, 551.

3. Carrie, L.E.S. (1990) Extradural spinal or combined spinal block for obstetric surgical anaesthesia. *Br. J. Anaesth.*, **65**, 225–33.

4. Morgan, B.M., Aulakh, J.M., Barker, J.P. *et al.* (1983) Anaesthesia for caesarean section. *Br. J. Anaesth.*, **55**, 885.

5. Lussos, S.A. and Datta, S. (1992) Anesthesia for cesarean delivery. Part I. General considerations and spinal anesthesia. *Int. J. Obst. Anaesth.*, **1**, 79–91.

6. Santos, A.C. and Pedersen, H. (1994) Current controversies in obstetric anesthesia. *Anesth. Analg.*, **78**, 753–60.

7. Raj, P.P., Pai, U. and Rawal, N. (1991) Techniques of regional anesthesia in adults, in *Clinical Practice of Regional Anesthesia* (ed. P. Raj), Churchill Livingstone, New York, pp. 271–364.

8. Patel, M. (1992) Combined spinal and extradural anesthesia. *Anesth. Analg.*, **75**, 640–1.

9. Stacey, R.G.W., Watt, S., Kadim, M.Y. and Morgan, B.M. (1993) Single space combined spinal–extradural technique for analgesia in labour. *Br. J. Anaesth.*, **71**, 499–502.

10. Rawal, N. (1995) European trends in the use of combined spinal–epidural technique – A 17-nation survey. *Reg. Anesth.*, **20**, A 162.

11. Rawal, N., Schollin, J. and Wesstršm, G. (1988) Epidural versus combined spinal epidural block for Caesarean section. *Acta Anaesthesiol. Scand.*, **32**, 61–6.

12. Holmström, B., Rawal, N., Axelsson, K. and Nydahl, P.-A. (1995) Risk of catheter migration during combined spinal epidural block: percutaneous epiduroscopy study. *Anesth. Analg.*, **80**, 747–53.

13. Crawford, J.S. (1985) Some maternal complications of epidural analgesia for labour. *Anaesthesia*, **40**, 1219.

14. Phillips, D.C., MacDonald, R. and Lyons, G. (1986) Possible subarachnoid migration of an epidural catheter. *Anaesthesia*, **41**, 653.

15. Ravindran, R., Albrecht, W. and Mckay, M. (1979) Apparent intravascular migration of epidural catheter. *Anesth. Analg.*, **58**, 252–3.

16. Zebrowski, M.E. and Gutsche, B.B. (1979) More on intravascular migration of epidural catheter. *Anesth. Analg.*, **58**, 531.

17. Kumar, C. (1987) Combined subarachnoid and epidural block for cesarean section. *Can. J. Anaesth.*, **34**, 329–30.

18. Dennison, B. (1987) Combined subarachnoid and epidural block for caesarean section. *Can. Anaesth. Soc. J.*, **34**, 105–6.

19. Thorén, T., Holmström, B. and Rawal, N. *et al.* (1994) Sequential combined spinal epidural block versus spinal block for cesarean section: effects on maternal hypotension and neurobehavioral function of the newborn. *Anesth. Analg.*, **78**, 1087–92.

20. Blumgart, C.H., Ryall, D., Dennison, B. and Thompson-Hill, L.M. (1992) Mechanism of extension of spinal anaesthesia by extradural injection of local anaesthetic. *Br. J. Anaesth.*, **69**, 457–60.

21. Bernards, C.M., Kopacz, D.J. and Michel, M.Z. (1994) Effect of needle puncture on morphine and lidocaine flux through the spinal meninges of the monkey *in vitro*. Implications for combined spinal–epidural anesthesia. *Anesthesiology*, **80**, 853–8.

22. Leach, A. and Smith, G. (1988) Subarachnoid spread of epidural local anesthetic following dural puncture. *Anaesthesia*, **43**, 671–4.

23. Hodgkinson, R. (1981) Total spinal block after epidural injection into an interspace adjacent to an inadvertent dural perforation. *Anesthesiology*, **55**, 593–5.

24. Suzuki, N., Koganemaru, M., Onizuka, S. and Takasaki, M. (1995) Dural puncture with a 26 G spinal needle affects epidural anesthesia. *Reg. Anesth.*, **20**, A118.

25. Rawal, N. (1986) Single segment combined spinal epidural block for cesarean section. *Can. Anaesth. Soc. J.*, **33**, 254–5.

26. Hughes, J.A. and Oldroyd, G.J. (1991) A technique to avoid dural puncture by the epidural catheter. *Anaesthesia*, **46**, 802.

27. Meiklejohn, B.H. (1987) The effect of rotation of an epidural needle: an *in vitro* study. *Anaesthesia*, **42**, 1180–2.

28. Hollway, T.E. and Tedford, R.J. (1991) Observations on deliberate dural puncture with a Tuohy needle:depth measurements. *Anaesthesia*, **46**, 722–4.

29. Carter, L.C., Popat, M.T. and Wallace, D.H. (1992) Epidural needle rotation and inadvertent dural puncture with catheter. *Anaesthesia*, **47**, 447–8.

30. Lyons, G., Macdonald, R. and Mikl, B. (1992) Combined epidural spinal anesthesia for caesarean section. Through the needle or in separate spaces? *Anaesthesia*, **47**, 199–201.

31. Holmström, B., Laugaland, K., Rawal, N. and Hallberg, S. (1993) Combined spinal epidural

block versus spinal and epidural block for orthopedic surgery. *Can. J. Anaesth.*, **40**, 601–6.

32. Randalls, B., Broadway, J.W., Browne, D.A. and Morgan, B.M. (1991) Comparison of four subarachnoid solutions in needle-through-needle technique for elective cesarean section. *Br. J. Anaesth.*, **66**, 314–8.

33. Simsa, J. (1990) Device to maintain the position of a 29-Gauge spinal needle. *Anaesthesia*, **45**, 593–4.

34. Westbrook, J.L., Donald, F. and Carrie, L.E.S. (1992) An evaluation of a combined spinal epidural needle set utilizing a 26-Gauge, pencil point spinal needle for caesarean section. *Anaesthesia*, **47**, 990–2.

35. Manchikanti, L., Hadley, C., Markwell, S.J. and Colliver, J.A. (1987) A retrospective analysis of failed spinal anesthetic attempts in a community hospital. *Anesth. Analg.*, **66**, 363– 6.

36. Tarkkila, P.J., Heine, H. and Tervo, R.R. (1992) Comparison of Sprotte and Quincke needles with respect to postdural puncture headache and backache. *Reg. Anesth.*, **17**, 283–7.

37. Katz, J. (1985) Spinal and epidural anatomy, in *Atlas of Regional Anaesthesia* (ed. J. Katz), Appleton-Century-Crofts, Norwalk, pp. 168–9.

38. Vandermeersch, E. (1993) Combined spinal–epidural anaesthesia. *Baillière's Clin. Anaesth.*, **7**, 691–708.

39. Husemeyer, R.P. and White, D.C. (1980) Topography of the lumbar epidural space. *Anaesthesia*, **35**, 7–11.

40. Joshi, G.P. and McCaroll, S.M. (1994) Evaluation of combined spinal–epidural anesthesia using two different techniques. *Reg. Anesth.*, **19**, 169–74.

41. Eldor, J. and Brodsky, V. (1991) Danger of metallic particles in the spinal–epidural spaces using the needle-through-needle approach. *Acta Anaesthesiol. Scand.*, **35**, 461.

DRUG ABUSE IN THE PREGNANT WOMAN

17

D.J. Birnbach and A. Van Zundert

INTRODUCTION

The drug-abusing mother presents many challenges to the anaesthetist. The unusual and clinically challenging situations that may arise in this patient population may be due to many factors including failure on the part of some of these patients to receive medical treatment during pregnancy, the effects of illicit drug use, unstable home environment, poor diet and the presence of untreated co-existing disease. Substance abuse in pregnancy is no longer a rare event. Obstetricians, paediatricians and anaesthetists are encountering an increasing number of pregnant women who use illicit substances, whether recreationally or as addicts [1]. In 1984, Frank *et al.* [2] reported that 17% of women delivering at Boston City Hospital had used an illicit drug at least once during pregnancy. In another study from the same hospital [3], it was reported that 18% of patients used cocaine during pregnancy.

THE WORLD

Substance abuse among women of childbearing age continues to be a major problem facing our society. The growing numbers of pregnant patients who are using illicit drugs are being reported from many sources throughout the world. For example, Chasnoff [4] reported that almost 15% of pregnant women in his study in the USA had a positive urine toxicology screen for cocaine, marijuana, alcohol or heroin. Recent data suggests that consumption of illicit drugs continues to increase in Europe, although cocaine use, which is being seen in epidemic proportions in the USA, is just starting to gain popularity in Western Europe and has not yet penetrated Eastern Europe [5]. Figure 17.1 shows the numbers of persons involved in illicit drugs in Belgium from 1983–1992. The Netherlands has also been seeing a growth of illicit drug use, and is now considered to be an important producer and exporter of synthetic drugs. In 1993 12 different laboratories which were synthesizing illicit drugs in the Netherlands were closed [6]. On one occasion in 1992, 2.5 million MDA (3,4-methylenedioxy-amphetamine) tablets were found by police during a raid and 1.6 million MDMA (*n*-methyl-3,4-methylenedioxy-amphetamine/XTC) tablets were found during a raid in 1993. Illicit drug use has increased throughout Europe as well. Although alcohol is the traditional substance abused in Eastern Europe, illicit drug use is also being seen. Recent figures project that there are 5.5 million drug addicts in the countries that comprised the former Soviet Union as

Clinical Problems in Obstetric Anaesthesia
Edited by Ian F. Russell and Gordon Lyons. Published in 1997 by Chapman & Hall, London. ISBN 0 412 71600 3.

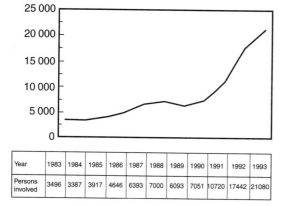

Year	1983	1984	1985	1986	1987	1988	1989	1990	1991	1992	1993
Persons involved	3496	3387	3917	4646	6393	7000	6093	7051	10720	17442	21080

Figure 17.1 Total number of people involved in illegal drugs in Belgium (National Statistics, Illegal Drugs in Belgium, National Police Department, Rijkswacht, Turnhout, Belgium, 1993).

compared to the approximately 20 million Americans using illicit drugs [7].

IN SOCIETY

Paternal as well as maternal behaviour, including drug abuse and domestic violence, may also impact on the well-being of the foetus. It has recently been argued that 'unconscious beliefs about gender appropriate behaviour have resulted in a skewed definition of foetal abuse, which focuses almost entirely upon socially inappropriate behaviours of the mother while ignoring the equally pernicious actions of their male partners' [8].

Of all the problems seen in inner-city pregnant woman, the use of illicit drugs can present one of the most difficult challenges to the anaesthetist. An illustrative example would be the anaesthetic management of a cocaine abusing patient admitted at 30 weeks' gestation in preterm labour with massive bleeding due to an abruptio placentae, foetal distress, and maternal cardiac arrhythmias, for an emergency caesarean section. The substance-abusing pregnant patient may also be seen in the main operating theatre in addition to labour and delivery, due to an acute injury. It

has recently been reported that recent substance abuse was documented in 48% of all injury deaths of pregnant patients in New York City [9].

Most pregnant drug abusers deny drug abuse, even when confronted with positive toxicology results. Among patients who do abuse illicit substances, polydrug use is the rule rather than the exception. This chapter will review the problems associated with the identification, treatment and anaesthetic management of women who abuse cocaine, narcotics, alcohol and cigarettes.

COCAINE ABUSE

Cocaine has been described in the USA as a major public health threat. While the use of most illicit drugs has remained stable or decreased in the USA over the past decade, the use of cocaine has increased dramatically, to the point where more than 5 million Americans abuse this drug regularly [10]. Approximately 60 tons of cocaine, worth upwards of $55 billion dollars are estimated to enter the USA each year [11]. Also large amounts of cocaine enter the Benelux countries. Figure 17.2 illustrates Belgian police activities involving cocaine, with more than two tons of cocaine being confiscated in Belgium in 1993.

The prevalence of cocaine use in the obstetric population is also increasing and anaesthetists, like obstetricians, paediatricians and emergency medicine physicians, are being exposed to patients under the effects of this potentially lethal drug. Positive cocaine toxicology results have been reported from across the USA and Europe, crossing geographic, socio-economic, and cultural boundaries. Because a majority of cocaine-abusing patients deny drug abuse [2], the exact extent of perinatal cocaine use is unknown. It has been estimated, however, that more than 50% of high-risk women cared for at urban teaching hospitals in the USA may be using cocaine [12]. Although patients who do not receive prenatal care ('unregistered') tend to have the highest

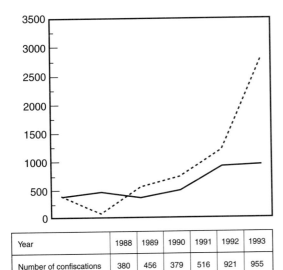

Year	1988	1989	1990	1991	1992	1993
Number of confiscations	380	456	379	516	921	955
Quantities confiscated (kg)	403	89	537	757	1221	2892

Figure 17.2 Belgian police activities involving cocaine (National Statistics, Illegal Drugs in Belgium, National Police Department, Rijkswacht, Turnhout, Belgium, 1993).

rates of cocaine use, registered private patients have also occasionally been found to be cocaine positive [13].

CLINICAL PHARMACOLOGY

Cocaine (benzoylmethylecgonine, $C_{17}H_{21}NO_4$) is an alkaloid derived from the plant *Erythroxylum coca* which is indigenous to Peru, Bolivia and Ecuador [14]. The alkalinized smokable form of cocaine is known as 'crack' and is presently the most widely used form of cocaine in the USA. Crack has become popular because it provides the abuser with an almost instant onset of intense euphoria at a low price. The pharmacologic effects of this drug are mediated through norepinephrine, dopamine and serotonin neurotransmitter systems [15]. By blocking the presynaptic reuptake of norepinephrine, cocaine produces an accumulation of this neurotransmitter and the expected clinical signs, including vasoconstriction, hypertension and tachycardia.

Despite the distinct clinical signs of cocaine abuse, one of the most difficult aspects of medical care for these women is the recognition of their cocaine use. A majority of cocaine abusers deny drug use when interviewed by physicians. Physical examination may lead to a suspicion of cocaine abuse, but in the pregnant patient, the differential diagnosis between preeclampsia and recent cocaine use may be difficult. Lack of prenatal care and cigarette smoking have been shown to be of predictive value in the recognition of a cocaine abuser and some authors have suggested that some of the foetal effects of cocaine may actually be due, at least in part, to other factors including cigarette smoking, alcohol intake and poor nutrition [16]. It has been suggested that the abuse of cocaine to the exclusion of all other psychoactive drugs is probably so rare that virtually all cocaine users are more accurately characterized as polydrug abusers who also use cocaine [17]. Perinatal cocaine abuse has been linked to many maternal and neonatal complications, which may tremendously impact on the patient's ability to withstand the stresses of anaesthesia and surgery. There is adequate data to demonstrate that cocaine use in pregnancy is dangerous to both mother and foetus [18].

It has been reported that pregnancy causes an increased sensitivity to the cardiovascular effects of cocaine [19]. Studies in pregnant and non-pregnant animals treated with progesterone to produce pregnancy levels have suggested that the metabolism of cocaine could be altered by the pregnant state [20]. The American College of Obstetrics and Gynecology has recognized that cocaine use has become a major public health concern and have published a review dealing with the ramifications of cocaine abuse in pregnancy [21]. They report that the medical complications which are found in association with cocaine use include the following:

- acute myocardial infarction, both with and without underlying coronary artery disease;

- cardiac arrhythmias, including life-threatening ventricular arrhythmias;
- rupture of the ascending aorta;
- stroke;
- seizures;
- bowel ischaemia;
- hyperthermia;
- malnutrition;
- sexually transmitted disease;
- hepatitis;
- endocarditis.

TESTING FOR COCAINE

Current laboratory screening methods for cocaine metabolites include gas chromatography, mass spectrometry and radioimmunoassay. The difficulty with some of these laboratory tests is the lag time between sending the sample and reporting of results. In some hospitals, it may take up to 72 hours to receive laboratory mass spectrometry toxicology results. These results may be of little benefit to the anaesthetist if the patient has undergone a cesarean section two days before! Although the reliability of urine testing depends on the time since the last exposure to the cocaine and the pharmacokinetics, an alternative testing method is available. An instant latex agglutination test for cocaine metabolites (OnTrak Assay ®, Roche Diagnostic Systems, Branchburg, NJ, USA) can provide an accurate result within four minutes and has been shown to be highly sensitive and specific when used by anaesthetists [9].

COCAINE AND THE PLACENTA

The use of cocaine in pregnancy has been associated with multiple adverse perinatal outcomes including an increased incidence of preterm labour, intra-uterine growth retardation, abruptio placentae, and pregnancy-induced hypertension [17, 22, 23]. Even after confounding variables such as age, race, alcohol abuse and smoking are taken into account, these complications are still seen and may be due to the vasoconstriction of uterine and umbilical vessels. It has recently been suggested that cocaine may do this by altering the placental production of prostaglandins, favouring thromboxane production, which may cause both vasoconstriction and decreased uteroplacental blood flow. There is evidence that cocaine may have a direct effect on several biochemical processes in the placenta [24]. Cocaine is rapidly transferred across the placenta by simple diffusion without metabolic conversion [25]. It has recently been suggested that the placental abnormalities which occur as a result of cocaine abuse may be the result of an impairment of the function of the placental serotonin transporter [26]. The effects of maternal cocaine use are thought to be incremental and cumulative [27]. Although there have been some conflicting reports, many authors have suggested that cocaine may have teratogenic effects including skeletal, urogenital, ophthalmologic and cardiac abnormalities [28].

ANAESTHESIA

The obstetric implications of maternal cocaine use include an increased incidence of spontaneous abortion, preterm labour, abruptio placentae and foetal distress [29]. Because these patients have a higher incidence of caesarean section due to 'foetal jeopardy', anaesthetists often meet these patients in an emergency setting. The choice of anaesthetic is occasionally dictated by the haemodynamic sequelae of cocaine use, as illustrated by abruptio placentae with massive haemorrhage. Even the strongest supporters of regional anaesthesia will select a general endotracheal anaesthetic for the hypotensive, hypovolaemic patient. In the more controlled situation, however, the anaesthetist will need to choose between the risks and benefits of regional and general anaesthesia in each individual patient. Epidural or spinal anaesthesia, unless contraindicated, is our first choice when administering an anaesthetic to the cocaine-abusing patient for caesarean section. Recently reported data on 'life-threatening' events that occurred under anaesthesia in the cocaine-abusing mother showed that these events were far more common during general anaesthesia than during regional anaesthesia [30].

The most frequently encountered problems under general anaesthesia were severe hypertension and arrhythmias. Since severe hypertension occurred most often after laryngoscopy, these patients should be treated prior to intubation. Propranolol is relatively contraindicated in the cocaine abuser since beta-blockade may cause unopposed alpha-adrenergic stimulation and therefore worsen the hypertension [31]. Labetalol, however, is very effective in treating the hypertension associated with acute cocaine intoxication [32]. Vertommen and coworkers evaluated hydralazine for the treatment of hypertension in these patients and concluded that it resulted in profound maternal tachycardia and did not restore uterine blood flow. Hughes compared this drug to labetalol and found that the latter did not increase heart rate and concluded that 'labetalol may be preferable to hydralazine for treatment of the acutely cocaine-intoxicated woman' [33]. Because these patients are at such a high risk for the development of arrhythmias, in the event that a general anaesthetic becomes necessary halothane should be avoided. Ketamine may also potentiate the cardiac effects of cocaine by further increasing catecholamine levels. There has also been a report of a prolonged block from succinylcholine in a cocaine-abusing patient, so caution should be taken if using this muscle relaxant [34]. Patients with a history of chronic cocaine use need to be monitored preoperatively, intraoperatively and postoperatively for signs of myocardial ischaemia. It has been reported that cocaine users frequently develop silent myocardial ischaemia manifesting as episodes of ST elevation during the first weeks of withdrawal [35].

The use of regional anaesthesia in the cocaine abuser may also be associated with

life-threatening risks, however. Thrombocytopenia has been reported as being associated with cocaine abuse and therefore these patients may be at risk of developing an epidural haematoma. Profound hypotension may occur after achievement of a sympathetic block and the cocaine-abusing patient may not respond appropriately to ephedrine. Should these patients develop ephedrine-resistant hypotension, they do respond to small doses of phenylephrine.

NARCOTIC ABUSE

Heroin, morphine, meperidine (pethidine) methadone and fentanyl have all been reported as being abused in pregnancy. Although a decrease is currently being seen in the incidence of patients in New York who present to the labour floor who are acutely abusing narcotics, it has been estimated that 250 000 women in the USA are intravenous drug abusers, with 90% of them being of childbearing age [36]. Perinatal abuse of narcotics may be associated with a host of medical problems including acquired immunodeficiency syndrome (AIDS), hepatitis, endocarditis, pulmonary, renal and cardiac disease. These patients may present with either narcotic overdose or withdrawal syndrome and often require caesarean section for foetal distress. Acute withdrawal syndrome may be recognized by tremors, anxiety, muscle pains, nausea, vomiting, anorexia, gastro-intestinal pain, tachycardia, hypertension and mydriasis. These signs peak at 48–72 hours after the last narcotic intake. The use of narcotic antagonists or agonist–antagonist drugs may precipitate acute withdrawal and therefore should not be used [37]. Narcotic overdose can be identified by coma, miosis or respiratory depression. When treating the patient with a narcotic overdose and a reduced conscious level, securing the airway should be performed immediately to decrease the risk of aspiration.

Regional anaesthetic techniques can provide comfort without the need for narcotic administration. The narcotic-abusing patient often has pain intolerance due to decreased endogenous opioid peptides and therefore is often intolerant of the pain of labour. In the rehabilitated narcotic abuser, the use of a regional anaesthetic allows for a comfortable patient without the administration of opioids. Local anaesthetics can also be used for post-operative pain management in these patients.

ALCOHOL ABUSE

It has been estimated that there are over 15 million alcoholics in the USA and that approximately a quarter of them are women [38]. It has been estimated that the percentage of the population who abuse alcohol is greater in Europeans with the largest percentage in the people of the former Soviet Union [7]. Over the past 40 years alcohol consumption rose 600% in the former USSR, whereas the population during that time period grew only 25%. Alcohol abuse can present numerous challenges to the anaesthetist since it can be associated with abnormalities of all body systems. For example, alcohol abuse has been associated with cardiomyopathy, decreased albumin concentration, coagulopathy, liver disease, ascites and electrolyte abnormalities.

Pietrantoni and Knuppel have defined a moderate drinker as one who consumes an average of three drinks a week to one drink a day and rarely more than three or four drinks at one sitting. They define a heavy drinker as one who has, on average, at least two drinks a day and sometimes five or six in one sitting. Heavy drinkers are in the group that can be expected to manifest multiple medical problems [39].

Alcohol is a known teratogen and its use in pregnancy is associated with the foetal alcohol syndrome. Signs and symptoms of this syndrome include craniofacial, cardiac, renal and musculocutaneous abnormalities. Children with complete foetal alcohol syndrome (FAS) are usually born to mothers who consume large amounts of alcohol throughout preg-

nancy. However, because a safe level of alcohol intake in pregnancy has not been established, abstinence is considered the safest course during pregnancy [40]. FAS is seen in 1% of all births in the Netherlands, which amounts to 350 babies born annually with FAS and another 350 babies with partial FAS.

In the absence of a coagulopathy or neuropathy, alcoholics can be safely and successfully anaesthetized using a regional anaesthetic. Occasionally, regional techniques in these patients may fail due to psychotic or combative behaviour. Should these patients require a general anaesthetic, a major consideration is prevention of aspiration since alcohol increases gastric acid secretion while decreasing protective reflexes. Because these patients may present with severe hypoalbuminaemia or cardiac manifestations of alcohol abuse, they may be sensitive to the myocardial depressant effect of anaesthetics. Due to tolerance and an expanded plasma volume, however, many alcoholics will require larger than normal doses of induction agents.

CIGARETTES

Pregnant patients probably abuse this substance more than any of the other substances previously described. In 1990, it was estimated that 29% of American women of childbearing age smoked cigarettes [41]. Despite the fact that there is no longer any doubt that cigarette smoking has adverse effects on mother and foetus, only 20% of women in the USA quit smoking during pregnancy [42]. Smoking during pregnancy has been associated with intra-uterine growth retardation, spontaneous abortion, premature rupture of membranes, placenta praevia, abruptio placentae and sudden infant death syndrome [43]. Because of these risks, Benowitz has suggested that nicotine replacement therapy be used on pregnant cigarette smokers [44].

Cigarette smoke is composed of over 1000 components, many of which affect the respiratory, cardiovascular and immune systems [45].

The respiratory effects of cigarette smoke include abnormalities in mucus secretion, ciliary transport and small airway function [46]. Postoperative respiratory morbidity is therefore a major risk of general anaesthesia in cigarette smoking patients. Although four to six weeks of abstinence are required to allow a decrease in the risk of postoperative respiratory complications, after as little as 48 hours of abstinence carboxyhaemoglobin levels fall and oxygen delivery increases. In addition, a few days of abstinence will improve mucociliary transport. The use of regional anaesthesia is particularly beneficial to the cigarette-smoking parturient undergoing cesarean section, by allowing an alternative to general anaesthesia and the risk of bronchospasm that may develop during airway manipulation.

REFERENCES

1. Knisely, J.S., Spear, E.R., Green, D.J. *et al.* (1991) Substance abuse patterns in pregnant women. *NIDA Research Monograph*, **105**, 280–1.
2. Frank, D.A., Zuckerman, B.S., Amaro, H. *et al.* (1988) Cocaine use during pregnancy: prevalence and correlates. *Pediatrics*, **82**, 888–95.
3. Zuckerman, B., Frank, D.A. Hingson, R. *et al.* (1989) Effects of maternal marijuana and cocaine on fetal growth. *New England Journal of Medicine*, **320**, 762–81.
4. Chasnoff, I.J., Landress, H.J. and Barrett, M.E. (1990) The prevalence of illicit drug or alcohol use during pregnancy and discrepancies in mandatory reporting in Pinellas County, Florida. *New England Journal of Medicine*, **322**, 1202–6.
5. Johns, A. (1990) Drug abuse in Eastern Europe. *Lancet*, **337**, 38–9.
6. Narcotica (1993) *Jaarbericht Central Recherch Info*, 8–11.
7. Davis, R.B. (1994) Drug and alcohol use in the former Soviet Union: Selected factors and future considerations. *International Journal of the Addictions*, **29**, 303–23.
8. Schroedel, J.R. and Peretz, P. (1994) A gender analysis of policy formation: the case of fetal abuse. *Journal of Health, Politics, Policy and Law*, **19**, 335–60.
9. Dannenberg, A.L., Carter, D.M., Lawson, H.W. *et al.* (1995) Homicide and other injuries as causes of maternal death in New York City, 1987–1991. *American Journal of Obstetrics and Gynecology*, **172**, 1557–64.
10. Rozenak, D., Diamant, Y.Z., Yaffe, H. *et al.* (1990) Cocaine: maternal use during pregnancy and its effect on the mother, the fetus and the infant. *Obstetric Gynecology Survey*, **45**, 348–59.
11. Gold, M.S. and Giannini, A.J. (1989) Cocaine and cocaine addiction, in *Drugs of Abuse* (eds A.J. Giannini and A.E. Slaby), Medical Economics Books, Oradell, pp. 83.
12. Birnbach, D.J., Stein, D.J., Thomas, K. *et al.* (1993) Instant recognition of the cocaine abusing parturient. *Anesthesiology*, **79**, A987.
13. Schutzman, D.L., Frankenfield-Chernicoff, M., Clatterbaugh, H.E. *et al.* (1991) Incidence of intrauterine cocaine exposure in a suburban setting. *Pediatrics*, **88**, 825–7.
14. Fleming, J.A., Byck, R. and Barash, P.G. (1990) Pharmacology and therapeutic applications of cocaine. *Anesthesiology*, **73**, 518–31.
15. Gold, M.S., Washton, A.M. and Dackis, C.A. (1985) Cocaine abuse: neurochemistry, phenomenology, and treatment. *National Institute of Drug Abuse Research Monograph Series*, **61**, 130–50.
16. Snodgrass, S.R. (1994) Cocaine babies: A result of multiple teratogenic influences. *Journal of Child Neurology*, **9**, 227–33.
17. Hutchings, D.E. (1993) The puzzle of cocaine's effects following maternal use during pregnancy: Are there reconcilable differences? *Neurotoxicology and Teratology*, **15**, 281–6.
18. Little, B.B., Snell, L.M., Klein, V.R. *et al.* (1989) Cocaine abuse during pregnancy: maternal and fetal implications. *Obstetrics and Gynecology*, **73**, 157–60.
19. Wood, J.R. Jr and Plessinger, M.A. (1990) Pregnancy increases cardiovascular toxicity to cocaine. *American Journal of Obstetrics and Gynecology*, **162**, 529–34.
20. Plesinger, M.A. and Woods, J.R. Jr (1993) Maternal, placenta and fetal pathophysiology of cocaine exposure during pregnancy. *Clinical Obstetrics and Gynecology*, **36**, 267–78.
21. ACOG Committee Opinion: Committee on Obstetrics (1993) Maternal and Fetal Medicine Number 114. *International Journal of Gynecology and Obstetrics*, **41**, 102–5.
22. MacGregor, S.N., Keith, L.G. and Chasnoff, I.J. (1987) Cocaine use during pregnancy: adverse perinatal outcome. *American Journal of Obstetrics and Gynecology*, **157**, 686–90.

23. Dombrowski, M.P., Wolfe, H.M., Welch, R.A. *et al.* (1991) Cocaine abuse is associated with abruptio placentae and decreased birth weight, but not shorter labor. *Obstetrics and Gynecology*, **77**, 139–41.

24. Ganapathy, V., Ramamoorthy, S. and Leibach, F.H. (1993) Transport and metabolism of monoamines in the human placenta. *Trophoblast Research*, **7**, 35–51.

25. Krishna, R.B., Levitz, M. and Dancis, J. (1993) Transfer of cocaine by the perfused human placenta: The effect of binding to serum proteins. *American Journal of Obstetrics and Gynecology*, **169**, 1418–23.

26. Prasad, P.D., Leibach, F.H., Mahesh, V.B. *et al.* (1994) Human placenta as a target organ for cocaine action: interaction of cocaine with the placental serotonin transporter. *Placenta*, **15**, 267–78.

27. Nair, B.S. and Watson, R.R. (1991) Cocaine and the pregnant woman. *Journal of Reproductive Medicine*, **36**, 862–7.

28. Fantel, A.G. and Macphail, B.J. (1982) The teratogenicity of cocaine. *Teratology*, **26**, 17–19.

29. Mastrogiannis, D.S., Decavalas, G.O., Verma, U.M.A. and Tejani, N. (1990) Perinatal outcome after recent cocaine use. *Obstetrics and Gynecology*, **76**, 8–11.

30. Birnbach, D.J., Stein, D.J., Thomas, K. *et al.* (1993) Cocaine abuse in the parturient. What are the implications to the anesthesiologist? *Anesthesiology*, **79**, A988.

31. Ramoska, E. and Sacchetti, A. (1985) Propranolol induced hypertension in the treatment of cocaine intoxication. *Annals of Emergency Medicine*, **14**, 1112–3.

32. Gay, G.R. and Loper, K.A. (1988) The use of labetalol in the management of cocaine crisis. *Annals of Emergency Medicine*, **17**, 282–3.

33. Vertommen, J.D., Hughes, S.C., Rosen, M.A. *et al.* (1992) Hydralazine does not restore uterine blood flow during cocaine-induced hypertension in the pregnant ewe. *Anesthesiology*, **76**, 580–7.

34. Jatlow, P., Barash, P.G., Van Dyke, C. *et al.* (1979) Cocaine and succinylcholine sensitivity: a new caution. *Anesthesia and Analgesia*, **58**, 235–8.

35. Nademanee, K., Gorelick, D.A., Josephson, M.A. *et al.* (1989) Myocardial ischemia during cocaine withdrawal. *Annals of Internal Medicine*, **111**, 876–80.

36. Hoegerman, G. and Schnoll, S. (1991) Narcotic use in pregnancy. *Clinical Perinatology*, **18**, 51–76.

37. Weintraub, S.J. and Naulty, J.S. (1985) Acute abstinence syndrome after epidural injection of butorphanol. *Anesthesia and Analgesia*, **64**, 452–3.

38. Williams, G.D., Grant, B.F., Harford, T.C. and Noble, B.A. (1989) Population projections using DSM-III Criteria. Alcohol abuse and dependence, 1990–2000. *Alcohol Health Research World*, **13**, 366–70.

39. Pietrantoni, M. and Knuppel, R.A. (1991) Alcohol use in pregnancy. *Clinical Perinatology*, **18**, 93–111.

40. Council on Scientific Affairs, American Medical Association (1983) Fetal effects of maternal alcohol use. *Journal of the American Medical Association*, **249**, 2517–21.

41. US Department of Health and Human Services (1991) *National Household Survey on Drug Abuse*, Washington DC, Public Health Service.

42. Prager, K., Malin, H., Spiegler, D. *et al.* (1984) Smoking and drinking behavior before and during pregnancy of married mothers of live-born infants and stillborn infants. *Public Health Report*, **99**, 117–27.

43. Feng, T. (1993) Substance abuse in pregnancy. *Current Opinion in Obstetrics and Gynecology*, **5**, 16–23.

44. Benowitz, N.L. (1991) Nicotine replacement therapy during pregnancy. *Journal of the American Medical Association*, **266**, 3174–7.

45. Stedman, R.L. (1968) The chemical composition of tobacco and tobacco smoke. *Chemical Review*, **68**, 153–207.

46. Pearce, A.C. and Jones, R.M. (1984) Smoking and anesthesia: preoperative abstinence and perioperative morbidity. *Anesthesiology*, **61**, 576–84.

18

CO-EXISTING NEUROLOGICAL DISORDERS

G. Lyons

BACKGROUND

In the 1984 edition of his textbook, the late J. Selwyn Crawford wrote 'A necessary preamble to the provision of a continuous lumbar epidural block for labour to a patient who is suffering from a chronic neurological disease is an explicit discussion of the inoffensiveness of the technique' [1]. Neurological disease had long been featured in the list of contraindications to regional blockade on the grounds that the latter has the potential to exacerbate the former, and that such a policy was a prudent way to circumvent litigation [2]. Evidence that either the provision, or the withholding, of regional blockade, has any influence on the risk of litigation, is lacking. Common sense on the one hand, and an accumulation of negative experience on the other, have inclined many practising anaesthetists to offer regional blockade to women suffering from chronic neurological conditions. Some of these conditions may be progressive, such as multiple sclerosis, and others, like poliomyelitis and cerebral palsy are not. Rarely the anaesthetist may be presented with progressive lesions that may have short histories and specific cautions with regard to regional blockade. The space-occupying lesion is one example of this. Some lesions arise acutely, and avoidance of regional blockade is often desirable, for example, when there is a disturbance of conscious level.

Obstetric general anaesthesia is less commonly associated with neurological sequelae than regional. The North American closed claims experience reveals that 50% of regional anaesthesia claims were paid out for 'maternal nerve damage' at a mean sum of US$ 38 000. However, 43% of regional anaesthesia claims were resisted, compared with only 27% of general anaesthesia claims. Regional anaesthesia resulted in fewer deaths and smaller payouts than general anaesthesia, and there were no clues to suggest that neurological diseases attracted litigation. However, seizures were the single most damaging event in association with regional blockade [3], and they and their significance will be considered below.

ACUTE DISORDERS

SEIZURES

When a seizure occurs peripartum the major problem presenting to the medical attendants is one of differential diagnosis [4]. When an epidural local anaesthetic top-up is the immediately preceding event, it is probably correct to

Clinical Problems in Obstetric Anaesthesia
Edited by Ian F. Russell and Gordon Lyons. Published in 1997 by Chapman & Hall, London. ISBN 0 412 71600 3.

Table 18.1 Incidence of seizures [2, 5–8, 10, 11]

	Incidence	Annual maternal mortality, UK
Intravenous bupivacaine	1 : 3500 to 1 : 23 800 epidurals	0
Eclampsia	1 : 2000 deliveries	4–5
Epilepsy	1 : 200 people	3–4

assume that the causative factor is inadvertent intravenous injection. Crawford classified this as a 'potentially life-threatening' complication, with an incidence in his practice of 1:13 500 epidurals, with no permanent damage [5]. Scott and Hibbard found an incidence of 1:23 800 in 500 000 epidurals in the UK with good recovery, though one suffered a transient cardiac arrest [6]. The US closed claims study reports 83% of seizures resulted in neurological injury or death to mother or foetus, or both. Almost all of these seizures were due to intravenous local anaesthetic, but two were due to eclampsia [3]. Clearly the inadvertent intravenous injection of local anaesthetic has been a more benign experience in the UK than the US. Seizures due to eclampsia can have a poor outcome. In the UK, four to five deaths occur every year in association with eclampsia. Approximately half have multiple convulsions [7, 8].

Distinguishing eclampsia from idiopathic epilepsy is not always easy because 38% of seizures occur before proteinuria and hypertension are documented. Case history and clinical examination remain essential to the differential diagnosis, and the electroencephalogram has been helpful in differentiating between eclampsia and epilepsy [9]. The incidence of eclampsia is 1:2000 deliveries, with three out of four women having their first seizure in hospital. One in fifty die, and 35% have at least one major complication. The still birth rate is 22:1000, and the neonatal death rate is 34:1000. Preterm pregnancies fare worst [10]. Epilepsy is the most common serious neurological problem encountered in obstetric practice, with an incidence of 0.3 to 0.5% of all pregnancies [11]. At least three maternal deaths per annum are attributed to epilepsy in the UK [8].

A seizure may also represent the primary manifestation of water intoxication or an intracranial catastrophe, or even hyperthyroidism. Whatever the cause, seizures have the potential to injure mother and child severely, and frequently initiate a move to caesarean delivery [4]. The prevention and management of epileptic seizures will be considered below. The incidence of seizures in the UK is given in Table 18.1.

Epilepsy

The effects of pregnancy on the individual epileptic are not predictable. While the choice and availability of anticonvulsants varies from region to region, they are, in general, a group of drugs that tend to be cleared more rapidly in pregnancy. Without a compensatory change in dosage, blood levels may become subtherapeutic, and relapses will occur. Even if blood levels are maintained 5–15% of women will experience an increase in their incidence of seizures during pregnancy, particularly those with longstanding epilepsy [12], but this is less likely to happen in those who are well controlled prepregnancy [11]. The *Report on Confidential Enquiries into Maternal Deaths in the United Kingdom 1988–1990* recommends that doses of anticonvulsants are increased in pregnancy, and, following a maternal death, that postmortem blood samples are analysed to assess the blood level of anticonvulsant [8].

Gestational epilepsy is the name given to the disorder when seizures occur only during pregnancy. It cannot be distinguished from the onset in pregnancy of idiopathic epilepsy, and is not thought to require any treatment [11].

Management of seizures

A seizure that is not associated with high blood levels of local anaesthetic, nor with preeclamptic changes in the placenta, should not necessarily be responsible for obstetric complications. However, if airway obstruction or inadequate ventilation due to muscle rigidity results in hypoxia and acidosis, decelerations in the foetal heart rate may become apparent [11], necessitating delivery using general anaesthesia. Failure to control seizures is an indication to expedite delivery, and in this unit the mother would remain intubated and ventilated after delivery until control is obtained. Initial management should be intravenous diazemuls 5 mg, repeated until convulsions cease [13]. The use of diazepam is associated with adverse effects on the foetus, but in a life-threatening situation, the risk is acceptable. Both the drug and its active metabolite, *n*-desmethyl diazepam, cross the placenta freely and accumulate in the foetus at serum levels up to three times those in the mother. Equilibrium between mother and foetus is established five to ten minutes after an intravenous injection. It is not harmful when given in labour, but loss of beat to beat variation of the foetal heart rate may be seen on the cardiotocograph, and a reduction in foetal movement may accompany its use. Neonatal effects are not seen until maternal doses in the region of 30–40 mg are given, when hypotonia, lethargy and feeding problems may be apparent. It appears in breast milk, and its use in lactating women is not recommended [14].

Three drugs that are commonly used in the long term prevention of epilepsy are phenytoin, carbamazepine and valproic acid. Their use in pregnancy is associated with a syndrome of congenital deformities incorporating craniofacial and digital abnormalities, and developmental delay. Overall the epileptic woman has a 2 to 3% greater risk of giving birth to a child with a congenital anomaly than her normal counterpart. Maternal folic acid deficiency is a special risk requiring close monitoring and treatment when indicated. A deficiency of vitamin K dependent clotting factors in the mother can give rise to haemorrhagic disease of the newborn if supplements are not given to the mother [14]. Because of the increased risk of neural tube defects associated with the use of valproic acid and carbamazepine, the Committee on the Safety of Medicines has advised that women already pregnant should be offered alpha-foetoprotein monitoring and a second trimester ultrasound scan [15]. Changing medication to avoid teratogenicity is another factor contributing to deterioration in pregnancy, and the risk of the former must be balanced with that of the latter [12]. All three drugs are compatible with breast feeding. Carbamazepine is given a lower risk category than phenytoin or valproic acid [14], but only time will tell if this is justified. Experience with new drugs such as clonazepam, clobazam, gabapentin, lamotrigine and vigabatrin is either insufficient or lacking altogether.

General anaesthesia

Thiopentone and propofol are credited with anticonvulsant properties, but the manufacturers warn against the use of propofol in epileptics. Etomidate is regarded as equivocal [16]. Isoflurane may be the volatile agent of choice, but although the use of enflurane is associated with epileptiform activity, this is unlikely at concentrations used in obstetric practice [17].

Regional blockade

Local anaesthetics are known convulsants, but seizures will only occur when blood levels are high. At levels associated with normal therapeutic activity however, their membrane-stabilizing effects may guard against seizure discharges. There are no special contraindications to the use of regional techniques [16], but there is a single case report of a first seizure occurring during a caesarean section under epidural anaesthesia [18].

Opioids

The administration of opioid analgesics is sometimes accompanied by myoclonic movement, but this has never been proven to be epileptiform in nature, and there are no special concerns over their use in epileptics. A metabolite of pethidine, norpethidine, has central excitatory effects, but given the wide choice in this field, there is no difficulty in avoiding its use [17].

Epilepsy and anaesthetic drugs

- There are no contraindications to regional blockade
- Thiopentone and isoflurane are recommended
- Diazemuls is the drug of choice for acute disorders

Water intoxication

The infusion of sodium-poor fluids such as 5% glucose as a vehicle for oxytocin to accelerate labour, has the potential to reduce plasma sodium. Large volumes, long periods of infusion, poor regulation and the antidiuretic effect of oxytocics, all predispose to hyponatraemia. When the plasma concentration of sodium falls below 120 mmol/l, a confusional state and seizures can occur. This may or may not be accompanied by fluid overload, the pulmonary effects of which can be monitored with a pulse oximeter. If renal function is normal, excess water is excreted and the electrolyte balance restored without the need for significant intervention. Prevention is the best treatment; use of sodium-containing fluids rather than pure glucose solutions, high concentrations of oxytocics to reduce infusion volumes and careful monitoring of input and output volumes will avoid this problem [11].

STROKE

Stroke can be defined as the sudden onset of motor and sensory deficit as the result of an ischaemic or haemorrhagic event. The incidence is 1:6000 pregnancies, comprising haemorrhagic (1:15 000) and non-haemorrhagic (1:10 000) [19]. In public hospitals in the Ile de France, the corresponding figures are 1:22 000 for haemorrhagic and 1:23 000 for non-haemorrhagic [20]. In the USA, the Maternal Mortality Collaborative gives 8.5% of 601 maternal deaths between 1980 and 1985 as being caused by stroke. When stroke is suspected a laboratory coagulation screen should always be performed. Examination of the cerebrospinal fluid has given way to computerized tomography and magnetic resonance imaging, and some will require angiography in addition. Whatever the nature of the lesion and its aetiology, outcomes range from recovery with no residual deficit, through permanent disability, to death. While the incidences of haemorrhagic and non-haemorrhagic stroke might be similar the causes and requirements are not, and these are discussed separately below.

Non-haemorrhagic stroke

Classically these are caused by arterial or venous thromboses, or emboli. Approximately one half will have had eclampsia diagnosed [20], and one quarter will have atherosclerosis, hypertension, diabetes or hyperlipidaemia [11]. Unusual causes must be investigated, and might include extracranial vertebral artery dissection, postpartum cerebral angiopathy, inherited protein S deficiency, or disseminated intravascular coagulation (DIC) associated with amniotic fluid embolism. Sharshar *et al.*, despite considerable investigation, failed to establish a cause in four out of 31 cases [20]. Embolic events might be due to valvular heart disease, atrial fibrillation or subacute bacterial endocarditis, and some women will require anticoagulation with heparin. Non-haemorrhagic strokes tend to present postpartum. The sudden onset of blindness, sometimes without a demonstrable occipital lesion, is generally associated with preeclampsia, but resolves in hours to days [21].

Anaesthesia and analgesia

With ischaemic strokes the principle of management is to avoid extremes of hypertension and hypotension, particular the latter when the possibility of impaired flow exists. When faced with established lesions, a high standard of care is required irrespective of the choice of technique. The latter may well be dictated by the aetiology of the stroke, since, for example, alterations in coagulation from either the prime disorder or its treatment might contraindicate regional blockade.

Haemorrhagic stroke

In the UK between 1988 and 1990, there were 35 maternal deaths following intracranial haemorrhage. Fourteen of these were complications of the hypertensive disorders of pregnancy and will not be discussed further, while 21 were due to primary disorders of the central nervous system. Of the latter, subarachnoid haemorrhage accounted for twelve and nine had other causes. Only two had symptoms prior to the fatal event, and perimortem caesarean section was performed in four. One of the former two cases had a twin pregnancy and presented at 38 weeks with headaches and neck stiffness requiring her admission to hospital. The decision to induce labour unleashed a cascade of undesirable events that ended with brain stem death. A berry aneurysm was found at autopsy [8]. When an aneurysm ruptures in pregnancy the risk of recurrent haemorrhage is 70%, with an 80% maternal mortality [22]. Intracranial aneurysms and arteriovenous malformations (AVM) are subject to bleeding and require a common approach.

Cerebral venous thrombosis

Although thrombotic in nature, cerebral venous thrombosis tends to produce a haemorrhagic form of stroke. Predisposing factors such as infection and dehydration are more likely to occur postpartum, and it can also arise as a complication of sickle cell disease [19].

Intracranial aneurysms and arteriovenous malformations

Subarachnoid haemorrhage (SAH) has an incidence between one and five cases per 10 000 pregnancies. For those under 25 years of age arteriovenous malformation (AVM) is more likely to be the cause of haemorrhage than berry aneurysm. The maternal mortality from AVM in pregnancy is 28% with depression of conscious levels in some 57%. One third of haemorrhages are due to causes which may not be identified: these include subacute bacterial endocarditis, vasculitis of systemic lupus erythematosus, cerebral venous thrombosis and spinal haemorrhage. Some patients will be admitted in coma, and all are likely to rebleed. While the conscious may complain of occipital and nuchal ache, nausea and vomiting and have a mild fever beware, since a fluctuating hypertension, tachyarrhythmias and leucocytosis might point erroneously to atypical eclampsia. Magnetic resonance imaging is useful and angiography can be performed with local anaesthesia using retrograde femoral arterial catheterization [23]. Surgery and embolization may have a place.

Moyamoya

Named in Japanese after the puff of smoke appearance at angiography, this rare condition is of unknown aetiology, but is not confined to Japan. Both intracranial carotid arteries are stenotic or occluded at the terminal bifurcation, and the resultant proliferation of small vessels, when filled with contrast, looks like smoke. Presentation during pregnancy is sometimes with seizures, following an intra-cerebral bleed [23–25].

Aneurysms tend to weaken in pregnancy, but are less likely to rupture during labour than AVMs. The latter enlarge during pregnancy, and then return to normal size within a few days of delivery. Postpartum bleeding is more likely to be from an aneurysm. SAH in pregnancy can precipitate labour, and once haemorrhage has occurred, a rebleed during labour is a high risk. Intrapartum cerebral haemorrhage is thought to be related to the Valsalva manoeuvre and second stage straining. The aim of anaesthetic management is the prevention of both hypertension and the elevation of intracranial pressure, and caesarean delivery using epidural anaesthesia is recommended [26]. Although labour can be avoided by caesarean section, the peripartum risks remain: a primipara who survived two episodes of bleeding from an AVM had a successful caesarean delivery – a single dose of ephedrine was given, and the avoidance of vomiting was stressed [27]. The same considerations for neurosurgical intervention apply as for the non-pregnant, and when an aneurysm is surgically treated the prognosis for the baby is excellent [11]. Even when an aneurysm has been clipped, an elective assisted vaginal delivery with an epidural is advised [22]. Surgical excision of AVM may be possible but carries a high risk. For survivors, the same approach to delivery suffices [28].

Simultaneous caesarean section and clipping of berry aneurysm

If surgery is indicated for a berry aneurysm, neurosurgical considerations take precedence, but aortocaval compression should be avoided and the foetal heart rate monitored [22]. If the gestation is appropriate, caesarean section can be performed simultaneously [29]. To spare the foetus the hazards of neuroanaesthesia, caesarean section is performed first. Dexamethasone may be given to reduce cerebral oedema [30], or it may be given for foetal lung matura-

tion [23]. If general anaesthesia is employed, beta-blockade has been used to blunt the hypertensive response to intubation, proceeding to caesarean delivery with established techniques. Craniotomy follows with mannitol, frusemide and induced hypotension [30, 31]. An alternative approach is to use epidural anaesthesia for caesarean delivery, followed by general anaesthesia for craniotomy: intubation, peaks of hypertension, beta-blockade and vasodilator drugs are thus avoided whilst the foetus is *in utero*, and the epidural can be used for postoperative analgesia without disturbance of conscious level. There is a theoretical risk of producing a rise in intracranial pressure as the epidural space is filled with local anaesthetic, but this can be prevented by slow injection or infusion. Both the described techniques have been used successfully [30–32]. Ergometrine should be avoided, and one group used an infusion of prostaglandin E_1 both to maintain uterine contraction, and induce hypotension, during craniotomy [31].

Persistent vegetative state

Intracranial haemorrhage may occasionally leave a young woman with severe permanent brain damage. Depending on the gestation, the goal of management will be either to support the mother for 48 hours until lung maturation can be improved with dexamethasone, or for a longer period until the foetus is viable. The clinical problem lies in the choice of drugs for maternal sedation during ventilation. Propofol is not recommended for sedating children in intensive care, but would allow periodic assessment of the mother's condition. Benzodiazepines have a longer elimination half-life and tend to accumulate. In a single report propofol was used for 48 hours before delivery, and, while the baby required intubation, there was no long-term problem [23]. In another case, an intracranial bleed at 15 weeks resulted in death at 22 weeks despite intensive therapy: problems with maternal maintenance and foetal growth proved insuperable during this longer period [33]. The best course of action is undecided.

BELL'S PALSY

Idiopathic facial paralysis is three times more likely to occur in pregnancy. One woman experienced it during each of her four pregnancies with complete postpartum resolution on each occasion [34]. In a ten-year review Dorsey and Camann found 36 cases of Bell's palsy associated with pregnancy in Brigham and Women's Hospital. Approximately two thirds of these occurred in the third trimester with the remainder being postpartum. There was no evidence to suggest that the incidence postpartum was related to any particular form of anaesthesia nor that, once established, the palsy was a reason for avoiding any form of anaesthesia. Preeclampsia was diagnosed in 19%, supporting an aetiology of fluid retention, but there is also a viral hypothesis [35]. Prognosis is poorer if taste is lost [11]. Steroids may be beneficial if given within 48 hours [11].

PROGRESSIVE DISORDERS

RAISED INTRACRANIAL PRESSURE

The stigmata of raised intracranial pressure include headaches, nausea and vomiting. The suspected presence of a space-occupying lesion invites careful examination of the fundi for papilloedema and, if present, all forms of anaesthesia are contraindicated except for general. When a space-occupying lesion exists without a disturbance of cerebrospinal fluid pressure, management must be directed at maintaining the status quo. Factors that might have adverse effects include respiratory depressants such as opioid analgesics, bearing down in the second stage, extreme changes in blood pressure, rapid epidural injection of fluid and dural puncture. Options for management include neurosurgery, elective caesarean section, perhaps in tandem, and epidural analgesia in labour. The latter has been used to control delivery in the second stage in the presence of both hydrocephalus and neoplastic growths, with good effect, but an inadvertent dural puncture would be a disaster [36]. This option is only for the very experienced [37].

Neoplasms

Intracranial neoplasms in pregnancy are very rare, with an estimated incidence of 3.6 per million live births. Fluid retention during pregnancy may promote peri tumour oedema formation, and pituitary tumours may enlarge during pregnancy [37]. Otherwise, concerns are managed along principles already established: neurosurgical considerations take precedence [38], and measures should be taken to avoid increases in intracranial pressure associated with labour.

Hydrocephalus

Wisoff *et al.* report a series of 21 pregnancies in 18 women with ventricular drainage shunts. Neurological complications occurred during pregnancy in 76%. More than half had symptoms related to increases in intracranial pressure, and 12% suffered exacerbations of seizure disorders. Surgery for shunt obstruction was required in 23%, but in two thirds all problems resolved postpartum. An early caesarean section using general anaesthesia is recommended if there is neurological instability. Antenatal monitoring of intracranial pressure and shunt patency is required, together with antibiotic prophylaxis against *Staphylococcus* species at delivery [36]. If the shunt is patent, there is no contraindication to regional anaesthesia. Antibiotic prophylaxis for this should be considered.

Raised intracranial pressure

Do

- Consider neurosurgery
- Consider elective caesarean section
- Have a low threshold for general anaesthesia
- Use epidural analgesia in labour
- Avoid extreme changes in blood pressure

Do not

- Use respiratory depressants, opioids and benzodiazepines
- Permit bearing down in the second stage
- Inject volumes of epidural drugs rapidly
- Puncture the dura

Benign intracranial hypertension

The diagnosis is generally made by exclusion. Periodic removal of cerebrospinal fluid is sometimes performed. Restrictions with regard to regional blockade are the same as for other causes of intracranial hypertension [11].

MULTIPLE SCLEROSIS

Multiple sclerosis (MS) is the most common crippling neurological disease of young adults. The greatest incidence of onset is between the ages of 20 and 35 and twice as many women as men are affected [39]. It is a patchy demyelinating disorder subject to relapses and remissions, and is characterized by weakness, inco-ordination, diplopia, blindness, sensory changes and vertigo. Uncomplicated MS does not have any effect on the outcomes of pregnancy, but pregnancy tends to have a protective effect on MS. However, onset and relapses are more common in the puerperium, and up to 40% of sufferers will experience a postpartum exacerbation within six months [11].

Anaesthesia and analgesia

Donaldson recommends that regional and general anaesthesia be administered in the usual fashion [11]. Certainly, there are reports of postpartum relapses both with and without epidural analgesia and anaesthesia, and general anaesthesia [40], and one report of epidural analgesia without relapse [41]. Warren *et al.* report a single case of recurrent sensory disturbance on the right thigh that occurred after epidural analgesia on two occasions, and lasted for six weeks [42]. Bader and colleagues question whether higher concentrations of epidural local anaesthetic are associated with a higher relapse rate [43], but as far as epidural and general techniques are concerned, most would regard them as perfectly compatible with MS. As regards spinal anaesthesia, in 1937, Macdonald Critchley said 'Spinal anaesthesia may be a precipitating agent in the evolution of such affections as disseminated sclerosis', and quoted a single instance of optic neuritis which occurred three days after spinal anaesthesia for a knee operation [2]. To this day, this single statement, carrying with it the inference that spinal anaesthesia may have some responsibility for both onset and exacerbation of the disease, has influenced the use of spinal anaesthesia. If spinal anaesthesia is associated with relapses it is likely to be due to an exaggerated effect of local anaesthetic, where high concentrations come into contact with areas of demyelination, and not due to any adverse effect of dural puncture [42]. In the past 60 years considerable advances have been made in the pharmacology and sterility of spinal drugs, but, given the high incidence of postpartum relapses, the impossibility of unravelling precipitated relapses from natural events, and the lack of scientific reports that could shed some light on this issue, the safety of modern spinal anaesthesia has yet to be documented. This problem illustrates the difficulty associated with the use of regional blockade in women with progressive disorders such as MS. One theoretical problem, yet to be encountered, is the postpartum neurological problem that is considered to be a complication of regional blockade, when in reality it is the first manifestation of MS.

Counselling

The key to successful management is to ensure that the appropriate advice is given to women with MS at a time antenatally when they are capable of absorbing the information. The discussion should outline the possibility of postpartum relapse, the potential for a contribution to this from regional blockade, the inability to distinguish one from the other, and the odds that modern practice with low concentrations of epidural local anaesthetics is likely to be particularly safe. For caesarean section, the validity that spinal anaesthesia may not represent the best option still awaits clarification, but one of the editors (IFR) has used spinal anaesthesia for caesarean section in the presence of MS since 1981 with no recognized problems.

Multiple sclerosis

- 40% experience postpartum relapse
- Epidural and general anaesthesia are safe
- Traditional doubts about spinal anaesthesia neither substantiated nor disproven

---

NEUROFIBROMATOSIS

Von Recklinghausen's neurofibromatosis is an inherited autosomal dominant condition of neuroectoderm with an incidence of 1:3000. Like multiple sclerosis it is a progressive disease with markedly variable manifestations, but it is possible for these to affect pregnancy adversely. The classical café au lait patches become more prominent during pregnancy, and neurofibromata may increase in size. Problems with neurofibromata depend on their site and size: spinal nerve root or peripheral nerve lesions may cause neurological problems, while intrapelvic growth may obstruct childbirth [11]. Vascular abnormalities include hypertension, aneurysmal dilatation and stenosis. Phaeochromocytoma is found in 1% of sufferers and scoliosis is frequently encountered.

General anaesthesia

Anatomical abnormalities caused by neurofibromata may make airway management difficult, and the hypertensive response to intubation should be anticipated and suppressed. Because of a single report suggesting that suxamethonium might not work, and that there might be extreme sensitivity to non-depolarizing muscle relaxants, the dose should be titrated against neuromuscular function.

Regional anaesthesia

When possible the presence of spinal neurofibromata should be detected by computed tomography or magnetic resonance imaging before confinement. Fear of puncturing a neurofibroma with a needle is probably unjustified, but dural puncture in the presence of an intracranial tumour and intracranial hypertension is hazardous. These must be excluded before spinal anaesthesia, but confident siting of an epidural catheter has worked well [44].

STABLE DISORDERS

SPINAL CORD TRANSECTION

Cord lesions above T5 result in loss of central regulation of the sympathetic nervous system below the level of the lesion. Nociceptive afferent activity below the transection can stimulate sympathetic overactivity, known as autonomic hyper-reflexia. Triggers for this include distension or contraction of the bladder, rectum, or uterus, as well as perineal manipulation, cervical dilatation, suprapubic pressure and incisions [45]. Sensory loss occurs and uterine contractions are painless if the lesion is at or above T10. Paraplegics are poikilothermic below the level of the lesion, and are unable to vasoconstrict. This reduces the likelihood of hypotension with regional blockade, but increases the chance of aorto-caval compression. When labour triggers autonomic hyper-reflexia, manifestations include sweating, blurred vision, warm skin, facial flushing, nasal congestion and headache [46]. Increases in blood pressure may be mild or extreme, with the potential to cause stroke. The foetal heart rate may quicken in response to maternal catecholamines, or slow in the presence of uteroplacental vasoconstriction. Other problems unrelated to the sympathetic system include chronic urinary infections, anaemia, thrombophlebitis, pressure sores, premature labour and respiratory embarrassment [45].

Anaesthesia

Consultation antepartum is required for an assessment of risk and discussion of options. An epidural performed prophylactically will prevent autonomic hyper-reflexia, and is recommended. Insertion might be difficult due to muscle spasm, and there may be previous back surgery [46]. Because of distal loss of motor and sensory function, testing for inadvertent subarachnoid injection is difficult, and caution is required. Dermatomal levels are difficult to assess in the presence of permanent loss of sensation, and failure of epidural analgesia must be assumed if the blood pressure is not controlled [45]. One way to assess block height is to elicit contractures with cutaneous stimuli, and note at what level they cease to occur. Caesarean section is more often employed for delivery than in the normal population [47], and spinal anaesthesia has been recommended for caesarean section [48].

CEREBRAL PALSY AND POLIOMYELITIS

Neither of these conditions is likely to give rise to a problem in its own right, and management should be along established lines. Occasionally acquired musculoskeletal abnormalities such as scoliosis may be a problem.

CONCLUSIONS

Because the acute lesions described here are rare, from time to time, symptomatology indicative of a serious pathology is passed off as a complication of regional anaesthesia: pre-occupation that a gradually progressive neurological deficit was due to a spinal anaesthetic delayed the diagnosis of meningioma of the cord for a year [49]; postpartum nausea and vomiting was attributed to an epidural bolus of sufentanil until cortical blindness ensued, when computerized tomography revealed a posterior fossa tumour [50]. Given that diagnostic imaging is non-invasive and capable of superb resolution, the threshold for using this service should be low. The support of colleagues in neurology and neuroradiology is of great value.

REFERENCES

1. Crawford, J.S. (1984) *Principles and Practice of Obstetric Anaesthesia*, 5th edn, Blackwell, Oxford.
2. Critchley, M. (1937) Discussion of the neurological sequelae of spinal anaesthesia. *Proceedings of the Royal Society of Medicine*, **30**, 1007–12.
3. Chadwick, H.S., Posner, K., Caplan, R.A. et al. (1991) A comparison of obstetric and nonobstetric malpractice claims. *Anesthesiology*, **74**, 242–9.
4. Mayer, D.C., Thorp, J., Baucom, D. and Spielman, F. J. (1995) Hyperthyroidism and seizures during pregnancy. *American Journal of Perinatology*, **12**, 192–4.
5. Crawford, J.S. (1985) Some maternal complications of epidural analgesia for labour. *Anaesthesia*, **40**, 1219–25.
6. Scott, D.B. and Hibbard, B.M. (1990) Serious nonfatal complications associated with extradural block in obstetric practice. *British Journal of Anaesthesia*, **64**, 537–41.

7. Department of Health, Welsh Office, Scottish Office Home and Health Department, Department of Health and Social Security, Northern Ireland (1991) *Report on Confidential Enquiries into Maternal Deaths in the United Kingdom 1985–1987*, HMSO, London.

8. Department of Health, Welsh Office, Scottish Office Home and Health Department, Department of Health and Social Security, Northern Ireland (1994) *Report on Confidential Enquiries into Maternal Deaths in the United Kingdom 1988–1990* (1994). HMSO, London.

9. Student, I., Niesert, S. and Ehrenheim, C. (1992) Differentialdiagnostik der Krampfanfalle im peripartalen Zeitraum. *Geburtshilfe und Frauenheilkunde*, **52**, 421–5.

10. Douglas, K.A. and Redman, C.W.G. (1994) Eclampsia in the United Kingdom. *British Medical Journal*, **309**, 1395–1400.

11. Donaldson, J.O. (1989) *Neurology of Pregnancy*, W.B. Saunders, London.

12. Kilpatrick, C.J. and Hopper, J.L. (1993) The effect of pregnancy on the epilepsies: A study of 37 pregnancies. *Australian and New Zealand Journal of Medicine*, **24**, 370–3.

13. Walker, J.J. (1993) The management of hypertensive disease in pregnancy. *Current Obstetrics and Gynaecology*, **3**, 82–7.

14. Briggs, G.G., Freeman, R.K. and Yaffe, S.J. (eds) (1990) *Drugs in Pregnancy and Lactation. A reference guide to fetal and neonatal risk*, 3rd edn, Williams & Wilkins, Baltimore.

15. Anon. (1994) Antiepileptics. *British National Formulary*, **28**, 193.

16. Modica, P.A., Tempelhof, R. and White, P.F. (1990) Pro and anticonvulsant effects of anesthetics (part ll). *Anesthesia and Analgesia*, **70**, 433–44.

17. Modica, P.A., Tempelhof, R. and White, P.F. (1990) Pro and anticonvulsant effects of anesthetics (part l). *Anesthesia and Analgesia*, **70**, 303–15.

18. Patel, A. and Hughes, K.R. (1995) Grand mal convulsion following epidural blockade. *International Journal of Obstetric Anaesthesia*, **4**, 254.

19. Simolke, G.A., Cox, S.M. and Cunningham, F.G. (1991) Cerebrovascular accidents complicating pregnancy and the puerperium. *Obstetrics and Gynecology*, **78**, 37–42.

20. Sharshar, T., Lamy, C. and Mas, J.L. (1995) Incidence and causes of strokes associated with pregnancy and the puerperium. A study in public hospitals of Ile de France. *Stroke*, **26**, 930–6.

21. Cunningham, F.G., Fernandez, C.O. and Fernandez, C. (1995) Blindness associated with preeclampsia and eclampsia. *American Journal of Obstetrics and Gynecology*, **72**, 1291–8.

22. van Buul, B.J.A., Nijhuis, J.G., Slappendel, R. *et al.* (1993) General anesthesia for surgical repair of intracranial aneurysm in pregnancy: Effects on fetal heart rate. *American Journal of Perinatology*, **10**, 183–6.

23. Bacon, R.C. and Razis, P.A. (1994) The effect of propofol sedation in pregnancy on neonatal condition. *Anaesthesia*, **49**, 1058–60.

24. Shimamoto, Y., Shimazaki, M., Ochiai, M. and Yamada, F. (1994) A juvenile onset case of moyamoya disease with intraventricular haemorrhage during pregnancy. *No Shinkei Geka – Neurological Surgery*, **22**, 867–70.

25. Amin-Hanjani, S., Kuhn, M., Sloane, N. and Chatwani, A. (1993) Moyamoya disease in pregnancy: a case report. *American Journal of Obstetrics and Gynecology*, **169**, 395–6.

26. Yau, G. and Lee, T.L. (1994) Repeat epidural caesarean section in a patient with a cerebral arteriovenous malformation. *Annals of the Academy of Medicine, Singapore*, **23**, 579–81.

27. Laidler, J.A., Jackson, I.J. and Redfern, N. (1989) The management of caesarean section in a patient with an intracranial arteriovenous malformation. *Anaesthesia*, **44**, 490–1.

28. Lanzino, G., Jensen, M.E., Capelletto, B. and Kassell, N.F. (1994) Arteriovenous malformations that rupture during pregnancy: a management dilemma. *Acta Neurochirurgica*, **126**, 102–6.

29. Kriplani, A., Relan, S., Misra, N.K. *et al.* (1995) Ruptured intracranial aneurysm complicating pregnancy. *International Journal of Gynaecology and Obstetrics*, **48**, 201–6.

30. Whitburn, R.H., Laishley, R.S. and Jewkes, D.A. (1990) Anaesthesia for simultaneous caesarean section and clipping of intracranial aneurysm. *British Journal of Anaesthesia*, **64**, 642–5.

31. Otaka, K., Enzan, K., Matsumoto, J. *et al.* (1993) Anesthetic management for cesarean section and clipping of aneurysm in a pregnant woman. *Masui – Japanese Journal of Anesthesiology*, **42**, 926–30.

32. Sury, M.R.J. and Barsoum, L.Z. (1991) Anaesthesia for simultaneous caesarean section and clipping of intracerebral aneurysm. *British Journal of Anaesthesia*, **66**, 145–7.

33. Antonini, C., Alleva, S., Campailla, M.T. *et al.* (1992) Morte cerebrale e sopravvivenza fetale prolungata. *Minerva Anestesiologica*, **58**, 1247–52.

34. Gbolade, B.A. (1994) Recurrent lower motor neurone facial paralysis in four successive pregnancies. *Journal of Laryngology and Otology*, **108**, 587–8.

35. Dorsey, D.L. and Camann, W.R. (1993) Obstetric anesthesia in patients with idiopathic facial paralysis (Bell's palsy): A 10 year survey. *Anesthesia and Analgesia*, **77**, 81–3.

36. Wisoff, J.H., Kratzert, K.J., Handwerker, S.M. *et al.* (1991) Pregnancy in patients with cerebrospinal fluid shunts: Report of a series and review of the literature. *Neurosurgery*, **29**, 827–31.

37. Finfer, S.R. (1991) Management of labour and delivery in patients with intracranial neoplasms. *British Journal of Anaesthesia*, **67**, 784–7.

38. Romansky, K., Arnandova, V. and Nachev, S. (1992) Hemangioblastoma during pregnancy. *Zentralblatt für Neurochirurgie*, **53**, 37–9.

39. Rudick, R.A. and Birk, K.A. (1992) Multiple sclerosis in pregnancy, in *Neurological Disorders in Pregnancy*, 2nd edn (eds P.J. Goldstein and B.J. Stern), Futura Publishing, New York.

40. Birk, K., Ford, C., Smeltzer, S. *et al.* (1990) The clinical course of multiple sclerosis during pregnancy and the puerperium. *Archives of Neurology*, 47, 738– 42.

41. Holdcroft A., Gibberd, F.B., Hargrove, R.L. (1995) Neurological complications associated with pregnancy. *British Journal of Anaesthesia*, 75, 522–6.

42. Warren, T.M., Datta, S. and Ostheimer, G.W. (1982) Lumbar epidural anesthesia in a patient with multiple sclerosis. *Anesthesia and Analgesia*, **61**, 1022–3.

43. Bader, A.M., Hunt, C.O., Datta, S. *et al.* (1988) Anesthesia for the obstetric patient with multiple sclerosis. *Journal of Clinical Anesthesiology*, **1**, 21–4.

44. Dounas, M., Mercier, F.J., Lhuissier, C. and Benhamou, D. (1995) Epidural analgesia for labour in a parturient with neurofibromatosis. *Canadian Journal of Anaesthesia*, **42**, 420–4.

45. Owen, M.D., Stiles, M.M., Opper, S.E. *et al.* (1994) Autonomic hyperreflexia in a pregnant paraplegic patient. *Regional Anaesthesia*, **19**, 415–7.

46. Crosby, E., St Jean, B., Reid, D. and Elliott, R.D. (1992) Obstetrical anaesthesia and analgesia in chronic spinal cord injured women. *Canadian Journal of Anaesthesia*, **39**, 487–94.

47. Cross, L.L., Meythaler, J.M., Tuel, S.M. and Cross, A.L. (1992) Pregnancy, labor and delivery post spinal cord injury. *Paraplegia*, **30**, 890–902.

48. Kaidomar, M., Raucoles, M., Ben Miled, M. *et al.* (1993) Epidural anesthesia and prevention of autonomic hyperreflexia in a paraplegic parturient. *Annales Françaises d'Anesthésie et de Réanimation*, **12**, 493–6.

49. Vandam, L.D. and Dripps, R.D. (1956) Exacerbation of pre existing neurologic disease after spinal anesthesia. *New England Journal of Medicine*, **255**, 843–9.

50. Shin, Y.K., Chapman, C.C. and Lees, D.E. (1992) Postpartum transient blindness probably related to undiagnosed brain tumour. *Southern Medical Journal*, **85**, 760–1

D. Benhamou, J. Hamza and H. Frizelle

INTRODUCTION

Epidural and spinal techniques are the most frequently applied forms of regional anaesthesia in obstetrics, being used for both labour and for caesarean section. Although these techniques are popular and usually work well, failure is an occasional event. In this chapter we will define 'failure' as any situation in which one of the three partners (anaesthetist, obstetrician or patient) is not fully satisfied with the regional technique. Delivery is different from other situations requiring analgesia, in that a high degree of satisfaction immediately postpartum is sometimes associated with long-term impression of failure.

MacArthur [1] found that 7% of women having requested epidural analgesia because of intense labour pain, and in whom analgesia was satisfactory, one week later admitted to dissatisfaction because they had been deprived of birth sensation. In most circumstances however, the cause of failure is that pain or discomfort persists during labour or surgery. We might classify these as technical failures, anaesthetic failures (failures during caesarean section) and analgesic failures (failure during labour).

TECHNICAL FAILURES

Technical failure may be defined as a situation in which the anaesthetist is unable to locate the epidural space or thread the epidural catheter. In some instances, the difficulty is due to individual variations in anatomy which may be either congenital, or acquired through previous surgery to the lumbar spine.

EXPERIENCE AND EPIDURAL TECHNIQUE

Technical skill is clearly related to experience. A learning curve has been described for epidural anaesthesia [2] in which it appears that experience of 50 epidurals is necessary before failure rates fall to an acceptable level. This result has been confirmed in a large series from Birmingham primarily aimed at examining long-term postpartum symptoms. In this study, the authors found that there was a statistically significant association between the occurrence of accidental dural puncture and the total number of epidurals performed by the anaesthetist. In cases where the number of previous epidurals was <30, the rate of dural puncture was $\geqslant 2\%$. In contrast, when the experience was of greater than 30 epidurals, the rate of dural puncture was close to 1.3% [3]. A significant correlation was also found

Clinical Problems in Obstetric Anaesthesia
Edited by Ian F. Russell and Gordon Lyons. Published in 1997 by Chapman & Hall, London. ISBN 0 412 71600 3.

between the incidence of dural puncture and the method used for identifying the epidural space, with the greatest proportion of taps occurring with the use of the Macintosh balloon. Loss of resistance using air has been associated with an increased risk of incomplete analgesia with air bubbles impeding the transfer of the local anaesthetic across the meninges [4]. Loss of resistance to saline would appear to be a better choice.

LUMBAR SPINE SURGERY

Previous lumbar spine surgery may adversely affect the efficacy of epidural anaesthesia. Several series have shown increased technical difficulty siting epidurals in patients following Harrington instrumentation. These include failure to identify the epidural space, vessel puncture, dural puncture and the need for multiple attempts [5–7]. However, given that these are essentially benign complications, the authors recommend that epidural anaesthesia is not denied to these women provided that it is undertaken by an experienced epiduralist, and provided that they have been apprised of these risks.

PATIENT POSITION

Tarkkila [8] showed that although inability to obtain a free flow of cerebral spinal fluid (CSF) during spinal anaesthesia was a rare event (0.1%), failure may occur despite successful CSF return (1%). He hypothesized that the needle may have moved during injection and that the anaesthetic agent may have been injected outside the CSF. The contribution of patient position to the incidence of failure remains controversial. Hodgson *et al.* [9] have recently shown that when lumbar puncture is performed with the patient in the lateral decubitus position, the needle usually deviates away from the midline to the non-dependent side, increasing the risk of failure. This finding is not supported by Tarkkila [8] who failed to find an increased rate of failure in the lateral

decubitus position as compared with the sitting position (3.1% versus 3.2% respectively).

NEEDLES

It has been suggested that the design of the needle tip also affects the failure rate. Crone and Vogel [10] found an increased overall failure rate with the use of the Sprotte needle as compared to other needle types (10.3% versus 4.3% respectively). They speculated that the dimensions and placement of the sideport of the Sprotte needle may be the cause. Since the length from the needle tip to the opening of the sideport is 1.2 mm and since length of the sideport ranges from 1.75 to 2.00 mm, it is possible for the side port to straddle the dura. As a result, part of the local anaesthetic solution may be deposited in the epidural space resulting in an inadequate block.

When a combined spinal–epidural (CSE) technique is used a higher failure rate can be expected. Collis *et al.* in her first series of 300 CSE punctures for labour described an 11% failure rate [11]. For most of these failures, difficulty obtaining free flowing CSF was a prominent feature. When this occurs, the suspicion is that the protruding tip of the spinal needle is too short to penetrate the dura. Joshi and Mac-Carroll have suggested that because the epidural space may be as large as 10–20 mm in the lumbar region, the spinal needle should protrude by at least 13 mm from the epidural needle [12]. Experience at the Hospital Antoine-Béclère, with several hundred patients, is that with sufficiently long spinal needles, the rate of technical failure with the CSE technique is similar to that seen with a standard spinal technique.

SUBDURAL PLACEMENT OF NEEDLE OR CATHETER

Finally, failure may occur because of needle or catheter placement within the subdural space. Subdural placement of an anaesthetic drug may well result in inappropriate spread. Failure may be secondary to asymmetrical spread of the local anaesthetic resulting in unabated pain [13]. On the other hand, since the subdural space is smaller than the epidural space, extensive spread may occur resulting in respiratory depression [14] or in hypotension. Finally, injection of too large a volume in this poorly compliant space may lead to arachnoid rupture [15]. Whatever the clinical picture, one should remember that once concern exists that an epidural catheter may in fact be subdural, it should be removed.

FAILURE OF ANAESTHESIA: REGIONAL ANAESTHESIA FOR CAESAREAN SECTION

INDIVIDUAL REQUIREMENTS FOR LOCAL ANAESTHETIC

Failure may arise due either to patient factors or anaesthetic factors. The selection of the appropriate dose of a given local anaesthetic is made difficult by wide individual variability in dose requirements. In this regard, a nice study was performed by Kestin *et al.* [16] who recorded the local anaesthetic needs in two groups of women scheduled for elective caesarean section. One group received continuous lumbar epidural anaesthesia and the other continuous spinal anaesthesia. The dose of local anaesthetic was titrated until an upper sensory level at T4 was achieved. They noticed that the range of dose required for either spinal or epidural anaesthesia was very large (from 1.4 ml to 7.8 ml of 0.5% bupivacaine in spinal anaesthesia and from 12 ml to 35 ml of 2% lidocaine in epidural anaesthesia). This helps us to understand why a single-shot spinal injection is likely to fail in a few patients and produce an excessive block in others.

At one extreme, the complete absence of block after spinal injection of lidocaine in spite of correct placement of the local anaesthetic into the CSF (as attested by clinically relevant concentrations of lidocaine in the CSF)

suggests that some patients have a physiologic resistance to lidocaine. This 'resistance' does not seem to be generic for all compounds of the amide local anaesthetic series since in these patients bupivacaine produced adequate anaesthesia [17].

Adaptation of the anaesthetic dose to each patient's needs may be achieved by a variety of means. The most popular is likely to be the use of a lumbar epidural catheter in which drugs are injected incrementally to obtain the desired effect, a T4 upper sensory level of anaesthesia. The major drawback of the epidural technique is the length of time required to achieve this effect. Time constraints may indeed prove problematic in large busy obstetric units. Failure of epidural anaesthesia for caesarean section is an additional problem. Crawford [18] found that analgesia was fair to poor in 7.2% of patients. Given that injection of a given dose of anaesthetic through the epidural catheter can result in patchy block, Laishley and Morgan [19] used an epidural technique based on the fractionated injection of 20 ml of bupivacaine through the Tuohy needle prior to the epidural catheter placement. Unfortunately they found that intraoperative supplementation was necessary in 40%. To overcome this relatively high rate of supplementation, the use of epidural opioids such as fentanyl 25–100 µg, or sufentanil 10–20 µg, in combination with the local anaesthetic has proved to be successful. Several studies have shown that this strategy consistently reduces the rate of visceral pain from a rate greater than 50% to less than 25% [20–23].

Other methods may be used to limit the incidence of inadequate anaesthesia during caesarean section. As previously mentioned, Kestin *et al.* [16] used incremental injection of local anaesthetic through a spinal catheter. However, adverse experiences related to toxicity from pooling of local anaesthetic have led to the withdrawal of very fine spinal catheters in the US, and continuous spinal anaesthesia is now only rarely used. Another means of adjusting the quality of anaesthesia is the use of a combined spinal–epidural technique. Fan *et al.* [24] have shown, for example, that patient satisfaction is better using moderate doses of spinal bupivacaine (5 or 7.5 mg) combined with a mean volume of epidural lidocaine 2% of 10 or 1.2 ml respectively. The flexibility obtained with incremental injections through the epidural catheter makes it an excellent technique for caesarean section.

MONITORING SENSORY BLOCKADE

Failure may also arise from an inadequate level of anaesthesia. Although all textbooks recommend that an upper sensory level of T4 be obtained before beginning caesarean section, they generally fail to define which sensation, and this could be critical. A sensory level at T4 as determined by the pinprick method is not similar to a T4 level obtained by loss of sensation to touch or loss of pain during electrical stimulation. Brull and Greene have shown that during epidural anaesthesia, a zone of differential sensory blockade exists with the upper sensory level, measured using pinprick, being one to two dermatomes higher than that measured with loss of touch [25]. Since loss of sharp pinprick sensation defines analgesia and loss of touch sensation defines anaesthesia, it can easily be understood that when the upper sensory level of analgesia is T4, the sensory level of anaesthesia will be only T5 or T6 and failure of the block to filter surgical stimulation may ensue. In support of this, Russell [26] has recently shown that no patient with a level of anaesthesia (loss of touch sensation) above T5 experienced pain. It may be concluded that pinprick testing may be misleading and if this method is used, an upper level (of analgesia) **above** T4 is required.

FAILURE WITH SPINAL ANAESTHESIA

The recent introduction of pencil-point needles with the promise of a reduction in dural puncture headaches, has led to the increasing use of spinal anaesthesia for caesarean section.

However, when a local anaesthetic (usually bupivacaine) is used alone, the incidence of visceral pain may be as high as 70%. Alahuhta *et al.* [27] showed that the incidence of visceral pain was similar with either epidural or spinal anaesthesia and Pedersen *et al.* [28] showed that increasing the dose from 7.5–10 to 10–12.5 mg of hyperbaric bupivacaine lowered the incidence of visceral pain from 70.5 to 31.6%. This reduced incidence of failure with increasing dosage has been confirmed several times [29, 30]. As for epidural anaesthesia, the failure rate may also be significantly decreased by the addition of opioids. Hunt *et al.* [31] showed that adding 6 to 12.5 μg of fentanyl to hyperbaric bupivacaine abolished visceral pain. Similar results have been found using the intrathecal combination of bupivacaine and sufentanil [32] or lidocaine and fentanyl [33]. The benefits of adding spinal morphine to bupivacaine are dose dependent. The addition of 0.2 mg morphine is associated with better intraoperative visual analogue pain scores than 0.1 mg (5 versus 25 mm) [34]. Similar improvement may result from adding other drugs. Clonidine is now known to produce efficacious visceral antinociception [35] and we have recently shown that the combination of clonidine with hyperbaric bupivacaine significantly decreases the pain score during caesarean section.

This effect is even greater when both clonidine and fentanyl are added to bupivacaine. Finally, although there are currently no data regarding the intraoperative efficacy of combining intrathecal neostigmine with bupivacaine for caesarean section, a synergistic effect of neostigmine with opioids and with α_2-adrenergic agonists represents a promising option for the future [36].

FAILURE OF ANALGESIA DURING LABOUR

INCIDENCE

Even among specialist groups of obstetric anaesthetists, the incidence of inadequate epidural block may be high. At the Brigham and Women's Hospital in Boston [37], a recent retrospective study has shown a replacement rate for epidural catheters of 12.3%. Repositioning the catheter was successful in 57% of cases. Many other studies have confirmed that satisfactory analgesia is not always obtained. Bleyaert *et al.* [38] were the first to use low concentrations of epidural bupivacaine (0.125% with epinephrine) in a large series of 3000 labouring women. Unsatisfactory analgesia was seen in 8% of cases of which 41% were due to unrelieved unilateral pain. Cruchley *et al.* have described a failure rate of 24%, defined as inadequate analgesia at some time during the course of labour [39] and our own experience is close to this [40]. Several studies have investigated the aetiologic factors involved in the failure of epidural block for labour and once again failures can be classified as patient, labour- or technique-related.

PROBLEMS WITH EPIDURAL CATHETERS

Patient or technique-related failures share several common aetiologies with those failures seen during caesarean section. For example, the use of air to identify the epidural space results in a greater frequency of unblocked segments [5,41]. Collier recently examined the role of epidural catheters by using contrast injection and subsequent radiographic screening ('epidurograms') [42]. He showed that the two major causes of inadequate block during labour were transforaminal escape of the catheter tip and persistent unilateral block associated with an obstructive barrier in the epidural space. Transforaminal escape of the catheter presents as a limited unilateral block confined to one or two segments. The radiograph usually shows a 'psoasgram' and this clinical picture is obviously related to the introduction of an excessive length of catheter in the epidural space. Several studies have recently reappraised the optimal length of catheter that should be threaded into the epidural space. Beilin *et al.* [43] showed that the incidence of

incomplete analgesia was minimized by a 5 cm insertion length of catheter as compared with either 3 or 7 cm. D'Angelo *et al.* found that when prolonged labour is likely, epidural catheters should be inserted 6 cm into the epidural space [44]. These two well-performed studies provide data which are both consistent and significantly different from current recommendations, i.e. insertion of only 1–3 cm. Interestingly, Beilin *et al.* used a multiorifice epidural catheter. This catheter has three lateral ports placed in close proximity to its closed end and the three side-ports are arranged around the circumference at 120% intervals spaced 4 mm from each other with the first hole originating 6 mm from the tip of the catheter. This seems important because the use of catheters with distal lateral eyes results in more satisfactory blocks than with catheters with terminal eyes [45].

Collier's epidurograms [42] attributed unilateral block or missed segment to a 'midline barrier'. Although the existence of a plica medialis has been disputed in several radiographic studies, Blomberg, using epiduroscopy, described a connective tissue structure in the dorsal midline of the lumbar epidural space of **each** subject. The appearance of the band varied from strands of connective tissue to a complete membrane (in 2% of cadavers) and extended vertically over at least two lumbar segments [46].

At the Hospital Antoine Béclère we evaluated the risk factors for incomplete analgesia in 456 women. We separated factors associated with failure during labour from failure during the delivery phase. Failure during labour was defined as either a visual analogue pain score >30 mm or a need for more than two top-ups during continuous infusion. Failure during delivery was defined as a pain score greater than 30 mm. We found a significantly greater incidence of failure during delivery than during labour (19.7 versus 6%). We suspect that the initial visceral pain of labour changes to a more somatic component which is more difficult to treat. However, the logistic regression used to analyse our data found that similar factors were responsible for failure during both labour and delivery: inadequate analgesia after the first analgesic dose, long duration of labour and occipitoposterior presentation. The occurrence of radicular pain during epidural puncture was also associated with the increased risk of asymmetrical block during labour. The question of whether combined spinal–epidural analgesia may reduce the failure rate during labour has yet to be answered. The excellent quality of analgesia obtained with intrathecal administration of opioid and/or local anaesthetic is known to improve patient satisfaction. This is in close agreement with our results showing that a successful first administration of analgesics is a good predictor of success.

MANAGEMENT OF A FAILED BLOCK

Management of inadequate block during labour may prove both difficult and time-consuming; partial catheter withdrawal combined with a further dose of local anaesthetic and/or the addition of opioid is often sufficient to obtain good analgesia.

Several studies have indeed shown that the addition of a lipid-soluble opioid (sufentanil 7.5 µg) to local anaesthetic results in an increased number of patients with good/excellent analgesia [47]. This beneficial effect has also been reported with fentanyl (100 µg) for perineal pain occurring during late labour [48]. When, in rare cases, the addition of opioid is not sufficient, the addition of epidural clonidine (150–300 µg) may solve the problem [49]. Repositioning the patient may sometimes be helpful but experience suggests that especially in high-risk labour, such manoeuvres may take up as much time and be less successful than resiting the catheter. When all is taken into account, it has been estimated that imperfect obstetric epidural analgesia can be resolved in 82%, leaving few real failures [50]. Moreover, we believe that antenatal counselling and consent improves the patient's understanding and

expectations, and can decrease the incidence of failed block and patient dissatisfaction.

CONCLUSION

Inadequate analgesia/anaesthesia is of great concern to obstetric anaesthetists. Many studies have been performed during both labour and caesarean section with a view to eliminating failure. Factors related to the patient, the stimulus and to the anaesthetic technique have been identified as causes of failure. This knowledge has led to technical and pharmacological improvements which have been successfully tried and introduced into practice. Together with attempts to improve the patient–physician relationship, this achieves a total quality-management programme. We anticipate a time when failure will be looked upon as a relic of the past.

REFERENCES

1. MacArthur, C. and Lewis, M. (1993) Evaluation of obstetric analgesia and anaesthesia: long-term maternal recollections. *International Journal of Obstetric Anaesthesia*, **2**, 3–11.
2. Kopacz, D.J. and Neal, J.M. (1994) Learning regional anaesthesia techniques: how many is enough. *Regional Anesthesia*, **19**, 37.
3. MacArthur, C., Lewis, M. and Knox, E.G. (1993) Accidental puncture in obstetric patients and long term symptoms. *British Medical Journal*, **306**, 883–4.
4. Dalens, B., Bazin, J.E. and Habere, J.P. (1987) Epidural bubbles as a cause of incomplete analgesia during epidural anaesthesia. *Anesthesia and Analgesia*, **66** 679–83.
5. Crosby, E.T. and Halpern, S.H. (1989) Obstetric epidural anaesthesia in patients with Harrington instrumentation. *Canadian Journal of Anaesthesia*, **36**, 693–6.
6. Sharrock, N.E., Urquhard, B. and Mineo, R. (1990) Extradural anaesthesia in patients with previous lumbar spine surgery. *British Journal of Anaesthesia*, **65** 237–9.
7. Daley, M.D., Rolbin, S.H., Hew, E.M. *et al.* (1990) Epidural anaesthesia for obstetrics after spinal surgery. *Regional Anesthesia*, **15**, 280–4.
8. Tarkkila, P.K. (1991) Incidence and causes of failed spinal anaesthetics in a university

hospital: a prospective study. *Regional Anesthesia*, **16**, 48–51.

9. Hodgson, P.S.A., Mack, B., Kopacz, D. *et al.* (1996) Needle placement during lumbar epidural anaesthesia deviates toward the non-dependent side. *Regional Anesthesia*, **21**, 26

10. Crone, L.A.L. and Vogel, W. (1991) Failed spinal anaesthesia with the Sprotte needle. *Anesthesiology*, **75**, 7171–8.

11. Collis, R.E., Baxandall, M.L., Srikantharajah, I.D. *et al.* (1994) Combined spinal epidural (CSE) analgesia: technique, management and outcome of 300 mothers. *International Journal of Obstetric Anaesthesia*, **3**, 75–81.

12. Joshi, G.P. and McCarroll, S.M. (1993) Combined spinal–epidural anaesthesia using needle-through-needle technique. *Anesthesiology*, **78**, 406–7.

13. Foster, P.N., Stickle, B.R. and Griffiths, J.O. (1995) Variable presentation of subdural block. *Anaesthesia*, **50**, 178.

14. Mizuyama, K. and Dohi, S. (1993) An accidental subdural injection of a local anaesthetic resulting in respiratory depression. *Canadian Journal of Anaesthesia*, **40**, 83–4.

15. Elliott, D.W., Voyvodic, F. and Brownridge, P. (1996) Sudden onset of subarachnoid block after subdural catheterization: a case of arachnoid rupture? *British Journal of Anaesthesia*, **76**, 322–4

16. Kestin, I.G., Madden, A.P., Mulvein, J.T. *et al.* (1991) Comparison of incremental spinal anaesthesia using a 32-gauge catheter with extradural anaesthesia for elective caesarean section. *British Journal of Anaesthesia*, **66**, 232–6.

17. Schmidt, S.I., Moorthy, S.S., Dierdorf, S.F. *et al.* (1990) A series of truly failed spinal anaesthetics. *Journal of Clinical Anesthesia*, **2**, 336–8.

18. Crawford, J.S. (1980) Experiences with lumbar extradural analgesia for caesarean section. *British Journal of Anaesthesia*, **52**, 821–4.

19. Laishley, R.S. and Morgan, B.M. (1988) A single dose epidural technique for caesarean section. A comparison between 0.5% bupivacaine plain and 0.5% bupivacaine with adrenaline. *Anaesthesia*, **43**, 100–3.

20. Gaffud, M.P., Bansal, P., Lawton, C. *et al.* (1986) Surgical analgesia for caesarean delivery with epidural bupivacaine and fentanyl. *Anesthesiology*, **65**, 331–4.

21. Paech, M.J., West More, M.D. and Speirs, H.M. (1990) A double blind comparison of epidural bupivacaine and bupivacaine–fentanyl for

caesarean section. *Anaesthesia and Intensive Care*, **18**, 22–30.

22. Preston, P.G., Rosen, M.A., Hughes, S.C. *et al.* (1988) Epidural anaesthesia with fentanyl and lidocaine for caesarean section: maternal effects and neonatal outcome. *Anesthesiology*, **68**, 938–43.

23. Capogna, G., Celleno, D. and Tomassetti, M. (1989) Maternal analgesia and neonatal effects of epidural sufentanil for caesarean section. *Regional Anesthesia*, **14**, 282–7.

24. Fan, S.Z., Susetio, L., Wang, Y.P. *et al.* (1994) Low dose of intrathecal hyperbaric bupivacaine combined with epidural lidocaine for caesarean section. A balance block technique. *Anesthesia and Analgesia*, **78**, 474–7.

25. Brull, S.J. and Greene, N.M. (1991) Zones of differential sensory block during extradural anaesthesia. *British Journal of Anaesthesia*, **66**, 651–5

26. Russel, I.F. (1995) Levels of anaesthesia and intraoperative pain at caesarean section under regional block. *International Journal of Obstetric Anaesthesia*, **4**, 71–7.

27. Alahuhta, S., Kangas-Saarela, T., Hollmen, A.I. *et al.* (1990) Visceral pain during caesarean section under spinal and epidural anaesthesia with bupivacaine. *Acta Anaesthesiologica Scandinavica*, **34**, 95–8.

28. Pedersen, H., Santos, A.C., Steinberg, E.S. *et al.* (1989) Incidence of visceral pain during caesarean section: the effect of varying doses of spinal bupivacaine. *Anesthesia and Analgesia*, **69**, 46–9.

29. De Simone, C.A., Leighton, B.L. and Norris, M.C. (1995) Spinal anaesthesia for caesarean delivery. A comparison of two doses of hyperbaric bupivacaine. *Regional Anesthesia*, **20**, 90–4.

30. Hirabayashi, Y., Saitoh, K., Fukuda, H. *et al.* (1995) Visceral pain during caesarean section: effect of varying dose of spinal amethocaine. *British Journal of Anaesthesia*, **75**, 266- -8.

31. Hunt, C.O., Naulty, J.S., Bader, A.M. *et al.* (1989) Perioperative analgesia with subarachnoid fentanyl–bupivacaine for caesarean section. *Anesthesiology*, **71**, 535–40

32. Courtney, M.A., Baden, A.M. and Hartwell, B. (1992) Perioperative analgesia with subarachnoid sufentanil administration. *Regional Anesthesia*, **17**, 274–8.

33. Palmer, C.M., Voulgaropoulos, D. and Alves, D. (1995) Subarachnoid fentanyl augments lidocaine spinal anesthesia for caesarean delivery. *Regional Anesthesia*, **20**, 389–94.

34. Cohen, S.E., Desai, J.B., Ratner, E.F. *et al.* (1996) Ketorolac and spinal morphine for postcesarean analgesia. *International Journal of Obstetric Anaesthesia*, **5**, 14–18.

35. Harada, Y., Nishioka, K., Kitahata, L.M. *et al.* (1995) Visceral antinociceptive effects of spinal clonidine combined with morphine, [D-Pen^2, D-Pen^5] enkephalin, or U50, 488H. *Anesthesiology*, **83**, 344–52.

36. Naguib, M. and Yaksh, T.L. (1994) Antinociceptive effects of spinal cholinesterase inhibition and isobolographic analysis of the interaction with and α2 receptor systems. *Anesthesiology*, **80**, 1338–48.

37. Eappen, S., Segal, S., Blinn, A. *et al.* (1995) Replacement rate and etiology factors associated with inadequate block during epidural analgesia in parturients. *Regional Anesthesia*, **21** (Suppl), 69.

38. Bleyaert, A., Soetens, M., Vaes, L. *et al.* (1979) Bupivacaine, 0.125 per cent, in obstetric epidural analgesia: experience in three thousand cases. *Anesthesiology*, **51**, 435–8.

39. Cruchley, P.M. and Rose, D.K. (1994) Supplemental analgesia requirements with continuous epidural infusion: patient profiles. *Canadian Journal of Anaesthesia*, **41**, A30A.

40. Langeron, O., Hamza, J., Narchi, P. *et al.* (1991) Risk factors associated with unilateral blockade during labour epidural analgesia. *Anesthesiology*, **75**, A832.

41. Valentine, S.J., Jarvis, A.P. and Shutt, L.E. (1991) Comparative study of the effects of air or saline to identify the extradural space. *British Journal of Anaesthesia*, **66**, 224–7.

42. Collier, C.B. (1996) Why obstetric epidurals fail: a study of epidurograms. *International Journal of Obstetric Anaesthesia*, **5**, 19–31.

43. Beilin, Y., Berstein, H.H. and Zucker-Pinchoff, B. (1995) The optimal distance that a multiorifice epidural catheter should be threaded into the epidural space. *Anesthesia and Analgesia*, **81**, 301–4.

44. D'Angelo, R., Berkebile, B.L. and Gerancher, J.C. (1996) Prospective examination of epidural catheter insertion. *Anesthesiology*, **84**, 88–93.

45. Collier, C.B., and Gatt, S.P. (1994) Epidural catheters for obstetrics. Terminal hole or lateral eyes? *Regional Anesthesia*, **19**, 378–85.

46. Blomberg, R. (1986) The dorsomedian connective tissue band in the lumbar epidural space of humans. An anatomical study using epiduroscopy in autopsy cases. *Anesthesia and Analgesia*, **65**, 747–52.

47. Vertommen, J.D., Lemmens, E. and Van Aken, H. (1994) Comparison of the addition of three different doses of sufentanil to 0.125% bupivacaine given epidurally during labour. *Anaesthesia*, **49**, 678–81.

48. Reynolds, F. and O'Sullivan, G. (1989) Epidural fentanyl and perineal pain in labour. *Anaesthesia*, **44**, 341–4.

49. Siegemund, M., Schneider, M.C., Kampl, K.F. *et al.* (1995) Epidural clonidine for relief from intractable labour pain. *Anaesthesia*, **50**, 663–4.

50. Mangin, R., Lalourcey, L., Aya, G. *et al.* (1995) Imperfections de l'analgésie péridurale obstétricale: quelles réponses? Quels résultats? *Annales Françaises d'Anesthésie- Réanimation*, **14** (suppl), R84.

J. Hamza, D. Benhamou and H. Frizelle

INTRODUCTION

Anaesthesia is a discipline that does not have a ready-made infrastructure for outpatient care, and before effective antenatal assessment can be provided, a number of organizational problems must be resolved. Should the clinic aim to see all pregnant women at some stage, or should the service be limited to those listed for elective procedures? Is it feasible to assess women who might otherwise request epidural pain relief in the throes of labour, at a convenient time before the onset of labour? Is it possible to run a clinic without significant waiting times, see all who might wish to attend, and make the best use of medical time? If this can be achieved, will the overall standard of care be improved? What are the main objectives of this consultation service?

We aim to consider these questions with particular attention to two main areas.

- Why should anaesthetists offer antenatal assessment of the pregnant woman?
- Can we provide this service to all mothers to be?

THE ROLE OF THE ANAESTHETIC ANTENATAL CLINIC

There are two main objectives of antenatal assessment by an anaesthetist. The first involves an assessment of risk, and takes advantage of the opportunity to fine tune any pre-existing medical condition. The second objective is to exchange information. The woman will wish to know where she stands with regard to risk, and the anaesthetist will wish to identify any particular concerns and potential areas of confusion, in order to allay anxiety. By such exchanges confidence is established, and informed consent is obtained.

WHAT ARE THE RISKS OF OBSTETRIC ANAESTHESIA?

The confidential triennial inquiry into maternal deaths in England and Wales [1] reminds us that anaesthesia was a major cause of maternal mortality. During the period 1976–1987, there were 76 deaths directly due to anaesthesia, of which 47% were related to problems at intubation, particularly during general anaesthesia for emergency caesarean section [2]. In obstetric practice, the risk of failed intubation has been reported to be as great as one in 300 patients undergoing caesarean section [3] which is eight times the rate in the general surgical population [4].

Can an antenatal assessment identify those at risk? Signs indicative of difficulty with intubation (evaluated in 1500 obstetrical patients

Clinical Problems in Obstetric Anaesthesia
Edited by Ian F. Russell and Gordon Lyons. Published in 1997 by Chapman & Hall, London. ISBN 0 412 71600 3.

just before general anaesthesia for caesarean section) were correlated with difficult intubation as judged during the subsequent laryngoscopy [5]. This study revealed that patients with a Mallampati grade 4 airway have an 11-fold increase in difficult intubation. The presence of a receding mandible multiplies the risk by five. When these two signs are present, the risk is multiplied by 55 as compared to a patient with a Mallampati grade 1 airway. As emergency general anaesthesia will always be required from time to time, it is imperative that anaesthetists preoperatively assess the risk of difficult tracheal intubation using these recognized criteria. When this is done just prior to inducing anaesthesia for emergency caesarean section, there is no scope for planned management of a difficult airway, and in the case of dire foetal asphyxia, there is little place for an alternative technique. Is it acceptable that, apart from elective caesarean section and induced labour, there is no opportunity for prior assessment by an anaesthetist? The reality of the urgent obstetric problem, such as cord prolapse or acute foetal distress, is that the anaesthetist must make the best of a situation that precludes a planned approach. This often means looking for complicating factors and hoping that despite their presence the outcome will be satisfactory.

While we must accept that unpredictable emergencies are the nature of obstetric practice, might we also accept that knowledge of the patient could reduce the incidence of anaesthesia-related accidents? Ignorance of, for example, a serious allergy or a problem intubation during a previous general anaesthetic, can have serious consequences. Prewarned is prearmed, and it seems logical that an opportune assessment of risk at a time when haste and anxiety do not feature, will permit a management plan with safety in mind. This will generally mean that an agreement is reached between the patient and anaesthetist on the best approach for analgesia or anaesthesia.

We think that the three most important aims are to detect potential airway problems since the greatest hazard associated with obstetric anaesthesia is failure to intubate; to identify contraindications, both relative and absolute, to regional blockade, since epidural analgesia tends to be the most popular procedure during labour; and to identify obstetric indications for urgent foetal delivery with a requirement for emergency anaesthesia. Also worthwhile are assessments of risk factors for thromboembolism, postpartum haemorrhage and allergic reactions, not forgetting backache and migraine, whose reappearance in the postpartum period could be confused with complications of epidural anaesthesia.

DOES AN ANTENATAL ANAESTHETIC ASSESSMENT ALLOW REDUCTION OF RISK?

The early identification of high risk for an emergency caesarean section or difficult intubation allows the anaesthetist to advocate epidural analgesia from the onset of labour. In this way antenatal evaluation might lead to a management plan where none previously existed. This use of 'preventive' epidural analgesia has been examined in several recent studies. Morgan *et al.* [6] have shown that evaluation of risk factors for emergency caesarean section correctly identified 87% of patients who subsequently needed an emergency caesarean section. An epidural catheter was placed in 77%, and of these, nine out of 10 had effective epidural anaesthesia for caesarean section. The remainder required general anaesthesia. If risk factors for caesarean section are actively sought during labour, early siting of an epidural catheter will avoid general anaesthesia in 90%. We recently conducted a prospective study of more than 3000 patients [7] seen in an outpatient obstetric anaesthesia clinic. We found that a number close to 10% of the clinic population had at least one predicting factor for difficult intubation. These women were strongly encouraged to accept early epidural catheter placement during labour. Subsequently, we showed that the percentage of patients having had an early

Table 20.1 Percentage of patients with or without a potentially difficult airway (PDA) having a functioning lumbar epidural analgesia (LEA) before a cervical dilation of 4 cm and at delivery [7]

	Early LEA (<4 cm)	LEA at delivery
Patients with PDA	168/313 53.7%*	276/313 88.2%*
Patients without PDA	1269/2878 44.1%	2322/2878 80.7%

*$P < 0.001$ versus patients without PDA.

epidural (cervical dilation <4 cm) was significantly higher in the group at risk for difficult intubation (Table 20.1) and that the percentage of patients requiring general anaesthesia in case of emergency caesarean section was significantly lower when an epidural catheter was already in place (Figure 20.1). Finally, intubation failure occurred (two cases) only in those without an epidural at the time of caesarean section [7]. This study underlines the advantage of foresight in the management of increased risk for general anaesthesia. Even in the emergency situation, forward planning can reduce the requirement for the latter.

When antenatal consultation allows evaluation of the 'risk profile' of the patient, this can subsequently be taken into account in the different 'scenarios' for labour analgesia and for occasional emergency delivery. But this is not its only goal.

IS CONSULTATION USEFUL FOR THE PATIENT?

If the anaesthetist finds unplanned emergency anaesthesia in an unprepared patient a stressful experience, some consideration is also due to the mother. Pregnant women are generally unaware of the true risks of general anaesthesia, and fear regional blockade [8, 9], in contrast to their anaesthetist who is likely to take the opposing view. The expectant nullipara sometimes believes that she can cope easily with labour-induced pain. If she wants to deliver without sensory and motor blockade

she might believe that the subsequent need for epidural analgesia during labour represents a personal failure. The opportunity to discuss the practical aspects of epidural pain relief, the pros and cons, the physiological effects, and at the same time correct the misinformation and half truths that abound in antenatal circles, will allow a woman to participate in her own care in a reasoned and effective manner. This kind of discussion forms the basis for informed consent. This is dealt with elsewhere.

If a written record of consent is required, this is the ideal time for this. Practices in North America [10], the UK [11] and other European countries may differ. While written consent is not required in France, an assessment performed several days before the administration of an anaesthetic is required by law. Not surprisingly, this poses a significant organizational problem, as it requires that all women booked to deliver in hospital must attend for outpatient consultation. We do not propose to discuss here specific medical problems as they have been adequately dealt with both in review articles [12, 13] and in other chapters of this book.

HOW CAN WE ORGANIZE AN OBSTETRIC ANAESTHESIA CONSULTATION FOR ALL?

A medical consultation can be defined as an exchange of information between a physician

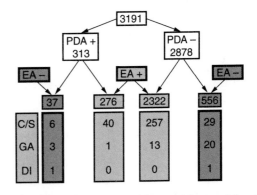

Figure 20.1 Number of patients with or without PDA and/or epidural analgesia (EA) having a caesarean section (C/S), general anaesthesia (GA), difficult intubation (DI) [7].

and patient, resulting in a mutually agreed management plan. This model applies perfectly to the obstetric anaesthesia consultation: the anaesthetist takes the history, risks are discussed and an approach agreed upon. In the absence of a serious medical problem, the discussion centres around the methods of pain relief during labour, enabling patient choice. All this contributes to the creation of confidence between the woman and her anaesthetist.

How can we make this consultation available to all, or nearly all? The first step is to consider the mechanics of the consultation, decide which clinical details are required from the history for risk assessment and what is the most suitable way of gathering this information.

WHAT DOES THE ANAESTHETIST REQUIRE?

The anaesthetist requires an understanding of what the consultation is expected to achieve. The broad objectives outlined earlier serve to provide direction as to what is useful, and what is not. For example, a history of tonsillectomy at two years of age, rubella at eight years of age and normal cardiopulmonary auscultation is of little value in the context of obstetric anaesthesia! This does not aid risk assessment. Key questions must be clearly identified before the interview and these should be targeted around the three basic objectives: identifying the risks associated with general anaesthesia, regional blockade and obstetric intervention.

ANSWERING KEY QUESTIONS

A self-rating questionnaire

A self-rating questionnaire for anaesthesia has several advantages. It costs little, it can be completed in the waiting room, and while tick boxes are very simple they allow interrogation to an adequate level. However, it may pose problems for those of limited understanding. We generally use a questionnaire (Appendix 20.A) before the consultation.

The traditional one-to-one consultation

The private one-to-one consultation enables a detailed and personalized history to be taken. It also allows physical examination, but a kind and sympathetic bedside manner is required for the timid patient. The disadvantage of this type of consultation is that it is not suitable for repetitive trawling of standardized data and it is less reproducible than the questionnaire. Human nature makes it difficult to ask all women identical questions. For example, specific questions related to bleeding disorders are often too time-consuming and rarely systematically asked. A specific questionnaire is more effective. However, the individual consultation does allow questioning to be tailored to each woman's requirements.

Questionnaire and one-to-one consultation

The time saved by filling in a questionnaire before the consultation can be used to advantage in the one-to-one consultation. It is not necessary to overhaul every point but only to confirm the positive responses and explore them. We examine for airway and back problems in all, and extend our examination when the questionnaire, the obstetric chart, or the woman herself, suggests the need. The framework of the anaesthesia file is a risk-orientated one (Appendix 20.B) and indicates the specific risk profile of the patient at one glance. We believe that this 'one-glance' risk evaluation is useful for the anaesthetist who will have to provide epidural analgesia or an emergency anaesthetic to a woman he/she has encountered for the first time in the labour ward.

WHAT INFORMATION SHOULD BE GIVEN TO THE PATIENT?

This can be considered in terms of the information that the anaesthetist wishes to convey to the woman, and what she, in turn, wishes to find out.

What does the anaesthetist want the patient to know?

In the presence of an identified risk it is important that a woman understands and complies with an agreed approach, for example, convincing the patient presenting with a difficult airway or severe asthma that early epidural analgesia is of benefit, because it limits the risks of possible general anaesthesia. In the calm environment of the clinic she is more likely to understand and absorb the case that is put to her. The reticent are more likely to be successfully swayed here than in the hurly burly of the labour ward

One important point to mention is that the anaesthetist is fallible, and that occasionally, even with the best of intentions, procedures can fail. Complications of epidural pain relief should also be mentioned along with unilateral and low blocks, and perineal sparing. The physiological effects that accompany regional blockade should also be explained. Specific anxieties should be sought and reassurance offered. Concerns are often inappropriate and are part of a public misperception of epidural analgesia. This might take the form of doom and gloom (paralysis, puncture of the spinal cord, severe headache, debilitating backache), or represent quite unrealistic expectations of perfection.

What does the patient want from the anaesthetist?

It is important that the woman is able to have her say. An inducive atmosphere can be provided in one of two possible ways.

- During collective antenatal classes
  In many hospitals, antenatal classes provide information on epidural analgesia. Satisfaction is dependent on the eventual experience matching the expectation, and to achieve this, we believe that, whenever possible, this information should be given by anaesthetists themselves [8]. The class should take the form of a talk, suitably illustrated, followed by a question and answer session. This has the advantage not only of allowing each woman to ask her own questions but also for others to hear the answers. This provides an opportunity for the primiparous woman to share the experience of those who have previously benefited from different forms of analgesia (including epidural) or who have undergone general anaesthesia. The disadvantage is that the timid and inarticulate, even when burning with a question, risk being overlooked.

- During an individual consultation
  This is the solution for the shy and reticent, but requires a patient and sympathetic approach. Hopefully this can be accomplished within the 15 minutes allowed per patient. The clinic cannot expand to find more time. The attitude of the physician dealing with the same queries from successive patients must not succumb to weariness during the sequence of consultations.

MAKING THE BEST USE OF MEDICAL TIME

Traditional individual consultation

This type of consultation is time-consuming. At least 15 to 20 minutes must be devoted to each patient to allow enough time for the necessary exchanges and notation. This limits a three-hour consultation session to ten patients.

Not only is this format less efficient than the self-rating questionnaire, it is also less precise and often incomplete, and may cover less ground than the collective meeting.

Nevertheless, when assessing serious medical or obstetrical problems that require a thorough airing, this remains the most appropriate approach. It may still be combined with a questionnaire.

Collective meeting

This permits access to the greatest number of patients in a given time, and promotes dialogue between the anaesthetist and the women, and between the women themselves.

However, several problems must be avoided.

- It is important not to shock: images of some of the less presentable aspects of labour and delivery can be off-putting. Slide or video representations that show an epidural needle entering a back, or a woman barely coping with the pain of labour, are likely to create anxiety. Schematic diagrams are not threatening, and can be used to get points across without undue fear.
- All questions must be answered. Enquiries about headaches, paralysis and death are predictable. Not only can the wording of the response be rehearsed, but also the reassuring tone used to deliver it. Another frequent query relates to the qualifications (resident or consultant) of the anaesthetists present during the night and we believe it important to answer these questions honestly. When patients are informed about manpower limitations, they are usually more understanding when an unexpected emergency causes them to wait for their epidural analgesia.

While useful, this type of meeting is unsuitable for assessing an individual's risk.

Collective meeting and individual consultation

This has the advantages of both approaches. For our own practice, we have adopted the following.

- Information about the antenatal anaesthetic clinic is circulated to women booked for delivery at the hospital through obstetric and midwifery staff.
- Registration of the patients for the consultation begins at the sixth month of pregnancy: patients are informed that, each week, a collective meeting (30 to 40 women) will be held from 2 to 3 pm and will then be followed by individual consultations between 3 and no later than 5 pm.
- A self-rating questionnaire (Appendix 20.A) is completed by the patients during their time in the meeting room before the presentation on epidural analgesia or in the waiting room before the individual consultation.
- A 30-minute presentation with visual aids on pain relief in labour, describing principles of action and discussing the practical considerations of epidural analgesia and alternatives, precedes a general debate.
- The presenter responds to questions about other methods of pain relief, including questions relating to caesarean section or to anaesthesia for episiotomy repair or manual removal of the placenta, for 30 minutes. We encourage women who have already had epidural analgesia or anaesthesia for a previous delivery to describe their experience, even if they experienced a failed epidural or a spinal tap. Explaining shortcomings is a challenging but very stimulating exercise for us. We reassure the women that each problem has a solution.
- Individual consultation follows and can be rapid (< 10 minutes) because the only remaining objective is the assessment of risk, and this is based on the completed questionnaire. Clinical examination allows the evaluation of the airway and of the back, which is often necessary for patient reassurance. These consultations take place in three different rooms with three anaesthetists but in no more than two hours, and allows the completion of an anaesthesia file (Appendix 20.B).
- Filing of the anaesthesia notes in the obstetric file allows instantaneous access during labour, whatever the day or the hour.

The response of the women to this type of meeting is encouraging, as judged by the continually growing number of registrations and the favourable opinions expressed in a postpartum questionnaire. One main criticism has been that not all patients appreciated the necessity to make an appointment (2–5 pm).

In terms of efficiency, this three-hour session allows transmission of precise information in an interactive fashion to 30 to 40 patients (one hour), while not compromising on the other objectives of the clinic. The main constraint is the difficulty involved in simultaneously mobilizing three members of the anaesthetic team for a period of two hours. This can be difficult but is rarely insurmountable.

CONCLUSION

We intended to provide the reader with some solutions to the organizational problems of holding a large-scale antenatal anaesthetic clinic. We hope we have demonstrated that the number of times an anaesthetist is presented with an unanticipated problem as part of an obstetric emergency can be reduced.

We believe that there are no acceptable reasons why patients regularly seen by the obstetric team could not benefit from at least one anaesthesia consultation during their pregnancy, or why obstetrics remains the only subspecialty in which anaesthesia is not systematically preceded by a consultation. Of course, unbooked, a patient whose pregnancy is not known to the obstetric team before labour cannot have an outpatient anaesthetic consultation and requires assessment on the labour ward.

Anaesthetic antenatal assessment can be accomplished efficiently in an outpatient context, with promise of improved safety. Informing patients attenuates their fears and enhances more realistic expectations concerning epidural analgesia and anaesthesia.

Finally, and not insignificantly, the patients no longer see the anaesthetist as a technician but rather a physician managing both the pain of delivery and the risks that are sometimes associated with urgent deliveries.

APPENDIX 20.A A SELF-RATING QUESTIONNAIRE

QUESTIONNAIRE | Département d'Anesthésie-Réanimation Hôpital St-Vincent-de-Paul | **Code** |

Madam,

This questionnaire is designed to explore your medical history in order to detect any problem that could interfere with your anaesthetic care. Please, try to answer all questions. Thank you.

Surname (block capitals) | First name

Age

Weight (before pregnancy)

Height

Parity — Number of spontaneous deliveries

Gravidity — Number of interrupted pregnancies (spontaneous or induced abortions)

Address

Tel:

Profession

Number of caesarean sections

tick the corresponding box

Have you ever had high blood pressure ?	☐ don't know	☐ no	☐ yes	B1
Have you ever had any cardiac problems ? (if yes, give details)	☐ don't know	☐ no	☐ yes	B2
Have you ever had venous thrombosis? after delivery, after surgery, other circumstances (give details)	☐ don't know	☐ no	☐ yes	C1
Have you ever had a pulmonary embolus ?	☐ don't know	☐ no	☐ yes	C2
Do you suffer from varicose veins ?	☐ don't know	☐ no	☐ yes	C3
Has one of your relatives had a deep vein thrombosis or pulmonary embolus (mother, father, sister, brother) ?	☐ don't know	☐ no	☐ yes	C4
Do you suffer from antithrombin III or protein C or S deficiencies ?	☐ don't know	☐ no	☐ yes	C5
Have you ever had general anaesthesia ? If yes, when and for what reason ?	☐ don't know	☐ no	☐ yes	D1
Do you have difficulties in extending your neck ?	☐ don't know	☐ no	☐ yes	D3
Have you ever had - asthma ? (give details)	☐ don't know	☐ no	☐ yes	E11
- eczema, urticaria, allergic coryza ? (underline)	☐ don't know	☐ no	☐ yes	E12
Do you have any drug or food-induced allergies? If yes, state the causal agent and the type of allergic reactions	☐ don't know	☐ no	☐ yes	E2
Has any family member ever had an allergic reaction ?	☐ don't know	☐ no	☐ yes	E4
Have you ever had a severe allergic reaction during an anesthetic ? (give details)	☐ don't know	☐ no	☐ yes	E5
Before pregnancy, have you ever had: large bruises after minimal trauma?	☐ don't know	☐ no	☐ yes	F11
epistaxis (nose bleeds)?	☐ don't know	☐ no	☐ yes	F12
menorrhagia?	☐ don't know	☐ no	☐ yes	F13
Have you ever had abnormal bleeding : after surgery?	☐ don't know	☐ no	☐ yes	F21
after delivery?	☐ don't know	☐ no	☐ yes	F22
Do you suffer from a known coagulation disease leading to abnormal bleeding?	☐ don't know	☐ no	☐ yes	F3
Has any family member had an abnormal bleeding tendency?	☐ don't know	☐ no	☐ yes	F4

Do you suffer from spinal column problems ?: - Scoliosis?..	don't know | no | yes		G11
- Sciatica, sciatalgia, backache ?............................	don't know | no | yes		G12
- Vertebral fracture ?...	don't know | no | yes		G13
Do you suffer from neurologic or muscular disease ? (give details)........................	don't know | no | yes		G2
Do you occasionally suffer from migraine ?.......................	don't know | no | yes		G31
Have you ever had a convulsive crisis ?............................	don't know | no | yes		G32
Have you ever had a lumbar puncture ? If yes, when ?........... Why ?............................	don't know | no | yes		G4
Have you ever had epidural analgesia or anesthesia ? When?	don't know | no | yes		
- Without any problem..	don't know | no | yes		G51
- With no or unilateral pain relief	don't know | no | yes		G52
- Complicated by dural tap and severe headache..................................	don't know | no | yes		G53
Have you ever had a caesarean section ? When? ....Why ?................................	don't know | no | yes		H1
Does your pregnancy result from *in vitro* fertilization ?................................	don't know | no | yes		H2
Have you ever had a forceps delivery ?	don't know | no | yes		H3
Do you suffer from genital herpes ?................................	don't know | no | yes		H4
Have you ever had an uterine curettage after spontaneous or elective termination of pregnancy or a manual exploration of the uterus after delivery ? (if yes, underline)........	don't know | no | yes		H5
Do you smoke more than five cigarettes a day ?	don't know | no | yes		I11
Have you ever had respiratory problems ? (give details)............................	don't know | no | yes		I12
Have you ever had renal or urinary problems ? (give details)....................................	don't know | no | yes		I2
Have you ever had hepatic problems ? (give details)................................	don't know | no | yes		I3
Have you ever had spasmophilia? (give details)............................	don't know | no | yes		I41
Do you suffer from diabetes?....................................	don't know | no | yes		I42
Have you ever had thyroid problems ? (give details)................................	don't know | no | yes		I43
Have you ever had a blood transfusion ? (give details)................................	don't know | no | yes		I51
Do you suffer from a blood disease ? (give details)................................	don't know | no | yes		I52
Have you ever had herpes labialis?	don't know | no | yes		I61
Have you ever had other diseases ? (give details)................................	don't know | no | yes		I62
Do you take any drug ? Underline or give details below............................	don't know | no | yes		J

J1. Antihypertensive drugs
J2. Betamimetics drugs
J3. Anticoagulants
J4. Aspirin and related drugs
J5. Immunosuppressive drugs: Corticoids, Cyclosporin,...
J6. Antibiotics:
J7. Other drugs:

Date   Signature

Adapted from J. Hamza and P. Jullien in, *Guide BECAR-Anesthésie-Réanimation Obstétricale* (eds C. Champagne and D. Benhamou), Arnette, Paris 1994

APPENDIX 20.B ANAESTHESIA FILE

Département d'Anesthésie-Réanimation- Hôpital St Vincent-de Paul
SURNAME **CODE**
D-DAY (expected) .. /.. /.. **CONSULTATION (date)** ../../..

A. IDENTITY :

1. Age
2a. Weight before pregnancy
2b. Weight today
3. Height
4. Parity   Gravidity
5. Gestational age today
6. Rhesus Group

B. HAEMODYNAMIC RISK :
1. Hypertension
  - Not associated with pregnancy — **B11**
  - During a previous pregnancy — **B12**
  - During the present pregnancy — **B13**
2. Cardiac disease
  - Valvular — **B21**
  - Rhythm disturbances — **B22**
3. Symptomatic aorto-caval syndrome — **B3**

C. THROMBOEMBOLIC RISK :
1. Previous thrombosis — **C1**
2. Previous pulmonary embolus — **C2**
3. Varicose veins in the legs
  - Before pregnancy — **C31**
  - During pregnancy — **C32**
4. Previous thromboembolism in family — **C4**
5. Deficit AT III, Prot C, Prot S — **C5**

D. DIFFICULT INTUBATION RISK:
1. Never previously intubated — **D1**
2. Obesity (BMI > 30) — **D2**
3. Cervical spine problems — **D3**
4. Uvula
  - Non-visible (Mallampati 3) — **D41**
  - Half-visible (Mallampati 2) — **D42**
5. Mouth opening <5 cm — **D5**
6. Distance glottis–chin <6 cm — **D6**
7. Limited neck extension — **D7**

E. ALLERGIC RISK :
1. Allergic disease
  - a) Asthma — **E11**
  - b) Eczema, Urticaria, Rhinitis — **E12**
2. Drug-induced allergy — **E2**
3. Food allergy — **E3**
4. Familial allergy — **E4**
5. Anaesthetic allergic accident — **E5**

F. HAEMORRHAGIC RISK :
1. Important and easy bruises — **F11**
  - Epistaxis — **F12**
  - Menorrhagia — **F13**
2. Post-operative haemorrhage — **F21**
  - Post-partum haemorrhage — **F22**
3. Coagulopathy — **F3**
4. Familial haemorrhagic history — **F4**
5. Early pregnancy haemostasis
  - Thrombocytopenia < 150 000/mm3 — **F51**
  - APTT prolonged (> 10" = M/T) — **F52**
  - Quick test <70% — **F53**
6. Anticoagulants — **F6**
7. Aspirin/persantin < 10 days — **F7**

G. NEUROLOGIC RISK:
1. Spinal column problems
  - Scoliosis — **G11**
  - Sciatica–sciatalgia before pregnancy — **G121**
  - during pregnancy — **G122**
  - Vertebral fractures — **G13**
2. Neurologic disease — **G2**
3. Migraine — **G31**
  - Epilepsy — **G32**
4. Previous lumbar puncture — **G4**
5. Previous epidural
  - Without problems — **G51**
  - With inadequate pain relief — **G52**
  - With dural tap and no blood patch — **G531**
  - With dural tap and blood patch — **G532**

H. OBSTETRICAL RISK:
1. Uterine scar from
  - previous caesarean section — **H11**
  - myomectomy — **H12**
2. Multiple pregnancy — **H2**
3. Dystocic risk previous forceps — **H3**
  - Height < 150 cm — **H31**
  - Malpresentations (breech, transv,..) — **H32**
4. Foetal risk Genital herpes — **H4**
  - Hypotrophy < 10th perc. — **H41**
  - Hypertrophy > 90th perc. — **H42**
  - Foetal anomaly — **H43**
5. Retained placenta risk — **H5**
  - (previous curettage or placental removal)
6. Postpartum haemorrhage risk
  - Placenta praevia or marginal — **H61**
  - Previous postpartum haemorrhage — **H62**

I. OTHER RISKS :
1. Respiratory problems
  - Tobacco (> 5 cig/day) — **I11**
  - Other — **I12**
2. Renal problems — **I2**
3. Hepatic problems — **I31**
  - Digestive problems (pyrosis, GE reflux) — **I32**
4. Spasmophilia — **I41**
  - Diabetes, — **I42**
  - Hypothyroidism — **I43**
5. Previous blood transfusion — **I51**
  - Haematologic or immunologic problems — **I52**
6. Herpes labialis — **I61**
  - Other problems — **I62**

CONCLUSION:

REFERENCES

1. Turnbull, A., Tindall, V.R., Beard, R.W. *et al.* (1989) *Report on Confidential Enquiries into Maternal Deaths in England and Wales 1982–1984*, HMSO, London, pp. 1–166.
2. Tindall, V.R., Beard, R.W., Sykff, M.K. *et al.* (1991) *Report on Confidential Enquiries into Maternal Deaths in the United Kingdom 1985–1987*, HMSO, London, pp. 1–164.
3. Lyons, G. (1985) Failed intubation: Six years' experience in a teaching maternity unit. *Anaesthesia*, **40**, 759–62.
4. King, T.A. and Adams, A.P. (1990) Failed tracheal intubation. *British Journal of Anaesthesia*, **65**, 400–14.
5. Rocke, D.A., Murray, W.B., Rout, C.C. *et al.* (1992) Relative risk analysis of factors associated with difficult intubating in obstetric anaesthesia. *Anesthesiology*, **77**, 67–75.
6. Morgan, B.M., Magny, V. and Goroszeniuk, T. (1990) Anaesthesia for emergency caesarean section. *British Journal of Obstetric Gynaecology*, **97**, 420–4.
7. Hamza, J., Ducot, B., Dupont, X. and Benhamou, D. (1995) Anaesthesia consultation can decrease the need for general anaesthesia for emergency caesarean section in parturients with difficult airway. *British Journal of Anaesthesia*, **74**, A353.
8. Mischel, E. and Brighouse, D. (1995) Does the primiparous woman have a realistic expectation of childbirth? *International Journal of Obstetric Anaesthesia*, **4**, 65.
9. Ranta, P., Spalding, M., Kangas-Saarela, T. *et al.* (1995) Maternal expectations and experiences of labour pain – options of 1091 Finnish parturients. *Acta Anaesthiologica Scandinavica*, **39**, 60–6.
10. Bush, D.J. (1995) A comparison of informed consent for obstetric anaesthesia in the USA and the UK. *International Journal of Obstetric Anaesthesia*, **4**, 1–6.
11. Lanigan, C. and Reynolds, F. (1995) Risk information supplied by obstetric anaesthetists in Britain and Ireland to mothers awaiting elective caesarean section. *International Journal of Obstetric Anaesthesia*, **4**, 7–13.
12. Schwalbe, S.S. (1990) Preanaesthetic assessment of the obstetric patient. *Anesthesiology Clinics*, 741–748.
13. Rosaeg, O.P. and Yarnell, R.W. (1993) The obstetrical anaesthesia assessment clinic: a review of six years experience. *Canadian Journal of Anaesthesia*, **40**, 346–56.

ANAESTHESIA FOR THE COMPROMISED FOETUS

21

P. Jouppila, S. Alahuhta and R. Jouppila

INTRODUCTION

Anaesthesia for caesarean section poses a novel challenge since the care of two patients must be taken into account: the mother and the foetus. In elective caesarean section the obstetrician will have chosen abdominal delivery for stable, elective foetomaternal indications (e.g. foetopelvic disproportion or breech presentation). When delivery is not preterm and there are no signs of foetal distress, the choice of anaesthetic depends on local practice, the experience of the anaesthetist and obstetrician, and on the preferences of the woman. In emergency situations, the choice of anaesthetic technique may be as important as the decision to perform operative delivery. This is especially true in cases of acute or chronic foetal asphyxia, extreme prematurity and severe preeclampsia. A significant insight into the pharmacophysiological effects of regional and general anaesthesia has been achieved through the use of ultrasound in human studies. Information from this source has made a significant contribution to our understanding of the effects of various forms of anaesthesia on the uteroplacental and foetal circulations, and is available to assist the clinician in deciding which technique to use for caesarean section.

FOETAL AND UTEROPLACENTAL PATHOPHYSIOLOGY

VASCULAR RESISTANCE

A sound knowledge of basic maternal and foetal physiology is necessary for selecting the right anaesthetic technique as well as for avoiding potential complications. Maternal blood pressure is one of the major determinants of acute changes in the uterine blood flow. Unlike the cerebral and coronary circulations, the uterine vascular bed lacks an autoregulatory mechanism. Vascular resistance in the uteroplacental arteries is low during the second half of normal pregnancy, due to maximal dilation of the spiral arteries which open into the intervillous space of the placenta. In hypertensive pregnancies and other disorders that lead to intra-uterine growth retardation, the trophoblastic invasion around the spiral arteries is deficient. This produces layers of contractile muscle that increase the vascular resistance in the maternal placental circulation. Quantitative determination of this resistance to blood flow in the main uterine arteries can be accomplished using Doppler or colour Doppler ultrasound.

Clinical Problems in Obstetric Anaesthesia
Edited by Ian F. Russell and Gordon Lyons. Published in 1997 by Chapman & Hall, London. ISBN 0 412 71600 3.

One of the main pathophysiological characteristics of preeclampsia is decreased blood volume and general peripheral vasoconstriction. On the foetal side of the placenta, the blood in the two umbilical arteries flushes through the villous capillaries allowing gas exchange between the maternal and foetal circulations. The vascular resistance in the umbilicoplacental circulation is often increased in hypertensive diseases due to the changes in the villous arteries. This arterial vascular resistance can be assessed using the Doppler method. The artery of interest is first localized by colour Doppler and the blood velocity waveforms are then recorded by pulsed Doppler method. Pulsality index (PI), the most commonly used parameter for quantifying vascular resistance, is determined from the waveforms by using the following formula: PI = (systolic peak velocity − end-diastolic velocity)/mean velocity during cardiac cycle. The increased vascular resistance is seen as a decrease in diastolic velocity and leads to increased PI values.

RESPIRATORY GAS EXCHANGE

A 70 mm Hg gradient exists between the pO_2 levels in the maternal uterine arteries and the umbilical vein. There are several mechanisms by which the foetus is able to adapt to oxygen tensions lower than maternal values. Foetal haemoglobin has a greater capacity for oxygen binding than adult haemoglobin, and levels of foetal haemoglobin are increased. Thus the total oxygen content is high in foetal blood and tissues. Within the foetal circulation are the ductus venosus at the level of the liver, and the ductus arteriosus between the pulmonary artery and the descending aorta. Through these two shunts oxygenated blood is passed directly to vital organs, and to the cerebral and coronary arteries in particular. Assessment of foetal blood flow can be selectively performed in the abdominal aorta, the middle cerebral and the renal arteries, using Doppler ultrasound.

CHOICE OF ANAESTHESIA: BASIC PRINCIPLES

In high-risk pregnancies, such as when severe preeclampsia, chronic foetal asphyxia or intrauterine growth retardation threaten premature delivery, early communication between obstetrician and anaesthetist is necessary. An appropriate preanaesthetic examination is required to ensure smooth induction of emergency anaesthesia. Preparation includes establishing effective intravenous access, the detection of potential airway problems, and the inspection and palpation of the lumbar spine. The administration of sodium citrate will increase gastric pH. Pre-existing epidural analgesia can be rapidly extended for operative delivery. The local protocol for emergency caesarean section should reflect a high standard and be tried and tested by regular practice. When the choice of anaesthetic technique is not simple, the discussion should include the obstetrician and the anaesthetist, and the wishes of the mother should be taken into account if at all possible. The anaesthetist must have the final and decisive word in this decision. Maternal medical, drug (e.g. beta-mimetics) and anaesthetic history, as well as laboratory findings will play an important role in this decision-making process.

Regardless of the anaesthetic technique chosen, high inspired oxygen concentrations should be administered to the mother in order to improve foetal oxygen reserve. Aortocaval compression must be avoided.

GENERAL ANAESTHESIA

The major advantage of general anaesthesia for caesarean delivery of the compromised foetus is speed. In many clinics the interval from decision to the delivery of baby, for an emergency caesarean section, is five to 10 minutes. Properly administered general anaesthesia provides excellent conditions for surgery, and is reliable and controllable.

Disadvantages include the unrecognized difficult airway, and failed tracheal intubation

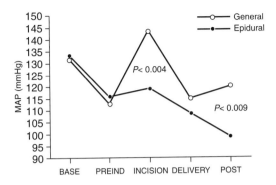

Figure 21.1 Changes in mean arterial pressure (MAP) in the study groups. BASE = baseline values; PREIND: in the general anaesthesia group = MAP obtained after pretreatment with labetalol or nitroglycerine and in the epidural anaesthesia group = MAP with T4 sensory block; INCISION = at skin incision; DELIVERY = at delivery of infant; POST = postpartum.

with subsequent hypoxaemia of the mother and foetus, and the risk of aspiration of gastric contents. At the induction of general anaesthesia and during surgical incision, the mean maternal blood pressure commonly increases from base levels by 40–70 mm Hg with a simultaneous rise in maternal stress hormones (adrenocorticotrophic hormone, endorphins) [1] (Figures 21.1 and 21.2). This may lead to vasoconstriction of the uteroplacental arteries and decreased placental blood flow [2], which can endanger the oxygenation of the compromised foetus.

The disadvantages and advantages of general anaesthesia are summarized in Table 21.1.

DRUGS

Barbiturates such as thiopental are the most commonly used agents for induction of anaesthesia. An intravenous dose of 4 mg/kg has minimal effects on the haemodynamics of a healthy mother, but may result in a decrease in cardiac output and blood pressure in hypovolaemic patients. Higher doses of thiopental (5–7 mg/kg) may be advisable in healthy

mothers to assure maternal unconsciousness. Light general anaesthesia not only risks awareness and recurrent nightmares, but can result in high maternal concentrations of catecholamines. Thiopental rapidly crosses the placenta. After a single maternal injection, peak concentrations in the umbilical venous blood are reached at one minute and in the umbilical arterial blood in two to three minutes. At delivery, the umbilical venous/maternal venous ratio is close to one. Factors such as rapid maternal redistribution

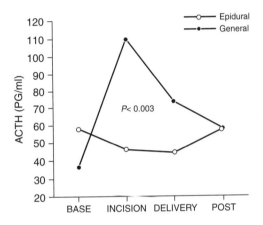

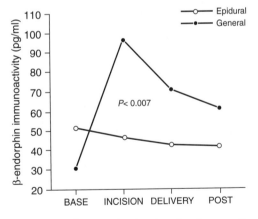

Figure 21.2 Changes in levels of adrenocorticotrophic hormone (ACTH) and β-endorphin-like immunoactivity in the two study groups: before induction of anaesthesia (BASE), at skin incision (INCISION), at delivery of infant (DELIVERY) and postpartum (POST).

Table 21.1 Choice of anaesthetic technique: general anaesthesia

Interval: 5 min	
For	*Against*
Speed	Airway problems
Reliable	Aspiration
Uterine relaxation	Hypertensive response
	Drug transmission
	Increase in acidosis

and tissue uptake of thiopental, the non-homogeneity of the blood flow in the intervillous space, dilution in the foetal inferior vena cava and foetal hepatic uptake, protect the foetal brain from exposure to high concentrations of thiopental. There is therefore no advantage in delaying delivery until thiopental concentrations decrease.

Ketamine is also a viable alternative induction agent with a rapid onset of action. Sympathomimetic properties make it a useful choice in cases of maternal haemorrhage or hypovolaemia, but it should not be used in the hypertensive patient. Induction doses of 1.0–1.5 mg/kg of ketamine do not alter uterine blood flow or increase uterine tone. It provides analgesia, limits maternal intraoperative awareness [3] and improves neurobehavioural scores of infants compared with thiopental [4]. Ketamine, however, may produce psychotropic reactions during awakening.

Succinylcholine in doses of 1.0–1.5 mg/kg to facilitate intubation is associated with minimal placental passage, and its neonatal effects are clinically insignificant.

Nitrous oxide crosses the placenta rapidly. The foetal uptake of nitrous oxide continues during the first 20 minutes after induction of general anaesthesia and a prolonged induction–delivery interval may lead to neonatal depression [5]. If the inspired nitrous oxide concentration is limited to 50% before birth, the chances of subsequent diffusion hypoxia are minimal. If prolonged maternal nitrous oxide exposure occurs before delivery the infant should be ventilated with 100% oxygen at birth for a short time.

It must be remembered that after general anaesthesia, signs of neonatal depression (low Apgars at one and five minutes) do not correlate with biological findings of hypoxia or acidosis. Low Apgar scores that are the result of drug-induced central depression are reversible and are not associated with any longer-term prognostic significance, unlike depression due to asphyxia. The induction–delivery time is not as critical to the neonate as is the time from uterine incision to delivery. Regardless of the anaesthetic technique, a prolonged uterine incision–delivery time seems to correlate with low umbilical blood pH values, low Apgar scores and increased catecholamine concentrations in the umbilical artery blood [6].

Although the mature and normoxic foetus can tolerate general anaesthetic drugs well, neurophysiological disturbance in newborns can still be detected for up to three hours [7]. Apgar scores at one and five minutes are significantly lower in premature infants after general anaesthesia compared with epidural block [8]. Sleepiness, and delay in the first contacts between mother and newborn are also undesirable features. This is not simply due to the higher maternal postoperative morbidity seen with general anaesthesia [9]. Neonatal neurobehavioural scores after general anaesthesia are lower for the first 24 hours of life [10]. The latter may be due to the exposure of the foetus to general anaesthetic drugs.

REGIONAL ANAESTHESIA

Contraindictations to epidural and spinal anaesthesia include maternal coagulopathy and infection at the site of injection. With epidural or spinal anaesthesia, airway problems and aspiration are unlikely. Regional anaesthesia blunts the hypertensive and neuroendocrine stress responses at induction and emergence from general anaesthesia [1] (Figures 21.1 and 21.2). Continuous epidural anaesthesia allows for the titration of local

Table 21.2 Choice of anaesthetic technique: epidural anaesthesia

Interval: 30 min

For	*Against*
Hypotension is controllable	Failure rate
Maintains foetal homoeostasis	Block quality

anaesthetic with a gradual onset of sensory analgesia and sympathetic blockade. Compensatory mechanisms have time to become established with a resultant reduction in the incidence of severe hypotension. With regional anaesthesia the awake mother can participate to some extent and, when foetal condition permits, be allowed to cuddle her baby immediately after delivery. Recovery from regional anaesthesia is relatively short and neurobehavioural scores of newborns after regional anaesthesia are similar to those of infants after normal vaginal delivery. Epidural anaesthesia is summarized in Table 21.2.

HYPOTENSION

Both spinal and epidural techniques require a thorough working knowledge of the prophylaxis and treatment of maternal hypotension. Several studies indicate that uterine and foetal haemodynamic stability can be maintained at caesarean section in both normal and preeclamptic mothers, if prophylaxis against hypotension is practised during epidural and spinal anaesthesia [11–13]. A significant decrease in maternal blood pressure despite preloading is common, especially in conjunction with spinal anaesthesia (30–50%), and in some cases may lead to a short-term increase in vascular resistance in the uterine arteries [13]. The onset of spinal anaesthesia is more rapid than epidural block, and while this may lead to a shorter decision to delivery time, the rapid onset of sympathetic blockade predisposes to hypotension. Despite this, we believe it should

not be routinely used in true emergencies (Table 21.3).

THE PREMATURE INFANT: ANAESTHESIA FOR CAESAREAN SECTION

Obstetric and anaesthetic problems tend to multiply in extreme prematurity, before the 32nd gestational week. In Finland, 1% of deliveries occur between the 22nd and 31st weeks, which compares well with other countries. Caesarean section rates are markedly increased due to special circumstances, such as the high incidence of multiple pregnancies, breech and other unusual presentations, premature rupture of membranes and chorioamnionitis. Early neonatal complications include respiratory distress syndrome (RDS), intraventricular haemorrhage, hypoglycaemia, hyperbilirubinaemia and structural abnormalities. The perinatal mortality rate in this subgroup is 30%, mainly concentrated in the 22nd–28th weeks and mostly associated with RDS and congenital abnormalities. The prognosis has improved markedly, however, during the last few years due to better foetal surveillance and timing of delivery, to the increased use of prophylactic corticosteroids for foetal lung maturation and especially to the expertise of the neonatologist. The use of surfactant has been of value, together with a range of sophisticated applications of intensive therapy.

Beta-adrenergic agonists are frequently employed as tocolytics in the treatment of premature labour. Their cardiovascular effects persist for 60 to 90 minutes after discontinuation, so it is therefore recommended that

Table 21.3 Choice of anaesthetic technique: spinal anaesthesia

Interval: 10 min

For	*Against*
Rapid	Failure rate
Dense block	Hypotension
Simple	Vasopressors

regional anaesthesia is not administered for at least 30 minutes after stopping. Women undergoing treatment are at an increased risk of developing fluid retention-induced pulmonary oedema, hypotension and tachycardia. These dangers appear to be increased when saline is used as a vehicle for beta-adrenergic agonists, particularly when there is multiple pregnancy with its increased plasma volume. The simultaneous use of corticosteroids for improving the foetal lung maturation may further increase the risk of pulmonary oedema [14].

The premature foetus has special physiological features which make it vulnerable to obstetric intervention and anaesthesia. It is more sensitive to asphyxia and traumatic delivery than the mature foetus, and cerebral bleeding often occurs as a consequence of birth hypoxia. The preterm foetus has less plasma protein available for drug binding and decreased protein-binding capacity compared to the full-term foetus. Furthermore, the premature foetus has a decreased ability to metabolize and excrete drugs. Because its blood–brain barrier is more permeable to drugs, they are capable of greater penetration into the central nervous system. When prematurity coincides with chronic asphyxia, the detrimental effects of transplacentally acquired anaesthetic drugs may be at their height. Foetal acidosis increases placental drug transfer and traps weak bases, such as amide local anaesthetics and opioids in the foetal circulation. Concentrations of drugs including anaesthetic agents may therefore be markedly higher in the premature than in the mature foetus.

Unsatisfactory relaxation of the uterus during regional anaesthesia may make operative delivery of the very premature difficult. This can cause a lengthening in the uterine incision–delivery time, which may be reflected in an increase in foetal acidosis [15].

LOCAL ANAESTHETICS

Expertly conducted epidural anaesthesia for caesarean section is not associated with toxic foetal concentration of local anaesthetic agents. According to Pedersen *et al.* [16], there are no differences in the pharmacokinetics of lignocaine between preterm and full-term foetal lambs and transplacental passage did not affect foetal haemodynamics or acid–base balance. In experimental asphyxia of premature foetal lambs, however, the maternal administration of lignocaine at doses required to achieve epidural anaesthesia in humans, resulted in a significant decrease in foetal blood pressure and pH, and an attenuation of the normal compensatory responses to asphyxia [17]. They did not balance these findings with an evaluation of the benefits of regional anaesthesia, particularly that of decreased levels of catecholamines. Oversights of this nature inhibit the universal extrapolation of results obtained in animal studies for clinical use.

Bupivacaine, the most commonly used local anaesthetic drug for regional anaesthesia in obstetrics, has a low potential for foetal toxicity due to its high maternal protein binding. It is, however, the unbound fraction of the drug that readily equilibrates across biological membranes. Foetal free concentration closely correlates with maternal free concentration, and high foetal/maternal concentration ratios of free bupivacaine have been reported following epidural administration [18]. However, the concentrations are well below the toxic range. Bupivacaine has cardiotoxic properties and may cause clinical problems after unintentional maternal intravascular injections. Concern over bupivacaine's cardiotoxicity has led to the development of new local anaesthetic drugs. Initial results have demonstrated that ropivacaine, which is less cardiotoxic than bupivacaine, is a possible suitable alternative for obstetric epidural anaesthesia as it does not appear to compromise the uterine of foetal haemodynamics in healthy mothers [19].

PRELOAD

Volume preloading in conjunction with left uterine displacement has been the cornerstone of prophylaxis against maternal hypotension during regional anaesthesia for caesarean section. Hypotension induced by regional anaesthesia may lead to uteroplacental hypoperfusion, and foetal hypoxia and acidosis. Maternal hypotension of short duration, however, does not seem to harm the full-term foetus if promptly recognized and treated [20]. This may not be the case during caesarean delivery of the premature foetus due to its sensitivity to hypoxic events. According to Karinen *et al.* [21] preloading with a crystalloid (15 ml/kg) or colloid (7.5 ml/kg) infusion prevents hypotension in healthy women with full-term pregnancy during epidural anaesthesia. Simultaneously vascular resistance in the uterine and foetal umbilical, cerebral and renal arteries is maintained. During spinal anaesthesia, on the other hand, preloading with one litre of crystalloid or half a litre of colloid infusion did not decrease the high incidence of hypotension in 62% (crystalloid) and 38% (colloid) of healthy women [13]. Nevertheless, the mean PI in the uterine arteries, reflecting the vascular resistance in these vessels, did not change during spinal blockade despite some short-term individual increases. Acute volume expansion with 20 to 25 ml/kg of a balanced electrolyte solution over 15 to 20 minutes before and during induction of spinal anaesthesia is recommended by basic texts on anaesthesia [22, 23]. Recently, the role of preloading in the prevention of spinal anaesthesia induced hypotension in the pregnant woman has been questioned, and the use of vasopressors encouraged [24]. Prophylactic ephedrine as small-dose infusion had no effect on uterine and foetal haemodynamics during spinal anaesthesia [25], whereas a bolus injection of 10 mg ephedrine and 1 mg etilefrine increased vascular resistance in the uterine arteries. Ephedrine also decreased PI values in the foetal middle cerebral and renal arteries and increased foetal right ventricular contractility in the heart [26]. A cautious and vigilant approach is therefore well justified in the prophylaxis and treatment of maternal hypotension with vasopressors. Lateral uterine displacement is of the utmost importance in maintaining stable maternal haemodynamics during regional anaesthesia. Doppler studies have demonstrated that disturbances in uterine haemodynamics can be best avoided if uterine displacement is accomplished with a wedge rather than with a mechanical device [27].

CHOICE OF ANAESTHETIC TECHNIQUE

What are the decisive criteria in the selection between extradural and spinal regional anaesthesia? The relative merits of both techniques have already been aired. If spinal anaesthesia, with its rapid, more certain, dense blockade could be achieved without hypotension, there would be little debate. Given the sensitivity of the premature foetus to maternal hypotension and its treatment, the less certain, incremental, haemodynamically stable nature of epidural anaesthesia could be the technique of choice. If preload, tilt and fractional doses of 0.5% bupivacaine (18 to 26 ml), alone or with 100 µg adrenaline are used in healthy women, the foetoplacental circulations are maintained [11, 28]. This requires 20 to 30 minutes to spare before surgery. Therefore, its use in the emergency situation is limited to those women who have had an epidural sited for labour.

Other risks exclusive to epidural anaesthesia are inadvertent injection of local anaesthetic, either intravenously or subarachnoid. Even without inadvertent intravenous injection, the relatively large amounts of local anaesthetic required for successful epidural anaesthesia can result in maternal blood levels sufficient to cause uterine arterial vasoconstriction and placental hypoperfusion. However, when the accepted practice is followed, no effects on neonatal behaviour are evident after bupivacaine anaesthesia [29].

The problem of choice between epidural and spinal anaesthesia must be largely solved at the individual patient level. Both methods have been used successfully for anaesthesia for caesarean delivery of premature infants, as has general anaesthesia. The latter is fast and reliable, and provides optimal conditions for rapid but gentle extraction of a small foetus. The only challenge for the anaesthetist is to minimize drug-induced depression.

UTERINE RELAXATION

Urgent uterine relaxation is occasionally required during caesarean section to assist the delivery of a small and premature foetus when the isthmic part of the uterus is not fully developed and the thickness and contraction of the uterine wall hampers the delivery of the foetus. The problem occurs mainly with abnormal foetal positions (breech, transverse lie) and premature twins, especially with the birth of the second infant's head. During general anaesthesia, halothane or another volatile agent can be used to relax the uterus. When the problem occurs in regional anaesthesia, intravenous nitroglycerin at doses of 100 250 and 1000 µg, has been used successfully [30, 31]. Uterine relaxation appears in 60–90 seconds and any maternal blood pressure decrease is easily controlled with intravenous ephedrine.

FOETAL DISTRESS

Foetal distress can be defined as the decompensation of foetal physiological responses to acute or chronic disturbance in the maternal or foetal organism. Foetal prognosis is greatly dependent on the aetiology of the distress and the length of gestation. Time is the critical factor that dictates the choice of anaesthesia. Extremely urgent caesarean sections due to umbilical cord prolapse, placental abruption, prolonged bradycardia, or severe foetal acidosis require the administration of general anaesthesia. If the available time interval is longer than 30 minutes (stable emergency, e.g. in dystocia, variable decelerations) regional anaesthesia should be considered as the primary alternative.

Maternal hypertensive disease resulting in vasoconstriction of the uteroplacental arteries and placental infarction is one of the aetiological factors which lead to chronic foetal asphyxia. Umbilical cord accidents, uterine hypertonus, acute maternal hypovolaemia and placental abruption are, on the other hand, typical causes of acute foetal hypoxia and acidosis. The foetus activates several adaptive responses in these situations. The release of catecholamines from the adrenal medulla increases the foetal heart rate and blood pressure. The foetus has the capacity to redistribute blood flow from peripheral to central organs. Blood flow through the musculoskeletal and splanchnic beds decreases due to vasoconstriction and is redirected to the brain, heart, adrenals and placenta. If the process is sustained, it will result in foetal intra-uterine growth retardation. The foetus also decreases its body movements and breathing activity. Oxygen utilization decreases and aerobic metabolism may be replaced by anaerobic. Finally, foetal heart rate variability decreases and the initial tachycardia is replaced by different forms of bradycardia which are evident in the cardiotocograph. The worst perinatal problems tend to accumulate when severe foetal distress occurs before the 32nd week.

REGIONAL ANAESTHESIA FOR EMERGENCY CAESAREAN SECTION

When foetal distress occurs, extending an epidural established earlier for labour analgesia is an excellent method of anaesthesia for emergency caesarean section if the foetal condition is stable. The early application of epidural analgesia should therefore be encouraged in labours at risk for foetal distress (preeclampsia, intra-uterine growth retardation, oligohydramnios, meconium-stained amniotic fluid). Morgan *et al.* [32] showed that extending epidural analgesia was successful in 70% of 360 consecutive emergency caesarean sections. With time as a critical factor, the use of chloroprocaine should be considered. Apart from having a prompt onset of action, it is also rapidly metabolized on either side of the placenta. Foetal acidosis does not enhance its placental transfer. A single bolus dose of 20 ml of 2% lignocaine with adrenaline has also been used with great success [33]. If there is time, epidural anaesthesia for the stable emergency caesarean can be instituted *de novo*. In these circumstances, the anaesthetic agent most often used is bupivacaine. Its advantages are a relatively slow onset and a lower incidence of severe maternal hypotension associated with a decreased risk of reduced uteroplacental perfusion. In order to minimize maternal hypotension, rapid volume loading with a dextrose-free balanced salt solution must be initiated immediately or the infusion begun during labour should be increased. In many retrospective comparisons of emergency caesarean sections, the infants managed at least as well after epidural as after general anaesthesia [34, 35]. As these are all non-randomized studies, however, the possibility for selection bias does exist.

It could be argued that sympathetic block induced by epidural anaesthesia is likely to reduce vasoconstriction of the uteroplacental small arteries, especially in preeclamptic mothers, by eliminating sympathetic innervation of the uterine vasculature. In preeclamptics, epidural blockade for labour pain indeed improves intervillous blood flow [36]. On the other hand, maternal hypotension induced by epidural blockade may superimpose on the reduced plasma volume which frequently characterizes severe preeclampsia, with a subsequent deterioration of existing foetal distress. Alahuhta *et al.* [12] studied the haemodynamic effects of epidural anaesthesia in 23 hypertensive mothers with signs of chronic foetal distress. By using bupivacaine or bupivacaine with adrenaline as the local anaesthetic agent, a slight but significant decrease in maternal blood pressure was observed despite initial preloading with one litre of crystalloid solution. The maternal haemodynamic state remained reasonably stable with further fluid loading and no vasopressors were required. There was no change in the vascular resistance of uterine and foetal arteries in the bupivacaine group, whereas vascular resistance increased in the uterine arteries after bupivacaine–adrenaline and some modification in the foetal circulation was observed. There was no difference between the groups, however, in the clinical condition of the newborns. It seems that the epidural administration of adrenaline with local anaesthetic cannot be recommended in preeclamptic mothers.

In summary, if time is not a critical factor, appropriately conducted epidural blockade is the anaesthetic technique of choice for emergency caesarean section in women with preeclampsia.

The use of spinal anaesthesia for emergency caesarean sections remains controversial. Its main advantages in comparison with the epidural technique include a more rapid onset of surgical anaesthesia, minimal foetal exposure to depressant medication and its technical simplicity. Maternal hypotension which occurs in 30–50% is the only major disadvantage, and for this reason it is best avoided when there is haemorrhage and hypovolaemia, placental abruption or placenta praevia. In stable situations it can be used successfully by experienced anaesthetists. Vasopressors, such as ephedrine, can be used either prophylactically or after a decrease in maternal blood pressure. Karinen *et al.* [37] found the mean maximal percentage decrease in maternal blood pressure was 19% in 12 preeclamptic patients during spinal anaesthesia for caesarean section, despite the use of 1000 ml crystalloid preload infusion. The vascular resistance in the uterine arteries, however, did not change during preload and spinal blockade.

GENERAL ANAESTHESIA IN FOETAL DISTRESS

Its rapid onset of action favours its use in truly urgent situations. The good relaxation of the abdominal muscles and the uterus are of especial benefit, particularly in caesareans for prematurity associated with foetal distress. Disadvantages include the depressant effects of anaesthetic drugs on the acidotic foetus. During experimental hypoxia and acidosis caused by uterine or umbilical artery occlusion in ewes and foetal lambs, general anaesthesia decreases foetal pH [38]. In another study, halothane exposure for 15 minutes had no effect on the cerebral blood flow or the cerebral oxygen supply of asphyxiated lamb foetuses [39]. In the same model, isoflurane has been shown to cause deterioration in foetal acidosis and reduce the compensatory increase in cerebral blood flow.

Ketamine produced less change in the circulation and oxygen metabolism of acidotic foetal lambs compared with thiopental [40]. One must be cautious, however, in extrapolating results from animal studies to clinical practice. The few studies on humans are retrospective and for ethical reasons it is impossible to perform controlled studies in which anaesthetic techniques for emergency caesarean section for foetal distress are randomized

HYPERTENSIVE RESPONSE TO INTUBATION

The risks associated with **acute hypertension** during the induction of general anaesthesia have long been appreciated. The hypertensive response is particularly exaggerated in the presence of a hypertensive disease of pregnancy. The increase in blood pressure results from greater sensitivity to pressor hormones and may lead to a rise in pulmonary artery pressure. Preeclamptics are at risk, and potential consequences can include cerebrovascular accidents and cardiac failure.

The antihypertensive agents most often used to control acute hypertensive responses during the induction of general anaesthesia are labetalol, sodium nitroprusside, nitroglycerin and nifedipine. Ramanathan *et al.* [41] administered labetalol intravenously in incremental doses up to 1 mg/kg to 25 women with mild to moderate preeclampsia before general anaesthesia. This resulted in a moderate reduction of maternal mean arterial pressure and heart rate with attenuation of the hypertensive and tachycardiac responses to intubation. No adverse effects of labetalol were observed in the newborns. Hood *et al.* [42] observed a 20% decrease in blood pressure after a nitroglycerin infusion was begun before the induction of anaesthesia in a controlled study of women with severe preeclampsia. The neonatal parameters in this group did not differ from those in the control group. Longmire *et al.* [43] studied the effects of intravenous nitroglycerin infusion on six patients with severe preeclampsia. The infusion rate was titrated until a 20% reduction in blood pressure was achieved. An increase in blood pressure of more than 20% over the baseline at intubation was successfully prevented in only two of the six cases. Nausea and vomiting was a frequent complication necessitating a reduction in the dose of nitroglycerin in four of six patients. The authors concluded that the previous preloading blunted the haemodynamic action of nitroglycerin.

All of the above mentioned agents are capable of inducing hypotension and the dosage must therefore be titrated according to the response. In acute hypertensive emergencies, abrupt and excessive decrements in blood pressure may decrease uteroplacental perfusion. This is important because preeclampsia is associated with chronic uteroplacental insufficiency. The direct determination of blood pressure via a radial artery catheter may be indicated if infusions of rapid acting antihypertensive agents are used.

Regardless of the choice of anaesthetic technique, it is vital that effective communication takes place between the obstetrician and anaesthetist, and the degree of urgency is agreed. This often makes the decision a simple matter. Foetal heart monitoring should continue up to the moment of delivery. Maternal considerations should never be overlooked, even if all concern is directed at the distressed foetus. Most maternal deaths due to anaesthesia are the result of emergency caesarean section.

REFERENCES

1. Ramanathan, J., Coleman, P. and Sibai, B. (1991) Anaesthetic modification of hemodynamic and neuroendocrine stress responses to cesarean delivery in women with severe pre-eclampsia. *Anesthesia and Analgesia*, **73**, 772–9.
2. Jouppila, P., Kuikka, J., Jouppila, R. *et al.* (1979) Effect of induction of general anaesthesia for cesarean section on intervillous blood flow. *Acta Obstetricia et Gynaecologica Scandinavica*, **58**, 249–53.
3. Schultetus, R.R., Hill, C.R., Dharamraj, C.M. *et al.* (1986) Wakefulness during caesarean section after anaesthetic induction with ketamine, thiopental, or ketamine and thiopental combined. *Anesthesia and Analgesia*, **65**, 723–8.
4. Hodgkinson, R., Marx G.F., Kim, S.S. *et al.* (1977) Neonatal behavioural tests following vaginal delivery under ketamine, thiopental, and extradural anaesthesia. *Anesthesia and Analgesia*, **56** 548–53.
5. Finster, M. and Poppers, P.J. (1968) Safety of thiopental used for induction of general anaesthesia in elective caesarean section. *Anesthesiology*, **29**, 190–1.
6. Bader, A.M., Datta, S., Arthur, G.R. *et al.* (1990) Maternal and foetal catecholamines and uterine incision-to-delivery interval during elective caesarean section. *Obstetrics and Gynecology*, **75**, 600–3.
7. Dick, W.F. (1995) Anaesthesia for caesarean section (epidural and general): effects on the neonate. *European Journal of Obstetrics and Gynaecology and Reproductive Biology*, **59** (suppl.), S61–S67.
8. Rolbin, S.H., Cohen, M.M., Levinton, C.M. *et al.* (1994) The premature infant: Anesthesia for caesarean delivery. *Anesthesia and Analgesia*, **78**, 912–7.
9. Morgan, B.M., Barker, J.P., Goroszeniuk, T. *et al.* (1984) Anaesthetic morbidity following Caesarean section under epidural or general anaesthesia. *Lancet*, **i**, 328–30.
10. Kangas-Saarela, T., Koivisto, M., Jouppila, R. *et al.* (1989) Comparison of the effects of general and epidural anaesthesia for caesarean section on the neurobehavioural responses of newborn infants. *Acta Anaesthesiologica Scandinavica*, **33**, 313–9.
11. Alahuhta, S., Rasanen, J., Jouppila, R. *et al.* (1991) Uteroplacental and fetal haemodynamics during extradural anaesthesia for Caesarean section. *British Journal of Anaesthesia*, **66**, 319–23.
12. Alahuhta, S., Rasanen, J., Jouppila, P. *et al.* (1993) Uteroplacental and fetal circulation during extradural bupivacaine adrenaline and bupivacaine for Caesarean section in hypertensive pregnancies with chronic fetal asphyxia. *British Journal of Anaesthesia*, **71**, 348--52.
13. Karinen, J., Rasanen, J., Alahuhta, S. *et al.* (1995) Effect of crystalloid and colloid preloading on uteroplacental and maternal haemodynamic state during spinal anaesthesia for Caesarean section. *British Journal of Anaesthesia*, **75**, 531–5.
14. Alahuhta, S., Karinen, J., Lumme, R. *et al.* (1994) Uteroplacental haemodynamics during spinal anaesthesia for caesarean section with two types of uterine displacement. *International Journal of Obstetric Anaesthesia*, **3**, 187–91.
15. Datta, S., Ostheimer, G.W., Weiss, J.B. *et al.* (1981) Neonatal effect of prolonged anaesthetic induction for caesarean section. *Obstetrics and Gynecology*, **58**, 331–35.
16. Pedersen, H., Santos, A.C., Morishima, H.O. *et al.* (1988) Does gestational age affect the pharmacokinetics and pharmacodynamics of lidocaine in mother and foetus. *Anaesthesiology*, **68**, 367–72.
17. Morishma, H.O., Pedersen, H., Santos, A.C. *et al.* (1989) Adverse effects of maternally administered lidocaine of the asphyxiated preterm foetal lamb. *Anaesthesiology*, **71**, 110–5.
18. Thomas, J., Long, G., Moore, G. *et al.* (1976) Plasma protein binding and placental transfer of bupivacaine. *Clinical Pharmacology and Therapeutics*, **19**, 426–34.
19. Alahuhta, S., Rasanen, J., Jouppila, P. *et al.* (1995) The effects of epidural ropivacaine and bupivacaine for caesarean section on uteroplacental and foetal circulation. *Anesthesiology*, **83**, 23–32.
20. Corke, S.E., Datta, S., Ostheimer, G.W. *et al.* (1982) Spinal anaesthesia for Caesarean section. The influence of hypotension on neonatal outcome. *Anaesthesia*, **37**, 658–62.
21. Karinen, J., Rasanen, J., Paavilainen, T. *et al.* (1994) Uteroplacental and foetal haemodynamics and cardiac function of the foetus and newborn after crystalloid preloading for extradural Caesarean section anaesthesia, *British Journal of Anaesthesia*, **73**, 751–7.

22. Shnider S. M. and Levinson, G. (eds) (1993) *Anaesthesia for Obstetrics*, Williams & Wilkins, Baltimore.

23. Chestnut, D.H. (ed.) (1994) *Obstetric Anaesthesia, Principles and Practice*. Mosby, St Louis.

24. Rocke, D.A. and Rout, C.C. (1995) Volume preloading, spinal hypotension and Caesarean section. *British Journal of Anaesthesia*, **75**, 257–9.

25. Alahuhta, S., Rasanen, J., Jouppila, P. *et al.* (1992) Ephedrine and phenylephrine for avoiding maternal hypotension due to spinal anesthesia for caesarean section. *International Journal of Obstetric Anaesthesia*, **1**, 129–34.

26. Rasanen, J., Alahuhta, S., Kangas-Saarela, T. *et al.* (1991) The effects of ephedrine and etilefrine on uterine and foetal blood flow and on foetal myocardial function during spinal anaesthesia for caesarean section. *International Journal of Obstetric Anaesthesia*, **1**, 3–8.

27. Clesham, G.J., Scott, J., Oakley, C.M. *et al.* (1994) Beta adrenergic agonists and pulmonary oedema in preterm labour. *British Medical Journal*, **308**, 260–2.

28. Alahuhta, S., Rasanen, J., Jouppila R. *et al.* (1991) Effects of extradural bupivacaine with adrenaline for Caesarean section on uteroplacental and foetal circulation. *British Journal of Anaesthesia*, **67**, 678–82.

29. Abboud, T.K., Nagabbala, S., Murakawa, K. *et al.* (1985) Comparison of the effects of general and regional anaesthesia for caesarean section on neonatal neurologic and adaptive capacity scores. *Anesthesia and Analgesia*, **64**, 996–1000.

30. Mayer, D.C. and Weeks, S.K. (1992) Antepartum uterine relaxation with nitroglycerin at Caesarean delivery. *Canadian Journal of Anaesthesia*, **39**, 166–9.

31. Rolbin, S.H., Hew, E.M. and Bernstein, A. (1991) Uterine relaxation can be life saving. *Canadian Journal of Anaesthesia*, **38**, 939–40.

32. Morgan, B.M., Magne, V. and Goroszeniuk, T. (1990) Anaesthesia for emergency caesarean section. *British Journal of Obstetrics and Gynaecology*, **97**, 420–4.

33. Price, M.L., Reynolds, F., Morgan, B.M. *et al.* (1991) Extending epidural blockade for emergency caesarean section: evaluation of 2%

34. Marx, G.F., Luykx, W.M. and Cohen, S. (1984) Foetal–neonatal status following caesarean section for foetal distress. *British Journal of Anaesthesia*, **56**, 1009–13.

35. Ramanathan, J., Ricca, D.M., Sibai, B.M. *et al.* (1988) Epidural vs. general anaesthesia in foetal distress with various abnormal foetal heart patterns. *Anesthesia and Analgesia*, **67**, 180.

36. Jouppila, P., Jouppila, R., Hollmen, A. *et al.* (1982) Lumbar epidural analgesia to improve intervillous blood flow during labour in severe pre-eclampsia. *Obstetrics and Gynecology*, **59**, 158–61.

37. Karinen, J., Rasanen, J., Alahuhta, S. *et al.* (1995) Maternal and uteroplacental haemodynamics in pre-eclamptic patients during preloading and spinal anesthesia for Caesarean section. *British Journal of Anaesthesia*, **75**, 531–5.

38. Schwartz J., Cummings M., Pucci, W. *et al.* (1985) The effects of general anaesthesia on the asphyxiated foetal lamb *in utero*. *Canadian Anaesthetic Society Journal*, **32**, 577–82.

39. Cheek, D.B.C., Hughes, S.C., Dailey, P.A. *et al.* (1987) Effect of halothane on regional cerebral blood flow and cerebral metabolic oxygen consumption in the foetal lamb *in utero*. *Anesthesiology*, **67**, 361–6.

40. Pickering, B.G., Palahniuk, R.J., Cote, J. *et al.* (1982) Cerebral vascular responses to ketamine and thiopentone during foetal acidosis. *Canadian Anaesthetic Society Journal*, **29**, 463–7.

41. Ramanathan, J., Sibai, B.M., Mabie, W.C. *et al.* (1988) The use of labetalol for attenuation of the hypertensive responses to endotracheal intubation in pre-eclampsia. *American Journal of Obstetrics and Gynecology*, **159**, 650–4.

42. Hood, D.D., Dewan, D.M., James, F.M. *et al.* (1985) The use of nitroglycerin in preventing the hypertensive response to tracheal intubation in severe pre-eclampsia. *Anesthesiology*, **65**, 329–32.

43. Longmire, S., Leduc, L., Jones, M.M. *et al.* (1991) The haemodynamic effects of intubation during nitroglycerin infusion in severe pre-eclampsia. *American Journal of Obstetrics and Gynecology*, **164**, 551–6.

22

ADULT RESPIRATORY DISTRESS SYNDROME IN PREGNANCY

A.C. Quinn

INTRODUCTION

Adult respiratory distress syndrome (ARDS) has been recognized since the first world war. It was first described in detail by Ashbaugh and coworkers in 1967 as 'acute respiratory failure in adults and adolescents with similar features to the respiratory distress pattern seen in infants' [1]. It is characterized by increased pulmonary capillary permeability, low-pressure pulmonary oedema and hypoxia, widespread diffuse pulmonary infiltrates on chest X-ray, reduced lung compliance and high airway pressures.

ARDS plays a significant part in maternal morbidity and mortality. The 1988–1990 report on the confidential enquiries into maternal death in the UK [2] cites ARDS as contributing to death in 18.5% of the direct and indirect maternal deaths reported (44 of a total of 238 women). However, this statistic illustrates only a small percentage of the overall incidence of the disease. In 1992, results of a six-year prospective study on ARDS in pregnancy in an American tertiary referral centre were published and the authors pointed out the paucity of data on the subject [3]. This was also highlighted in the UK maternal mortality enquiry. This lack of data, together with a lack of uniformity in the diagnosis and management of the disease, makes it difficult to assess the aetiology, pathophysiology and response to different treatment regimes.

DEFINITION AND AETIOLOGY

ARDS is a severe form of acute lung injury which is commonly scored according to the chest X-ray picture, degree of hypoxaemia, reduction in respiratory compliance and amount of positive end-expiratory pressure (PEEP) required. ARDS is strictly defined as a Murray score greater than 2.5 (Table 22.1) [4]. The joint European–American consensus conference on ARDS [5] has recently produced a narrower definition (Table 22.2), but a further proposal is that ARDS be defined more specifically by scoring the degree of alveolar damage and increase in pulmonary vascular permeability, e.g. by using radiolabelled albumin or positron emission tomography studies [6].

ARDS in pregnancy is a complication of many conditions (Table 22.3). The main initiating factors in the 1994 UK mortality report were haemorrhage or hypotension, chest infection, gastric aspiration and sepsis. In addition, 40% of these patients had a hypertensive disorder of pregnancy. There was a high incidence of multiorgan failure in these patients which is associated with a high mortality.

Clinical Problems in Obstetric Anaesthesia
Edited by Ian F. Russell and Gordon Lyons. Published in 1997 by Chapman & Hall, London. ISBN 0 412 71600 3.

Table 22.1 Components of the lung injury score

	Value	Score
1. Chest X-ray score		
No alveolar consolidation	–	0
Consolidation in one quadrant	–	1
Consolidation in two quadrants	–	2
Consolidation in three quadrants	–	3
Consolidation in four quadrants	–	4
2. Hypoxaemia score		
PaO_2/FiO_2	⩾300	0
PaO_2/FiO_2	225–229	1
PaO_2/FiO_2	175–224	2
PaO_2/FiO_2	100–174	3
PaO_2/FiO_2	<100	4
3. Respiratory system compliance score (ml/cm H_2O)		
Compliance	⩾80	0
Compliance	60–79	1
Compliance	40–59	2
Compliance	20–39	3
Compliance	⩽19	4
4. PEEP score (cm H_2O)		
PEEP	⩽5	0
PEEP	6–8	1
PEEP	9–11	2
PEEP	12–14	3
PEEP	⩾15	4
Final value = Total/no of components used		
No lung injury	0	
Mild–moderate	0.1–2.5	
Severe (ARDS)	>2.5	

PaO_2/FiO_2 = arterial oxygen tension (mm Hg)/fractional inspired oxygen concentration.
PEEP = positive end-expiratory pressure.

PATHOLOGY

There are many theories regarding the pathogenesis of ARDS including direct endothelial and epithelial damage from bacteria or endotoxin leading to a reduction in both the production of surfactant and the removal of oedema fluid. The plasma colloid osmotic pressure (COP) in pregnancy is reduced (a dilutional effect from the increased circulating volume and reduced albumin synthesis). This may be a factor predisposing the pregnant patient to pulmonary oedema. Activation of the complement cascade in sepsis has been implicated as a cause of endothelial injury, as has the activation of neutrophils and monocytes with the release of toxic free radicals, arachidonic acid metabolites and proteolytic enzymes [7–9]. Tumour necrosis factor (TNF), released from mononuclear cells in response to endotoxin stimulation, may play a role in the lung injury, and platelet activation and

Table 22.2 Definition proposed by the joint European–American Consensus conference on ARDS

Definition	Severe respiratory failure
Oxygenation	$PaO_2/FIO_2 \leqslant 200$ (regardless of the PEEP level)
Chest X-ray	Bilateral infiltrates seen on frontal chest X-ray
PAWP	$\leqslant 18$ mm Hg when measured or no clinical evidence of left atrial hypertension based on chest X-ray and other clinical data

PaO_2/FIO_2 = arterial oxygen tension (mm Hg)/fractional inspired oxygen concentration.
PEEP = positive end-expiratory pressure.
PAWP = pulmonary artery wedge pressure.

coagulation abnormalities may also contribute by stimulating the deposition of fibrin in the alveoli [10, 11].

The early histopathological changes are endothelial and epithelial damage leading to marked capillary leakage, severe alveolar and interstitial oedema and pleural effusions. The oedema fluid contains large numbers of inflammatory cells (mainly neutrophils, but also proteins). The protein concentration of the oedema fluid has been shown to correlate with survival; early resolution of the high protein concentration in the pulmonary oedema fluid indicates higher survival rates [12]. In this phase the patient requires a high inspired oxygen concentration and responds well to PEEP.

Table 22.3 Causes of ARDS in pregnancy

Infection
• Pneumonia
• Pyelonephritis
• Sepsis/abscess
• Septic abortion/chorioamnionitis
Preeclampsia/eclampsia
Gastric aspiration
Drugs
• Beta-agonists
Hypovolaemia
• Abruption
• DIC
Massive blood transfusion
Pancreatitis
Emboli
• Amniotic fluid
• Septic/trophoblastic disease
• Air/fat
Intra-uterine death

Once the ARDS has become more established, the interstium of the lung changes. This is thought to result from the release of various factors which lead to collagen growth and epithelial cell proliferation [13].

The final stage of the process involves destruction of the pulmonary architecture resulting in emphysema, pulmonary fibrosis and vascular obliteration. Here the characteristic ventilatory requirements are high minute volumes to counteract the increased dead space and high inspired airway pressures to overcome the reduced lung compliance. Superinfection by nosocomial organisms is also common at this stage, a consequence of the destructive airway changes. Figure 22.1 is a chest X-ray from a postpartum patient with faecal peritonitis and sepsis following bowel perforation during an elective caesarean section. The X-ray shows bilateral diffuse pulmonary infiltrates and an air bronchogram.

RESPIRATORY PHYSIOLOGY IN PREGNANCY

There are many changes in respiratory physiology throughout pregnancy. These peak at term and may have a bearing on the ventilatory management of patients with ARDS [14]. The expanding uterus pushes the diaphragm upwards resulting in a reduction in functional residual capacity of 10–25% by term (see Figure 22.2) [15]. The minute volume (MV) increases some 20–40% at term due to a rise in tidal volume of 30–45%. This respiratory stimulation is thought to result from the combined effects of increasing CO_2 production,

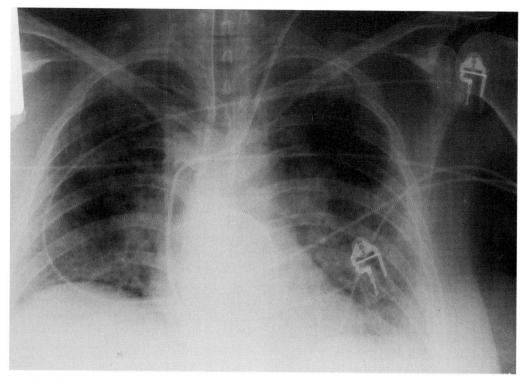

Figure 22.1 Chest X-ray. The X-ray demonstrates diffuse bilateral infiltrates and an air bronchogram in a postpartum patient with septicaemia and faecal peritonitis following bowel perforation during elective caesarean section.

starting at conception, and a progesterone-effect on the respiratory centre. This latter effect may be due either to direct respiratory stimulation or increased sensitivity of the respiratory centre to the PCO_2. The MV rises in excess of CO_2 production leading to a respiratory alkalosis and compensatory renal excretion of bicarbonate (HCO_3^-). The residual volume and expiratory capacity are slightly reduced but, owing to the increase in antero-posterior and transverse thoracic diameters, the vital capacity is unchanged despite diaphragmatic elevation. In normal pregnancy, neither the forced expiratory capacity in the first second (FEV_1) nor the lung compliance measurements differs from prepregnancy, although there is a reduction in total compliance owing to reduced chest wall compliance.

During pregnancy the oxygen cost of breathing increases with the rise in minute ventilation (by as much as 40% by the end of pregnancy) but this does not lead to a decrease in mixed venous oxygen saturation SvO_2) because of the increase in cardiac output. The relationship between oxygen requirement and cardiac output may be more finely balanced in cardiopulmonary disease and may deteriorate in the presence of labour pain [16]. Arterial oxygen partial pressure is generally around 13 kPa, but pregnant women have less oxygen reserve due to their increased oxygen consumption and reduced functional residual capacity (FRC). Severe labour pain may cause shallow breathing and, if very marked, may lead to hypoxaemia. Conversely, and more commonly, severe pain in labour results in hyperventilation leading to hypocarbia and

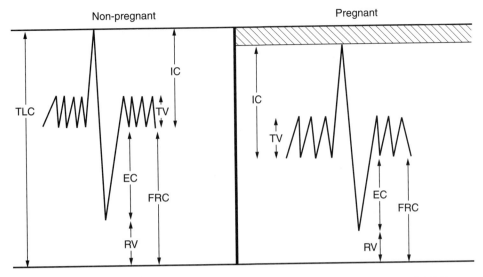

Figure 22.2 Effects of term pregnancy on ventilation parameters [15, with permission]: TLC = total lung capacity; EC = expiratory capacity; IC = inspiratory capacity; TV = tidal volume; FRC = functional residual capacity; RV = residual volume.

respiratory alkalosis and this can reduce the uterine blood flow. Both the hypoxaemia and the reduced uteroplacental function can be restored by adequate analgesia [16]. Typical arterial blood gas measurements at term are: PCO_2 3.7–4.3 kPa, PO_2 13.3 kPa, pH 7.4–7.47, HCO_3^- 18–21 (mEq/l). In addition to these physiological changes, the respiratory mucosa becomes more oedematous and hypersecretory, especially in the third trimester.

CURRENT TREATMENT AND OUTCOME OF ARDS

The current treatment of ARDS is focused on the provision of adequate gas exchange and the limitation of complications. Reports over the last 20 years have indicated that the overall prognosis of the disease may be improving [17]. This may be due to a variety of changes in the management of the disease. There is increased emphasis of good control of fluid balance and better treatment of nosocomial pneumonia. High minute ventilation, high PEEP and a high inspired oxygen percentage are the mainstays of respiratory support, all of which worsen the pulmonary injury. Various modes of ventilation have been evaluated in attempts to improve gas exchange and limit barotrauma: pressure controlled ventilation with reversed inspiratory:expiratory ratios and permissive hypercapnia; extracorporeal CO_2 removal; high frequency jet ventilation; high-frequency oscillatory ventilation. The effects of positional changes have also been studied. However, it is unclear whether any of these manoeuvres affect outcome [18].

Many pharmacological approaches have been evaluated. These modify the activation of humoral factors, inflammatory cells, platelets and endothelial cells (see Table 22.4) but most results have been inconclusive [19]. Of recent interest are the results following the use of ketoconazole: in a small, prospective, blinded placebo-controlled clinical trial there was a reduction in mortality in the treatment group [20]. Corticosteroids have also been shown to be effective in the late phase of the disease.

Exogenous surfactant has significantly reduced the mortality of infant respiratory

Table 22.4 Recent drug regimens for ARDS

Pathway	Drug
Arachidonic acid metabolism	**Methyl prednisolone**
Lipo-oxygenase–leukotrienes	Ibuprofen
Cyclo-oxygenase–prostaglandins	PGE_2
Thromboxane synthase–thromboxanes	Ketoconazole
Neutrophil activation–chemotaxis	
	Pentoxyfylline
	Antiproteases
	Antioxidants, e.g. *N*-acetyl cysteine
Anti complement therapy	
	C1 inhibitor
Antibodies to cytokines and receptors	
	TNF alpha antibody
	Interleukin-1 receptor antagonist

distress syndrome (IRDS). Although preliminary reports of exogenous surfactant in ARDS have been encouraging [21], it is unlikely to be as effective as in IRDS because of the difficulties in administration and in achieving a homogeneous dispersion of the large volume required. There have also been preliminary studies on the efficacy of liquid ventilation using perfluorocarbons [22]. These fluids have low surface tension and high oxygen and carbon dioxide solubilities, properties which facilitate gas exchange in the alveoli.

INHALED NITRIC OXIDE THERAPY

Over the past few years, inhaled nitric oxide (NO) gas has been shown to be effective in the treatment of ARDS. In 1987 this small gaseous molecule was shown to be responsible for the action of so-called endothelial-derived relaxing factor (EDRF). Nitric oxide has subsequently been shown to be synthesized in many cells throughout the body. In the respiratory tract, nitric oxide is thought to be largely formed in the nasopharynx [23] and is normally present in low basal concentrations in the lungs. In pregnancy, nitric oxide levels are thought to play a role in attenuating labour contractions and glyceryl trinitrate patches (a NO donor) have been shown to inhibit preterm labour [24]. Inhalation of exogenous NO has been used in a variety of cardiorespiratory disorders, including ARDS [25], but its exact mode of action is unclear: either correction of an absolute reduction in NO levels in the lungs or raised NO concentrations to compensate for a relative insensitivity to the normal endogenous NO concentrations.

Inhaled nitric oxide gas enters ventilated lung segments only and is thought to diffuse from the alveoli directly onto the smooth muscle of pulmonary resistance vessels where it combines with guanylate cyclase to produce cyclic guanylate monophosphate (cGMP) (Figure 22.3) and thus vasodilatation. By this mechanism it improves perfusion of the ventilated segments only and thus leads to a reduction in the ventilation/perfusion (V/Q) mismatch with a corresponding improvement in oxygenation. Because NO has a high affinity for haemoglobin (forming methaemoglobin) its duration of action is only the few seconds it takes to contact blood in the pulmonary capillaries. Consequently, it does not reduce the systemic vascular resistance, which is often already low in septic states. A recent

Exogenous NO

Alveolus

Endogenous NO

Endothelial cell

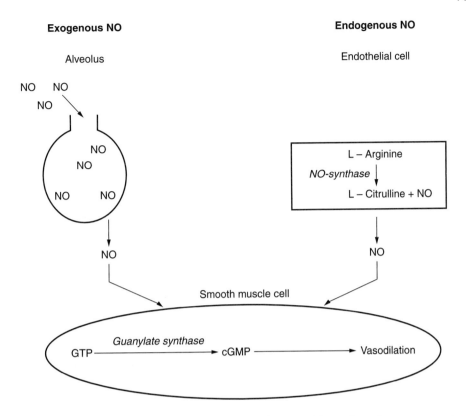

Figure 22.3 Schematic representation of the effects of inhaled nitric oxide on the pulmonary vascular smooth muscle: nitric oxide (NO), guanosine triphosphate (GTP), cyclic guanosine monophosphate (cGMP).

dose–response curve of inhaled NO for improving oxygenation in ARDS has shown an ED_{50} (dose producing 50% of the desired effect) of only 100 parts per billion (ppb) which is a typical level of NO in the urban environment [26]. Higher concentrations (up to 40 ppm, parts per million) are often required to lower pulmonary artery pressures.

In severe ARDS, many studies have shown inhaled NO to reduce pulmonary artery pressure, reduce right ventricular strain and improve oxygenation: the latter permits a reduction in airway pressure in severe ARDS thus decreasing the chance of barotrauma [27]. However, although commonly used in many centres, NO treatment is still undergoing evaluation as there are several significant potential side-effects. These include direct

toxicity from NO or its metabolites, (e.g. nitrogen dioxide or peroxynitrite), methaemoglobinaemia formation resulting in reduced oxygen carriage, and dependence, particularly after prolonged treatment. Moreover, NO has been shown to be mutagenic and this factor is therefore a particular consideration when used in pregnancy before the foetus has been delivered [28].

Many different criteria may be used to assess suitability for inhaled nitric oxide therapy. An example might be $PO_2 \leq 8\,\text{kPa}$ and $PCO_2 > 5.3$ kPa with a fraction inspired oxygen concentration (FiO_2) > 0.5, plus at least one of the following: PEEP > 10 cm H_2O, peak inspiratory pressure > 45 cm H_2O and mean airway pressure > 30 cm H_2O. Pulmonary artery systolic pressure > 50 mm Hg (previously normal) and extravascular lung water value > 7 ml/kg would reflect a severe form of the disease and justify a trial of treatment, but there are no hard-and-fast rules and these criteria will vary between centres.

Devising NO delivery, scavenging and monitoring apparatus poses additional problems: both inspired NO, and inspired and expired NO_2 concentrations should be monitored as well as NO pollution in the working environment.

As NO treatment is still undergoing evaluation, it is usually reserved for severe cases of ARDS refractory to conventional treatment. Although inhaled NO is available in many centres it is of great importance that the response and complications of the therapy be carefully monitored until more information on its long term effects, incidence of tolerance and dependency, and the effects, if any, on outcome are elucidated.

ECMO AND IVOX

Extra corporeal membrane oxygenation (ECMO) is accepted treatment for severe infant respiratory distress syndrome but has been less successful in the treatment of ARDS. It was hoped that the technique would permit a reduction in ventilation, inspired O_2 concentration and airway pressure. Complications of this technique include bleeding, sepsis, thromboembolism, renal failure and multiorgan failure. The National Institute of Health Trial results [29] were unimpressive and ECMO has not gained universal acceptance. Intravenacaval membrane oxygenation and carbon dioxide removal (IVOX) was also proposed as a method of providing partial respiratory support in severe respiratory failure. This gas exchange device consists of hollow fibres, with gas flowing through their lumina, surrounded by a coaxial cylinder of blood travelling in the opposite direction to the gas flow. The technique requires surgical cannulation of the superior or inferior vena cava and anticoagulation. Complications such as haemorrhage,

infection and thrombus formation [30] have precluded its use.

Inhaled NO therapy provides a simpler, less invasive option than either of these procedures in many critically ill patients.

FLUID MANAGEMENT IN THE PREGNANT PATIENT WITH ARDS

The cornerstones in the treatment of pulmonary oedema in severe preeclampsia are effective vasodilation with fluid restriction and diuresis. Severe preeclampsia is a common problem found in association with ARDS [31] but determining the goals of fluid management in this situation is complicated by the multifactorial nature of the disease: many of these patients have multiorgan failure and require optimal oxygen transport and delivery, both of which may depend on adequate blood volume. Thus a delicate balance between fluid loading and restriction exists in each situation. Quantifying the extent of low-pressure pulmonary oedema is difficult: pulmonary artery wedge pressure (PAWP) measurements are often unhelpful. Mitchell and coworkers showed that the measurement of extravascular lung water was superior to PAWP measurements as a guide to the response to diuretic therapy and resulted in reduced ventilator-days and intensive care unit-days [32]. Echocardiography has also been shown to provide useful information for the management of pulmonary oedema in pregnancy. A prospective six-year study in an obstetric intensive treatment unit [33] identified three distinct groups on the basis of echocardiographic findings: (i) normal heart function requiring acute therapy only, (ii) myocardial systolic dysfunction which responded to diuretics, digoxin and angiotensin-converting enzyme inhibitors, and (iii) those with diastolic dysfunction and increased left ventricular mass who responded to diuretics and then long-term antihypertensive treatment. The authors recommended that echocardiography be used to evaluate all pregnant women with pulmonary oedema.

Fluid management in these patients is often complicated by the presence of renal failure requiring haemodialysis or haemofiltration. This treatment may have the advantage of removing inflammatory mediators, which exacerbate the pulmonary injury.

CLINICAL EXPERIENCE OF ARDS IN PREGNANCY

Information about the incidence, aetiology, treatment, and maternal and foetal outcomes of ARDS in pregnancy is scarce owing to its rare occurrence, the lack of specialist centres dealing with the problem and poor classification of the disease. However, some trends emerge from the information available. In the 1994 UK maternal mortality figures [2] the incidence and aetiology of ARDS was documented. The main causes of ARDS were haemorrhage or hypotension in 12 cases, chest infection in 11, aspiration in 10 and sepsis in six.

To date, the largest prospective study of ARDS in pregnancy [3] has examined a series of 16 pregnant patients (Murray score >2.5). They found the incidence of ARDS to be one in 1893 deliveries and it occurred primarily in the third trimester. Eight patients had a documented infective process and four had preeclampsia–eclampsia. Eleven of these patients were multiparous, 10 of Afro-Caribbean origin, 12 were antepartum. Overall seven patients died (44% mortality). Of the 13 viable pregnancies, six had a caesarean section.

Another case-control study examined acute lung injury as a complication of appendicitis in 49 pregnant patients in a tertiary referral centre [34]. Of these, nine developed pulmonary insufficiency (two ARDS) but there were no deaths. All patients with lung injury were more than 20 weeks' gestation and a multi-variate analysis with stepwise logistic regression showed that a model combining together an intravenous fluid overload of greater than four litres, respiratory rate of greater than 24, body temperature of greater than 38°C (100.4°F) and the use of tocolytics was predic-tive of lung injury in 99% of these patients. There was also a higher incidence of lung injury in patients when general anaesthesia, rather than regional anaesthesia, was used for surgery.

A series of 15 cases of pulmonary injury complicating antepartum pyelonephritis was published in 1987 [35]. The authors suggested a link between endotoxaemia and acute lung injury, especially in pregnancy of greater than 28 weeks [35]. One patient died due to multi-organ failure initiated by the endotoxaemia and ARDS was a contributory factor.

Over a five-year period, in an English tertiary referral intensive care unit, there were 23 obstetric admissions: three patients were diagnosed as having ARDS and two of these patients died [36].

Hypertensive disease in pregnancy is also a risk factor in the development of ARDS, although the exact pathophysiology of the alveolar–capillary damage is unclear. The triennial reports of UK mortality published in 1991 and 1994 show ARDS to be implicated in nine of 27 deaths [2, 37] in the 'hypertensive disease in pregnancy' groups. In the most recent report [38], 8 of 20 deaths in this group had ARDS. In a series of 37 patients with severe preeclampsia–eclampsia there were four deaths: ARDS was implicated in one [39].

GASTRIC ASPIRATION AND ARDS

During pregnancy the rise in intragastric pressure predisposes to the well-recognized risk of inhalation of stomach contents when airway reflexes are obtunded (e.g. general anaesthesia). Aspiration is still implicated in many deaths, but usually without direct evidence of gastric contents in the trachea and lower airways. In the UK triennial mortality report covering 1985–1987 [37] and 1991–93 [38] gastric aspiration was the **direct** cause of death in only one woman. In the latest report [2], it was again **directly** responsible for only one death but strongly implicated in another death. Details of the circumstances where gastric aspiration features as a **contributing** factor in maternal death are given in the 1988 –1990 maternal mortality report [2]:

- Deaths attributed to anaesthesia
  There were five deaths in this group with evidence of aspiration in two.
- Anaesthesia contributing to death
  There were a further 10 deaths in this group: in only two patients, was there evidence of gastric aspiration.
- ARDS
  Of the 44 patients developing fatal ARDS 10 were thought to have aspirated: in three cases there were strong implicating factors, but in the remaining seven, aspiration was presumed because of the rapid onset of respiratory failure following a situation where aspiration could have occurred [2]. The authors underlined the problem of aspiration in pregnancy, and concluded with recommendations about the use of antacid prophylaxis during labour and intraoperative gastric emptying. Perhaps this increased vigilance will reduce the incidence of ARDS but, alternatively, there may be another pathophysiological reason for the respiratory failure.

PRACTICAL MANAGEMENT OF ARDS – PROBLEMS SPECIFIC TO PREGNANCY

There are surprisingly few differences unique to the practical management of ARDS in the obstetric patient. Joint decisions, involving the intensivists, the obstetricians and the paediatricians, should be made about the optimal time of the delivery for either the mother or baby or both. Delivery of the foetus will result in reduced maternal oxygen requirements and improved ventilation. The foetus should be closely monitored, particularly if the mother is hypoxic, and may require to be delivered. Similarly, if continuation of the pregnancy poses a significant threat to the mother, as may occur in preeclampsia, the foetus will need to be delivered.

Measurement of PAWP through a pulmonary artery flotation catheter has been recommended to guide fluid restriction [37]. However, as PAWP is usually low, this is often a poor indicator of fluid overload but the catheter does enable measurement of oxygen delivery and mixed venous oxygen saturation. These latter values may be useful in determining the level of tissue oxygenation, often significantly compromised in ARDS, sepsis, physiological anaemia of pregnancy or by aortocaval compression.

As previously mentioned, in pregnancy (especially if the pregnancy continues past the estimated date of delivery), there is greater likelihood of atelectasis and decreased respiratory compliance resulting in increased airway pressures and barotrauma during ventilation. An added consideration is the congested respiratory mucosa: nasotracheal intubation or the insertion of nasogastric tubes must be performed with care to avoid epistaxis.

Whether by enteral or parenteral routes, maternal nutrition will also require particular attention.

In intensive care there is inevitably a large consumption of various drugs crucial to the treatment of the pregnant patient. These drugs may affect uteroplacental function and most will pass to the foetus (e.g. sedatives, opioids, antibiotics, inotropes). Foetal acidosis will augment the toxic effects on the foetus of many of the basic drugs. Prolonged drug administration will challenge the foetus' ability in drug handling [40] and pharmacological as well as teratogenic effects are dose-dependent. Little work is available on the extent of placental transfer and long-term foetal effects of the sedatives, opioids and muscle relaxants used in the intensive treatment unit. It is known that the transfer of polar compounds is placental membrane permeability-limited, whereas with lipophilic compounds, placental blood flow and rate of equilibrium (a reflection of plasma protein binding) are more important.

Patients with sepsis and ARDS often require vasopressors, which have the potential to reduce uterine and intervillous blood flow. Doppler studies have indicated that in low doses, ephedrine (mixed α and β-effects) is preferable to phenylephrine, a pure α_2-agonist [41].

It is of paramount importance that these patients are referred early to a specialist unit. There is anecdotal evidence to suggest that these young women with good physiological reserve are, unfortunately, often referred to the intensivist at an advanced stage of the disease when severe cardiorespiratory failure has occurred: studies have shown the ARDS mortality in pregnancy to be as high as in other groups of older less healthy patients [3].

CONCLUSION

The obstetric patient with severe ARDS provides a major challenge to the intensivist. Pregnancy results in a number of physiological and anatomical changes in the mother which alter the response to many disease processes. This rare subgroup of critically ill patients will present the intensivist with unique therapeutic and ethical decisions. Furthermore, this distinct group of patients do not exhibit normal disease patterns, as is reflected by the inability of the APACHE II scoring system to predict outcome in an obstetric population [42]. Available literature on this particular subgroup of ARDS patients is lacking and, until more detailed research is performed, we can only make an educated guess as to the aetiology, the prognosis and the best treatment regimen.

REFERENCES

1. Ashbaugh, D.G., Bigelow, D.B., Petty, T.L. and Levine, B.E. (1967) Acute respiratory distress syndrome in adults. *Lancet*, **2**, 319–23.
2. Department of Health Welsh Office, Scottish Office Home Health Department, Department of Health and Social Security Report on Health and Social Subjects (1994) *Report on Confidential Enquiries into Maternal Deaths in the United Kingdom 1988–1990*, HMSO, London, pp. 80–91.
3. Mabie, W.C., Barton, J.R. and Sibai, B.M. (1992) Adult respiratory distress syndrome in pregnancy. *American Journal of Obstetrics and Gynecology*, **167**, 950–7.
4. Murray, J.P., Matthay, M.A., Luce, J. and Flick, M.R. (1988) An expanded definition of the adult respiratory distress syndrome. *American Review of Respiratory Disease*, **138**, 770–3.
5. Bernard, G.R., Artigas, A., Brigham, K.L. *et al.* (1994) Report of the American–European consensus conference on ARDS: definitions, mechanisms, relevant outcomes and clinical trial coordination. The Consensus Committee. *Intensive Care Medicine*, **20**, 225–32.
6. Schuster, D.P. (1995) What is acute lung injury? What is ARDS? *Chest*, **107**, 1721–26.
7. Hunter, D.N., Keogh, B.F., Morgan, C.J. and Evans, T.W. (1990) The management of adult respiratory syndrome: 1. *British Journal of Hospital Medicine*, **42**, 468–71.
8. Wiener-Kronish, J.P., Glopper, M.A. and Matthay, M.A. (1990) The adult respiratory distress syndrome. Definition and prognosis, pathogenesis and treatment. *British Journal of Anaesthesia*, **65**, 107–29.
9. Hallgren, R., Barg, T. and Venge, P. (1984) Signs of neutrophil and eosinophil activation in adult respiratory distress syndrome. *Critical Care Medicine*, **12**, 14–8.
10. Fein, A., Lippman, M., Holtzmann, H. *et al.* (1983) The risk factors, incidence and prognosis of the adult respiratory distress syndrome following septicaemia. *Chest*, **83**, 40–2.
11. Moalli, R., Doyle, J.M., Tahhan, H.R. *et al.* (1989) Fibrinolysis in critically ill patients. *American Review of Respiratory Disease*, **140**, 287–93.
12. Wiener-Kronish, J.P. and Matthay, M.A. (1989) Sequential measurements of protein edema concentration provide a reliable index of alveolar epithelial function and prognosis in patients with the adult respiratory distress syndrome. *Clinical Research*, **37**, 165A..
13. Villar, J. and Slutsky, A.S. (1994) Stress proteins and acute lung injury, in *Yearbook of Intensive Care and Emergency Medicine* (ed. J.L. Vincent), Springer Verlag, Berlin, Heidelberg, New York, pp. 430–40.
14. Lapinsky, S.E., Kcuczynski, K. and Slutsky, A.S. (1995) Critical care in the pregnant patient. *American Journal of Respiratory Critical Care Medicine*, **152**, 427–55.

15. Alaily, A.B. and Carrol, K.B. (1978) Pulmonary ventilation in pregnancy. *British Journal of Obstetrics and Gynaecology*, **85**, 518–24.

16. Ackerman, W.E., Molnar, J.M. and Juneja, M.M. (1993) Beneficial effect of epidural anesthesia in a parturient with adult respiratory distress syndrome. *Southern Medical Journal*, **86**, 361–64.

17. Lemaire, F. (1996) The prognosis of ARDS; appropriate optimism? *Intensive care Medicine*, **22**, 371–3.

18. Keogh, B.F., Hunter, D.N., Morgan, C.J. and Evans, T.W. (1990) The management of adult respiratory distress syndrome: 2. *British Journal of Hospital Medicine*, **43**, 26–34.

19. Hudson, L.D. (1995) New therapies for ARDS. *Chest*, **108**, 79S–91S.

20. Mihae, Y. and Tomasa, G. (1993) A double-blind, prospective, randomised trial of ketoconazole, a thromboxane synthase inhibitor, in the prophylaxis of the adult respiratory distress syndrome. *Critical Care Medicine*, **21**, 1635–42.

21. Gregory, T.J., Gadek, J.E., Weiland, J.E. *et al.* (1994) Survanta supplementation in patients with acute respiratory distress syndrome (ARDS). *American Journal of Respiratory Critical Care Medicine*, **149**, A567.

22. Hirschl, R.B., Pranikoff, T., Overbeck, M.C. *et al.* (1995) Pulmonary distribution and elimination of perfluorocarbon (PFC) during partial liquid ventilation in adult patients with respiratory failure *Critical Care Medicine*, **23**, A121.

23. Gerlach, H. (1995) Inhaled nitric oxide in ARDS: Just a replacement therapy?, in *Yearbook of Intensive Care and Emergency Medicine* (ed. J.L. Vincent), Springer-Verlag, Berlin, Heidelberg, New York, pp. 358–67.

24. Lees, C., Campbell, S., Jauniaux, E. *et al.* (1994) Arrest of preterm labour and prolongation of gestation with glyceryl trinitrate, a nitric oxide donor. *Lancet*, **343**, 1325–6.

25. Rossaint, R., Falke, K.J., Lopez, F. *et al.* (1993) Inhaled nitric oxide for the adult respiratory distress syndrome. *New England Journal of Medicine*, **328**, 399–405.

26. Gerlach, H., Rossaint, R., Pappert, D. and Falke, K. (1993) Time course and dose-response of nitric oxide inhalation for systemic oxygenation and pulmonary hypertension in patients with adult respiratory distress syndrome. *European Journal of Clinical Investigation*, **23**, 499–502.

27. Haake, R., Schlichtig, R., Ulstad, D.R. and Henschen, R.R. (1987) Barotrauma: Pathophysiology, risk factors and prevention. *Chest*, **91**, 609–13.

28. Nguyen, T., Brunson, D., Crespi, C.L. *et al.* (1995) DNA damage and mutation in human cells exposed to nitric oxide in vitro. *Proceedings of the National Academy of Sciences of the United States of America*, **89**, 3030–34.

29. Zapol, W.M., Snider, M.T., Hill, J.D. *et al.* (1979) Extra corporeal membrane oxygenation in severe acute respiratory failure. *Journal of the American Medical Association*, **242**, 2193–6.

30. Murdoch, L.J., Boyd, O.F., Mackay, J. *et al.* (1993) The perioperative management of surgical insertion and removal of the intravenous oxygenation device (IVOX). A report of nine cases. *Anaesthesia*, **48**, 845–58.

31. Pearson, J.F. (1992) Fluid balance in severe pre-eclampsia. 1992. *British Journal of Hospital Medicine*, **48**, 47–51.

32. Mitchell, J.P., Schuller, D., Calandro, F.S. and Schuster, D.P. (1992) Improved outcome based on fluid management in critically ill patients requiring pulmonary artery catheterisation. *American Review of Respiratory Disease*, **145**, 990–8.

33. Mabie, W.C., Hackmann, B.B. and Sibai, B.M. (1993) Pulmonary edema associated with pregnancy: echocardiographic insights and implications for treatment. *Obstetrics and Gynecology*, **81**,227–34.

34. de Veciana, M., Towers, C.V., Major, C.A. *et al.* (1994) Pulmonary injury associated with appendicitis in pregnancy: Who is at risk? *American Journal of Obstetrics and Gynecology*, **171**, 1008–13.

35. Cunningham, F.G., Lucas, M.J. and Hankins, G.D.V. (1987) Pulmonary injury complicating antepartum pyelonephritis. *American Journal of Obstetrics and Gynecology*, **156**, 797–805.

36. Graham, S.G. and Luxton, M.C. (1989) The requirement for intensive care support for the pregnant population *Anaesthesia*, **44**, 581–4.

37. Department of Health Welsh Office, Scottish Office Home Health Department, Department of Health and Social Security Report on Health and Social Subjects (1991) *Report on Confidential Enquiries into Maternal Deaths in the United Kingdom 1985–1987*, HMSO, London.

38. Sibai, B.M., Mabie, B.C., Harvey, C.J. and Gonzalez, A.R. (1987) Pulmonary edema in severe preeclampsia–eclampsia. Analysis of thirty seven consecutive cases. *American Journal of Obstetrics and Gynecology*, **156**, 1174–9.

39. Department of Health Welsh Office, Scottish Office Home Health Department, Department of Health and Social Services, Northern Ireland

(1996) *Report on the Confidential Enquiries into Maternal Deaths in the United Kingdom 1991–93,* HMSO, London.

40. Reynolds, F. (1993) Principles of placental drug transfer: its measurement and interpretation, in *Effects on the Baby of Maternal Analgesia and Anaesthesia* (ed. F. Reynolds), W.B. Saunders, London, pp. 1–28.

41. Hollmen, A.I. (1993) The effects of regional anaesthesia on utero- and feto-placental blood flow, in *Effects on the Baby of Maternal Analgesia and Anaesthesia*), (ed. F. Reynolds), W.B. Saunders, London, pp. 67–87.

42. Lewinsohn, G., Herman, A., Leonov, Y. and Klinowski, E. (1995) Critically ill obstetric patients: outcome and predictability. *Critical Care Medicine,* **23,** 1449–50.

INDEX